Exploring Cultural Responsiveness

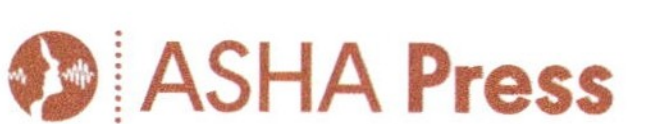

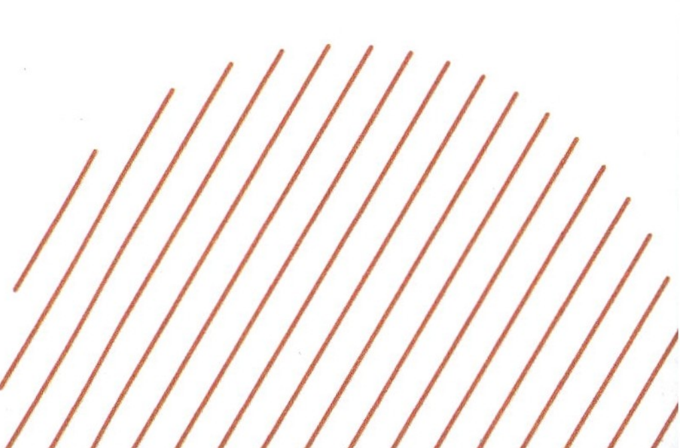

Published by

ASHA Press

An imprint of the American Speech-Language-Hearing Association (ASHA)

The American Speech-Language-Hearing Association (ASHA) is the national professional, scientific, and credentialing association for audiologists; speech-language pathologists; and speech, language, and hearing scientists. ASHA works to promote the interests of these professionals and to advocate for people with communication disorders.

ASHA adheres to the style guide of the American Psychological Association in using person-first language to describe attributes and diagnoses of individuals or groups of people. When there is a preference for identity-first language, ASHA honors that preference.

The opinions contained herein are the views of the contributors and are not to be construed as reflecting official policies or recommendations of ASHA.

All web links were active at time of publication.

ISBN: 978-1-58041-121-9

Copies may be ordered from:

ASHA Product Sales

2200 Research Boulevard

Rockville, MD 20850-3289

Tel: 888-498-6699

Fax: 301-296-8590

www.asha.org

ASHA Content Consultant: Karen L. Beverly-Ducker, MA, CCC-A, CAE

Product Manager: Catharine Gray

Graphic Designer: Christine Baumgarten

Copyeditor: Tyler Krupa

Printed in the U.S.A.

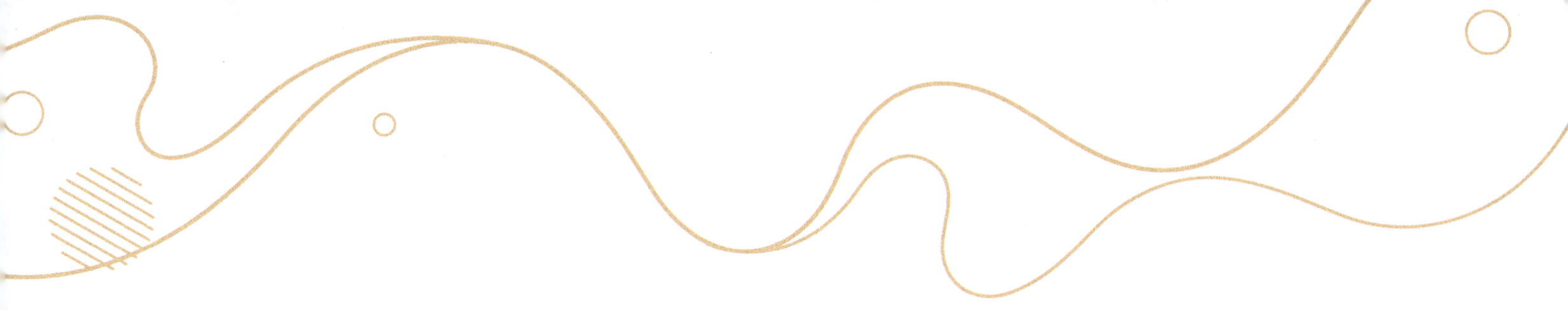

DEDICATION

This workbook is dedicated to our clients and their families who honor us with their lives and through their stories. Your courage and persistence have broadened our understanding of culture and inspire us to be better practitioners. We also dedicate this workbook to our colleagues who never tire in their desire to become more culturally responsive.

For Charlie, Grace, and Maura: You are my masterpieces.

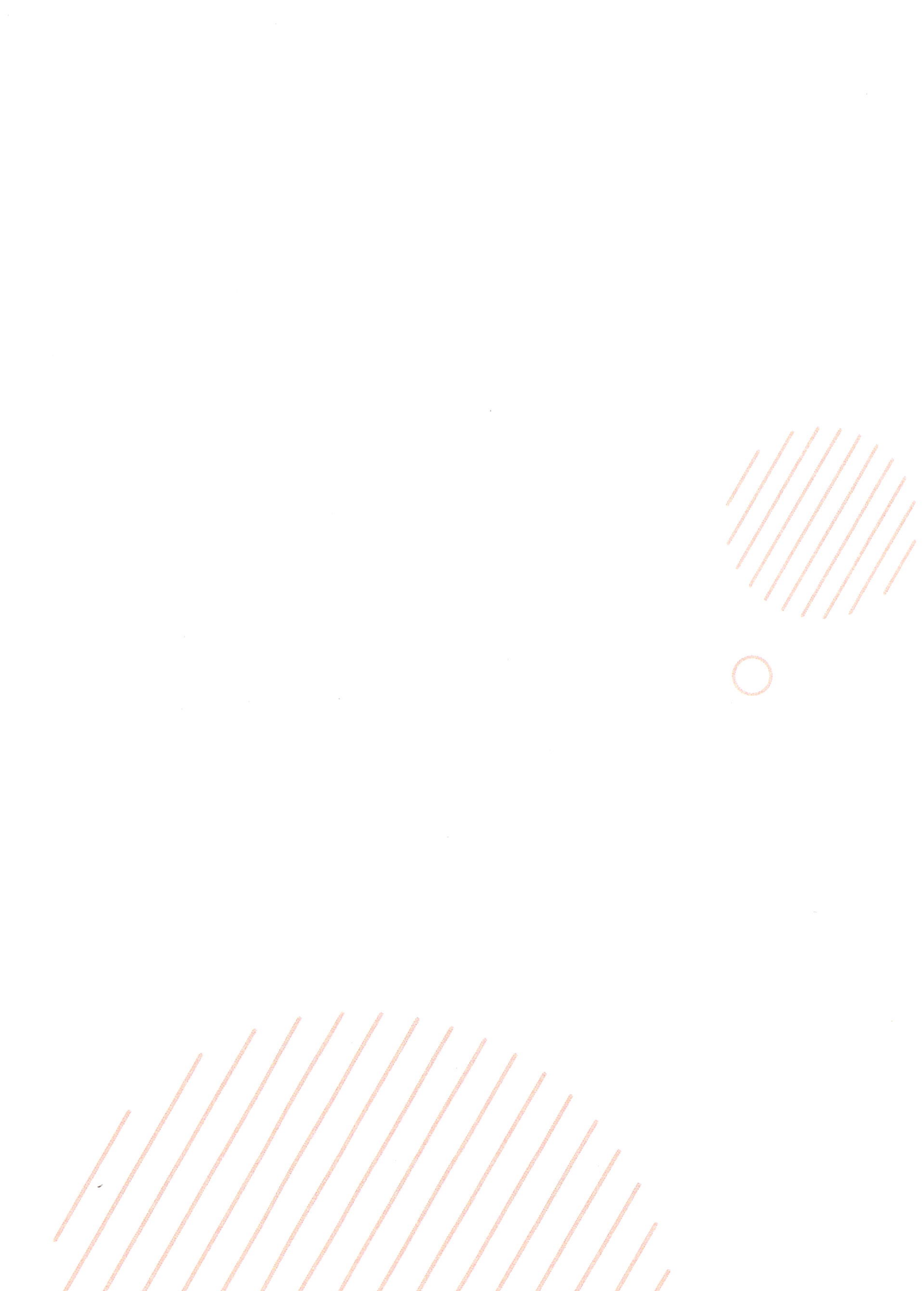

Table of Contents

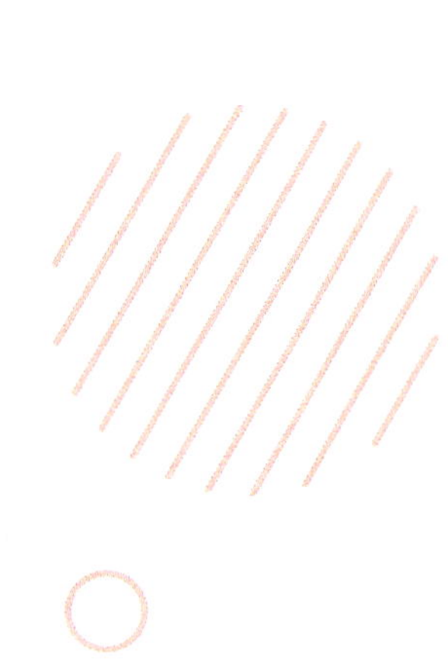

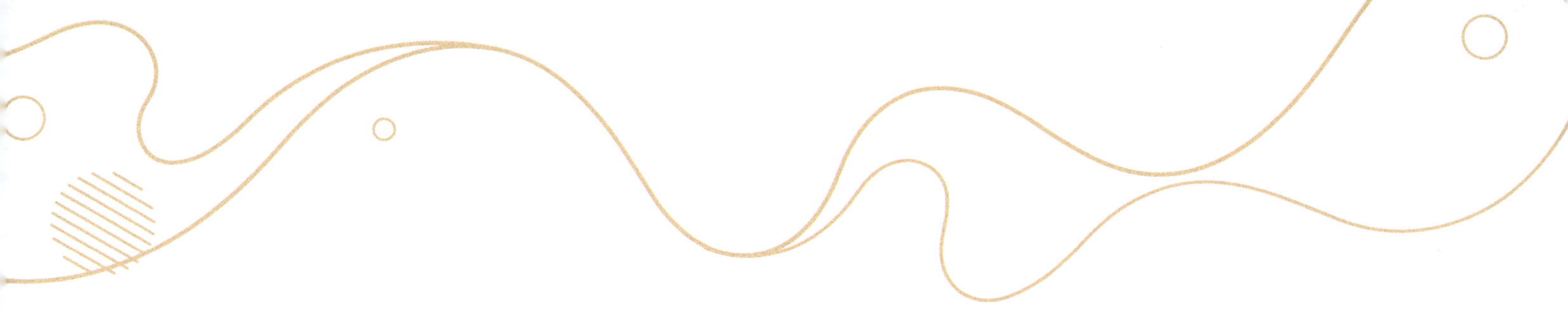

ACKNOWLEDGMENTS

THE EDITORS

We thank our families and friends for their support and patience. This process has evolved and expanded across its lifetime, and without your understanding and encouragement, it would not have been possible.

THE AMERICAN SPEECH-LANGUAGE-HEARING ASSOCIATION'S MULTICULTURAL ISSUES BOARD MEMBERS

We thank our colleagues, students, clients, and families who inspired us. Your stories and insights became the foundation for these guided scenarios. Without the collaboration and professional relationships of our colleagues, we would have never been able to produce such a work. We also acknowledge our clients and families for sharing their stories. Finally, we give a heartfelt thanks to Karen Beverly-Ducker, Catharine Gray, and the staff at the American Speech-Language-Hearing Association for their insight, feedback, and energy throughout this lengthy process. We are forever grateful. This work has been a true labor of love, and we are proud of the end result. We hope that it inspires clinicians and educators to persist on their journey of cultural competence.

ABOUT THE EDITORS

Alicia Fleming Hamilton, MS, CCC-SLP, (she/her/hers) is a bilingual (Spanish-English) speech-language pathologist who works with the Minneapolis Public Schools. She specializes in bilingual assessment in early childhood populations, bilingual clinical education, and multicultural assessment and intervention. She was the 2019 president of the Minnesota Speech-Language-Hearing Association.

Carmen Ana Ramos-Pizarro, PhD, CCC-SLP, (she/her/hers) is a bilingual (Spanish-English) speech-language pathologist. She is faculty at the University of the District of Columbia Speech-Language Pathology program where she also supervises student clinicians providing gender-affirming voice services to the transgender and gender-diverse community in the Greater Washington, DC, region.

Jean Franco Rivera Pérez, PhD, CCC-SLP, (he/him/his) is a bilingual (Spanish-English) assistant professor of communication sciences and disorders at Texas Christian University. His academic interests and areas of expertise include the use of technology to promote vocabulary in bilingual (Spanish-English) preschool children with and without language disorder and multicultural perspectives.

Wendyliza González, MS, CCC-SLP, TSSLD-BE, (she/her/hers) is a New York City school-based, bilingual (Spanish-English) speech-language pathologist. She specializes in assessment and curriculum-aligned treatment approaches for bilingual children and currently works with prekindergarten through eighth-grade students in the South Bronx.

Karen L. Beverly-Ducker, MA, CCC-A, CAE, (she/her/hers) is the director of multicultural practices at the American Speech-Language-Hearing Association and the ex-officio to the Multicultural Issues Board.

THE AMERICAN SPEECH-LANGUAGE-HEARING ASSOCIATION'S 2019 MULTICULTURAL ISSUES BOARD MEMBERS:

Mariam M. Abdelaziz, PhD, CCC-SLP, (she/her/hers) is a bilingual (Arabic-English) speech-language pathologist. Her areas of research interest include language and literacy development and multicultural topics within the fields of education and communication sciences and disorders. She is currently an assistant professor at Radford University.

Ivan Campos, MS, CCC-SLP, (he/him/his) is a bilingual speech-language pathologist fluent in English and Spanish. His areas of interest include multilingual language development, equitable assessment practices, and service delivery for students from culturally and linguistically diverse backgrounds.

Alison Marie Dungca, (she/her/hers) is a graduate student studying speech-language pathology at San Francisco State University. Her interests include working with underrepresented populations, specifically the Asian community, and augmentative and alternative communication users. She currently serves as the vice president for planning of the National Student Speech Language Hearing Association.

Puja Goel, MA, CCC-SLP, (she/her/hers) is a multilingual school-based speech-language pathologist (SLP) who has worked for the Chicago Public Schools and currently works in New Mexico as a supervising SLP. She has experience in early intervention, private practice, acute care, skilled nursing facilities, and outpatient settings. She completed the American Speech-Language-Hearing Association's Leadership Development Program and Minority Student Leadership Program. She is a first-generational South Asian born in the United States and holds dual citizenship in India.

Mark Guiberson, PhD, CCC-SLP, is a professor and the department chair at the University of Wyoming Division of Communication Disorders. He is Spanish-English bilingual and teaches coursework in child language, speech disorders, and stuttering. His areas of research include clinical approaches with dual language learners and other children from diverse cultural backgrounds, with a focus on preschool-age children and children with hearing loss.

Pei-Fang Hung, PhD, CCC-SLP, (she/her/hers) is a trilingual (Mandarin Chinese, Taiwanese, and English) speech-language pathologist with dual licenses and certificates in the United States and Taiwan. She is an associate professor and interim chair in the Department of Speech-Language Pathology at the California State University, Long Beach. Her professional interests include aphasia management and cognitive-communication disorders.

Perry Flynn, MEd, CCC-SLP, is a professor in the Department of Communication Sciences and Disorders at the University of North Carolina Greensboro and is the consultant to the North Carolina Department of Public Instruction in the area of speech-language pathology. He served as the Board of Directors liaison to the Multicultural Issues Board.

Ishara Ramkissoon, PhD, CCC-A, is an associate professor at Gallaudet University where she teaches graduate audiology classes, and conducts research in multicultural issues, aging and age-related hearing loss, evoked potentials, and environmental variables. Her background experience as an audiologist and speech therapist included providing clinical services for multilingual clients. She currently serves on the ASHA Ad Hoc Committee to Develop Guidance for Engaging Globally, and has developed a collaborative student study abroad experience in South Africa.

Dorian Lee-Wilkerson, PhD, CCC-SLP, (she/her/hers) is an American Speech-Language-Hearing Association fellow. Her areas of scholarship include cultural competence, substance abuse, and scholarship of teaching. As an associate professor and chair of the Department of Communicative Sciences and Disorders at Hampton University, she manages an undergraduate program in communicative sciences and disorders and a graduate program in speech-language pathology. She teaches courses in anatomy and physiology, phonetics, and family intervention practices and manages the Saturday Social Skills Group for the Hampton University Speech-Language-Hearing Clinic.

Rachel M. Williams, PhD, CCC-SLP, (she/her/hers) is an American Speech-Language-Hearing Association fellow. She is an associate professor and the director of the Doctor of Speech-Language Pathology Program at Nova Southeastern University. As an associate professor, she teaches multicultural issues and fluency disorders courses and as a graduate clinical supervisor, she specializes in working with individuals who stutter. Her research areas of interest include assessment and treatment of fluency disorders in culturally and linguistically diverse populations, diversity training in clinical education, and supervision and leadership in higher education.

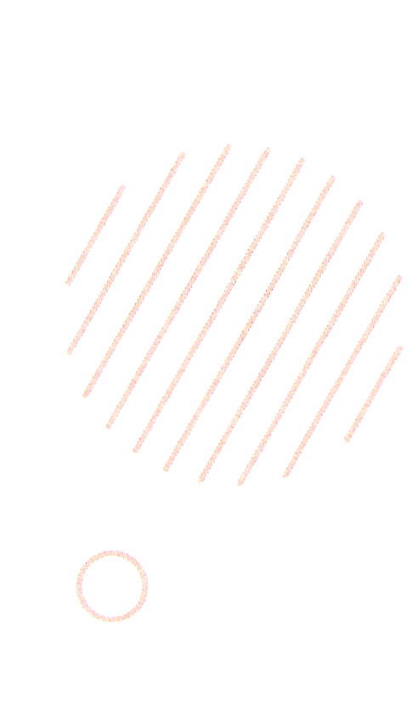

Foreword

— Vicki R. Deal-Williams, MA, CCC-SLP, FASAE, CAE

What if we were all the same?

What if we all said or did things the same way?

What if all our clients/patients/students were the same?

The reality is that our clients/patients/students are not all the same, nor are all audiologists and speech-language pathologists. And, if we were all the same, and said and did things in the same manner, what richness our professions would lack, and what an uninspiring existence for our discipline!

Part of the beauty of the practice of our professions is the intrinsic variety. No client/patient/student is exactly like a former one. The uniqueness and challenge of diversity is part of the calling and attraction to our chosen vocations. The vast scope of practice across the lifespan and along every possible dimension of diversity is part of the appeal. But with that diversity of clientele comes the challenge of appropriately identifying the range of differences and disorders—and addressing those differences and disorders that can occur in speech, language, hearing, swallowing, and balance. The very thing that pulled many of us into these professions keeps us awake at night.

Nearly every respected and credible audiologist or speech-language pathologist has had a humbling experience where they've questioned their ability, second-guessed their training, and wondered whether they picked the right profession. When that experience occurred in conjunction with a cross-cultural exchange gone wrong, often we were left to our own devices. Our ability to appropriately address culture and language in service delivery hinges on our recognition of the beauty and complexity of the intersection of language and culture in daily life—and the extent to which we've had practice addressing those complexities.

What makes a good audiologist or speech-language pathologist *good* in the first place, though, is that nagging in the back of our minds about whether the course of action we're about to take is right. That dose of humility can make an even bigger difference than we often realize. (I would argue that a healthy dose of humility is always a requisite skill, especially when we realize that we are one part of a larger ecosystem that will influence any one individual's success in achieving their personal goals—of which communication may be just a part). What is it that increases our comfort and quiets that questioning voice, to some extent? It's familiarity—it's the sense that we've seen something like this before.

If we're only as good as the collection of experiences upon which we can draw, our success will be severely limited. The guided scenarios included in this workbook expand our exposure and provide access to a more diverse pool of cases than we're likely to have seen or experienced in our professional training—and, in some cases, in years of service delivery. The insight that this workbook provides offers professional challenges that may have been missing in your clinical education and will help you think through circumstances that you may not have been exposed to or seen before. These scenarios can provide you with a bit of familiarity upon which to draw when you encounter something similar in your future clinical interactions.

Finding ways to enhance our skills and continue to grow in our ability to address culture and language in service delivery is every clinician's imperative. This resource is a valuable tool for the necessary self-reflection, learning, and growth that we as clinicians need in order to consider the unfamiliar and enhance our knowledge, skills, and clinical judgment—and to do so in a manner that values diversity and serves all clients/patients/students appropriately and effectively.

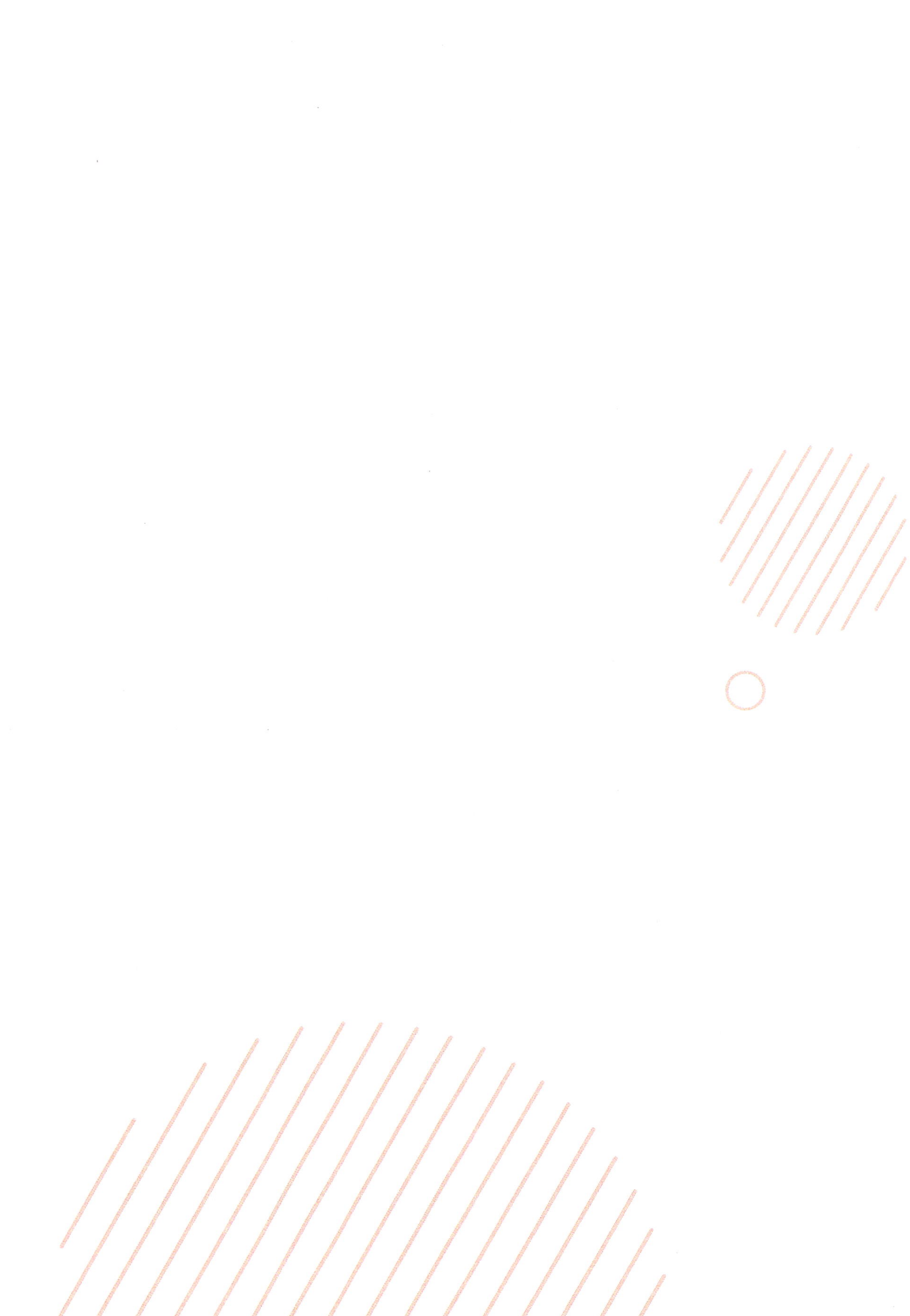

Prologue

Not everything you do is going to be a masterpiece, but you get out there and you try and sometimes it really happens. The other times you're just stretching your soul.

—Maya Angelou

This workbook began as a tiny idea, inspired by conversations of the American Speech-Language-Hearing Association (ASHA) Multicultural Issues Board (MIB). The MIB consists of 12 ASHA members, one National Student Speech Language Hearing Association representative, a Board of Directors liaison, and a staff ex officio. The MIB is charged with

> *facilitating the ability of all ASHA members and certificate holders to enhance human communication by providing culturally competent services and to provide leadership, guidance, and strategic planning in reviewing, recommending, and developing ASHA policies, procedures, and programs that are responsive to cultural and linguistic influences, particularly those impacting historically underserved and underrepresented populations. These populations include but are not limited to individuals identified by race, ethnicity, culture, language, dialect, national origin, gender, gender identity or expression, sexual orientation, age, religion, socioeconomic status, and/or ability. (ASHA, n.d., para. 1)*

Each guided scenario was inspired by real situations. Thus, they reveal one experience of a situation with multiple perspectives. Although the members have diverse experiences in multicultural issues, these experiences do not and cannot represent the views of all the cultures or clients represented in the scenarios. They are simply one perspective and are not presented as the only possible approach. As members of the MIB, we take our charge thoughtfully and seriously and hope this resource inspires others to enhance human communication in all areas.

REFERENCE

American Speech-Language-Hearing Association. (n.d.). *Multicultural Issues Board.* Retrieved from https://www.asha.org/About/governance/committees/CommitteeSmartForms/Multicultural-Issues-Board/

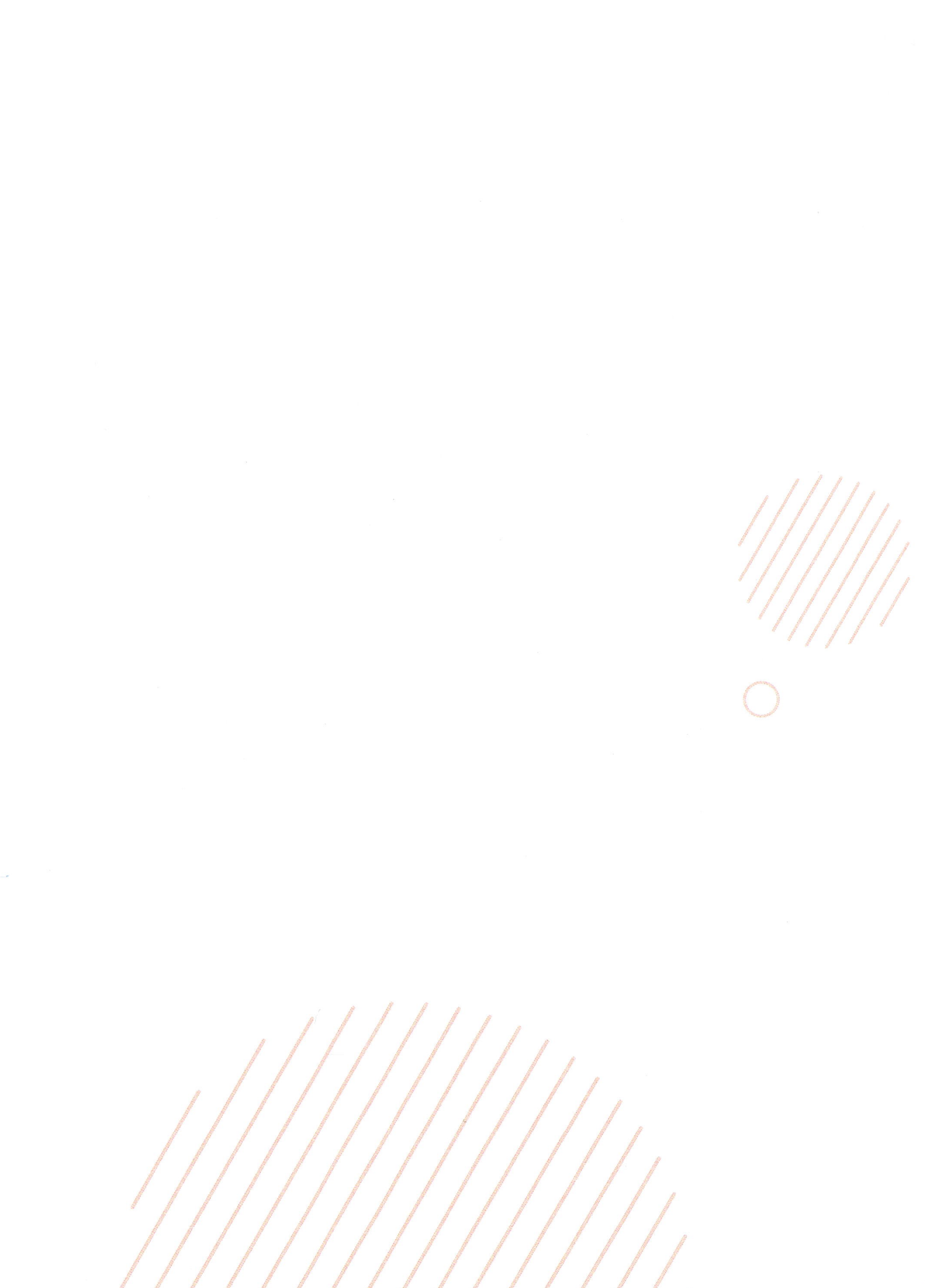

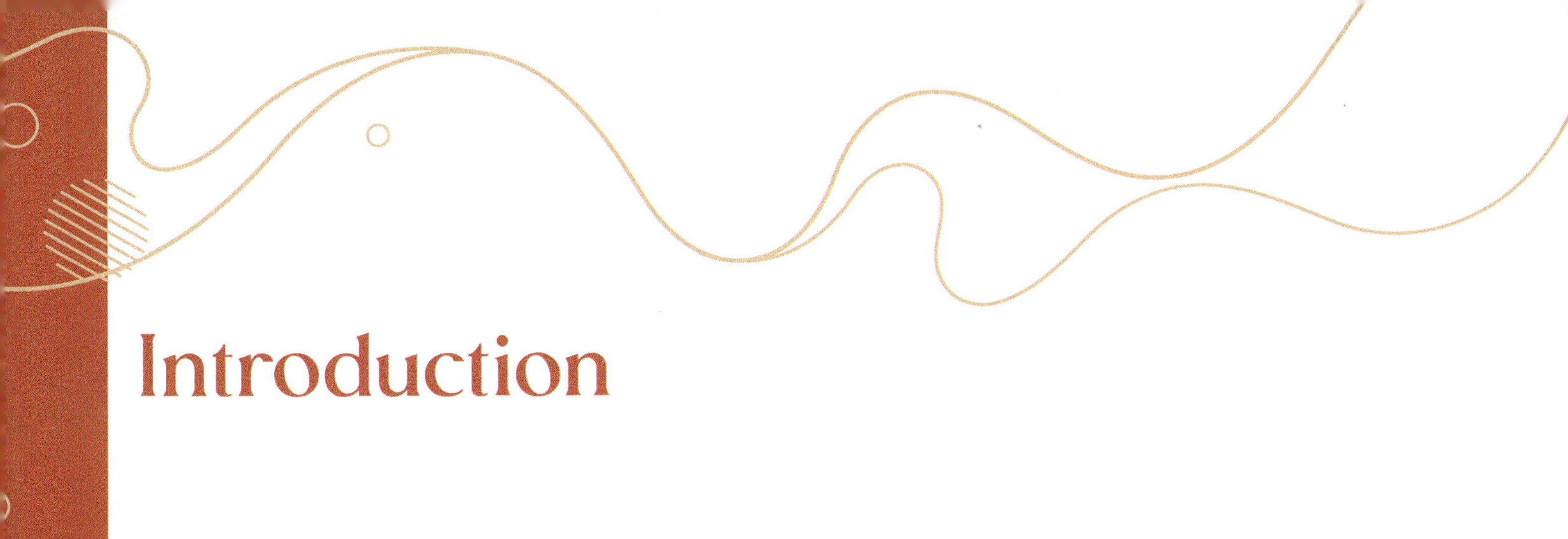

Introduction

WHAT IS CULTURAL COMPETENCE?

notes:

Developing cultural competence across one's professional career is a dynamic process that requires ongoing, critical self-assessment and the continuous expansion of one's cultural knowledge (American Speech-Language-Hearing Association [ASHA], 2017). *Cultural competence* refers to a provider's ability to deliver effective services that meet the social, cultural, and linguistic needs of clients (Betancourt, Green, & Carrillo, 2002). ASHA guides its members to be aware of discrimination on the basis of race or ethnicity, gender, gender identity and gender expression, age, religion, national origin, sexual orientation, and disability while providing services and conducting scholarly research activities. Communication sciences and disorders (CSD) professionals are also encouraged to follow the cultural and linguistic competence guidance outlined in ASHA's (2016a) *Code of Ethics.*

To cultivate cultural competence, practitioners should first examine their own cultural practices and personal biases before they attempt to understand and acquire knowledge about another culture. Culturally competent professionals appreciate the cultural patterns and individual variations in their clients. They engage in cultural self-scrutiny to assess personal bias and to improve cultural self-awareness (Kohnert, 2008). Personal bias can be both explicit and implicit. *Explicit bias* refers to outward beliefs and attitudes, whereas *implicit bias* refers to attitudes or stereotypes that unconsciously affect our understanding, actions, and decisions (Arora, 2017), which is often unconscious and may go against the values we openly profess or believe.

Clinicians have several tools available to them that may be used for self-assessment and monitoring throughout the development of cultural competence. Georgetown's National Center for Cultural Competence (n.d.) offers online tools useful in determining strengths in cultural competence as well as potential areas of growth. Another resource from Harvard University offers an Implicit Association Test to help professionals understand their beliefs and attitudes surrounding certain topics (https://implicit.harvard.edu/implicit/takeatest.html). After completing a self-assessment, a professional may analyze the results and take specific steps to expand their cultural knowledge in areas that require further growth. These steps can include learning about a client's culture, developing a fluid definition of "culture" for one's own clinical practice, understanding the evolving nature of culture, and integrating a client's culture into assessment and treatment, among others.

STAGES OF CULTURAL COMPETENCE

Cultural competence is often described using the concept of a continuum, including several stages: cultural destructiveness, cultural incapacity, cultural blindness, cultural pre-competence, cultural competency, and cultural proficiency (Cross, Bazron, Dennis, & Isaacs, 1989). Cross et al. (1989) described the stages below:

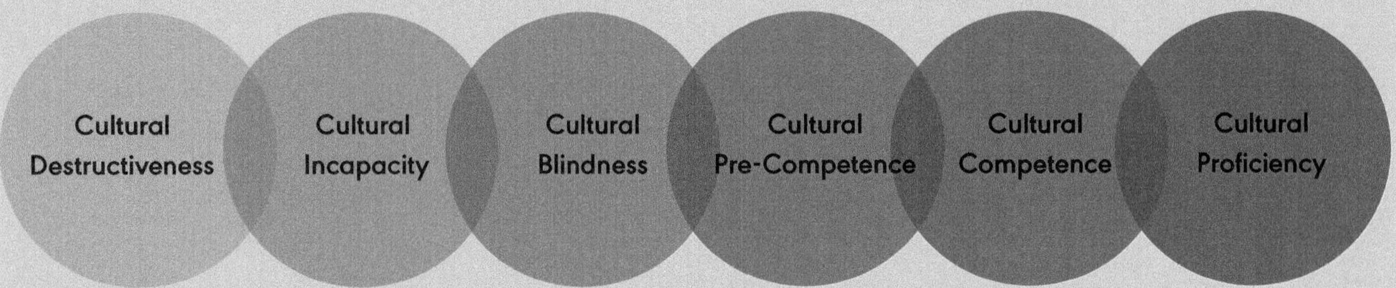

Cultural destructiveness is characterized by overt behaviors aimed at destroying other cultures.

Cultural incapacity is characterized by ethnocentric attitudes and biases but not necessarily overt negative behaviors toward those from other cultural, racial, or ethnic backgrounds.

Cultural blindness refers to not believing one has bias related to racial or cultural differences, or that culture has a primary influence on their own values and behaviors, or that culture plays a role in the attitudes and actions of others. They may attribute cultural differences to individual preferences rather than broad cultural patterns of socialization. Cultural blindness is not uncommon with individuals who have limited contact with others outside of their primary cultural group.

Cultural pre-competence is characterized by increased appreciation of the symbiotic nature of behaviors and values as well as increased recognition of the implicit aspects of culture. People at this stage have engaged in self-assessment, studied cultures of other groups, and participated in cross-cultural learning opportunities.

Cultural competence is characterized by thinking, feeling, and acting in ways that acknowledge, respect, and build on social, cultural, and linguistic diversity (Lynch & Hanson, 2004). Cultural competence establishes positive helping relationships, engages the client in the intervention process, and improves the quality of services provided.

Cultural proficiency is characterized by advocating for systemic changes that address inequities based on cultural differences. Cultural proficiency leads to broadly implemented inclusive practices that affect clinical service delivery, professional policies and training, and the diversity of CSD professions.

Culturally competent CSD professionals are able to demonstrate professional and clinical competence. Professional competence includes practicing in a manner that considers the impact of the unique combination of cultural variables as well as the language exposure and acquisition of their clients and their families. ASHA's *Scope of Practice in Speech-Language Pathology* (2016b) and *Scope of Practice in Audiology* (2018) identify what speech-language pathologists and audiologists are able to do on the basis of their knowledge, skills, training, and further experiences. The Audiology and Speech-Language Pathology certification standards identify the knowledge, skills, and training that audiologists and speech-language pathologists must have to earn certification and be recognized as qualified professionals. Part of these documents note that clinicians are responsible for providing competent services, including cultural responsiveness to clients, patients, and families during all clinician interactions. Moreover, clinically competent professionals should use multiple resources, including client experience and opinion, evidence-based practice, and clinical judgment while working with all culturally and linguistically diverse clients to ensure high-quality service delivery (ASHA, 2016b). Cultural competence, clinical competence, and professional competence are part of an ongoing pursuit across one's career.

CULTURAL RESPONSIVENESS

Cultural responsiveness is a congruous approach to cultural competence in which the provider recognizes the importance of including the client's cultural references in all aspects of their treatment and learning (Ladson-Billings, 1994). Cultural responsiveness sees the client as the expert of their own life and engages with them to help create solutions that are effective and impactful in their treatment. Cultural responsiveness is often described as a pedagogy and is cited as an effective method of instruction for educators, but it can also be applied across other professional settings. Childers-McKee (Burnham, 2019) has suggested five culturally responsive teaching strategies for educators that may be applied to clinical work during assessment and treatment:

1. **Activate a client's prior knowledge.** This activity anchors new learning to an already familiar task.
2. **Make learning contextual.** Connect strategies and skills to real-life scenarios in an attempt to provide a broader, more meaningful context for your client.
3. **Encourage clients and families to leverage their cultural capital.** Let clients and families serve as the cultural experts of their own lives while using personal experiences to shape and set their own goals.
4. **Reconsider your classroom/office/clinic setup.** Ensure that your environment is a welcome place for all. Consider reviewing the groups found in the anti-discriminatory statement of the Multicultural Issues Board's charge found in the prologue and work through each group to identify how they may feel included or excluded by the physical space at your practice.
5. **Build relationships by demonstrating to your clients and families that their goals and unique cultural experiences are valued by you.** Ensure that clients and families feel respected.

CULTURAL HUMILITY

Cultural humility is defined as the "ability to maintain an interpersonal stance that is other-oriented in relation to aspects of cultural identity that are most important to the person" (Hook, Davis, Owen, Worthington, & Utsey, 2013, p. 354). It promotes valuing a client as the expert in their own life. Cultural humility also encourages providers to evaluate their own biases and privileges while developing a curiosity to learn about the cultural background of their clients. Cultural humility can be described as self-reflective, other-oriented, and power-attenuating with an openness to clients as multicultural beings. It places high value on the client-patient as the expert of their lives and places the professional as an active collaborator. Cultural humility further values respect, openness, lack of ego, and consideration of the many facets of a client's background. In other fields, it involves developing mutual partnerships that address power imbalances and creates another-oriented stance that is open to learning new cultural information (Mosher, Hook, Farrell, Watkins, & Davis, 2017).

Cultural humility is similar to cultural competence in that it involves a lifelong commitment to self-evaluation and self-critique (Tervalon & Murray-Garcia, 1998). This view supports the idea that one is never truly done learning and that an endpoint in cultural knowledge is never truly achieved. In addition to becoming culturally competent, the practice of cultural humility encourages the participant to be humble in admitting there are always more perspectives to seek out and that part of our professional responsibility is to continue that journey. A second feature of cultural humility described by Tervalon and Murray-Garcia (1998) is a desire to correct power imbalances where none ought to exist. A practitioner must value the knowledge that clients bring to the clinical process and then use scientific approaches and clinical training to collaborate with the client to create the best clinical outcomes within a balanced client-practitioner relationship.

The final feature of cultural humility involves developing partnerships with people and groups who advocate against systemic imbalances. Pairing clinical practice with advocacy helps to create clinical processes and relationships that center on the client. Cultural humility also reminds practitioners that regardless of cultural affiliation, each client is unique in their experiences and practices. In honoring each client's unique experiences and allowing ourselves to be respectfully curious about them, we learn that individuals from the same place or with the same beliefs may view the same experience differently and may experience different outcomes. Framing our clinical interactions with humility and genuine curiosity provides us the privilege to learn something new and to see our clients for the full, unique people who they are.

In honoring each client's unique experiences and allowing ourselves to be respectfully curious about them, we learn that individuals from the same place or with the same beliefs may view the same experience differently and may experience different outcomes.

CHARACTERISTICS OF CULTURALLY RESPONSIVE CSD PROFESSIONALS

Culturally competent professionals approach each step of the clinical experience by analyzing appropriate ways to make sure clients feel culturally included. Initially, clinicians can create clinical environments that are culturally inclusive by displaying images and materials that are representative of all cultural groups served. CSD professionals implement clinical processes such as scheduling appointments, greeting and contacting clients, adapting intake questionnaires and interviews, and requesting information in ways that reflect the cultural practices and values of the groups that are served. Culturally competent clinicians use their professional and clinical expertise, knowledge of culturally appropriate evidence-based practices, and application of empirical evidence through the client's cultural lens when making clinical decisions. Culturally competent clinicians consider the communicative contexts and social needs of clients and their families when providing clinical services (Kohnert, 2008).

ASHA's (n.d.) *Cultural Competence* provides a list of suggestions to assist professionals in being responsive to cultural variables during the identification, assessment, treatment, and management phases of the intervention process:

- Completing self-assessment to consider the influence of one's own biases and beliefs and the potential impact on service delivery
- Identifying and acknowledging limitations in education, training, and knowledge and seeking additional resources and education to develop cultural competence via continuing education, networking with community members, and so forth
- Seeking funding for and engaging in ongoing professional development of cultural competence throughout one's career
- Demonstrating respect for an individual's age, disability, ethnicity, gender identity, national/regional origin, race, religion, sex, sexual orientation, and veteran status
- Integrating clients'/patients'/families' traditions, customs, values, and beliefs in service delivery
- Identifying the impact of assimilation and acculturation on communication patterns during identification, assessment, treatment, and management of a communication disorder/difference
- Assessing/treating each client/patient/family as an individual and responding to his/her unique needs, as opposed to anticipating cultural variables based on assumptions
- Identifying appropriate intervention and assessment strategies and materials that do not violate the client's/patient's/family's unique values and/or create a chasm between the clinician and client/patient/family and his/her community
- Using culturally appropriate communication with clients/patients, caregivers, and family so that information presented during counseling is provided in a health literate format consistent with clients'/patients' cultural values
- Referring to/consulting with other service providers with appropriate cultural and linguistic proficiency, including using a cultural informant or broker
- Upholding ethical responsibilities during the provision of clinically appropriate services.

Clinicians should note the differences between seeking cultural competence and engaging in cultural stereotyping. Seeking cultural competence involves obtaining information about a client while recognizing that each client should be treated as a unique individual and not as a reflection of cultural assumptions or generalizations.

Clinical competency requires clinicians to use their training and cultural knowledge to distinguish between differences in communication practices and communication disorders. It encourages clinicians to seek more information about cultural practices and linguistic patterns, when it is needed, and to use multiple resources to investigate the social, regional, and other factors that shape an individual's communication behavior. This approach to clinical practice moves away from *ethnocentrism*, or the belief that there is only one valid set of values beliefs and practices, and from *essentialism*, which does not account for variations within a culture. Cultural competence in practice leads a clinician to form a true partnership with their

Cultural competence in practice leads a clinician to form a true partnership with their client, valuing the unique variables they bring to each clinical encounter.

client, valuing the unique variables they bring to each clinical encounter. Culturally competent professionals establish positive helping relationships, engage the client, and—as a result—improve the quality of services provided. Culturally competent professionals think, feel, and act in ways that acknowledge, respect, and build on social, cultural, and linguistic strengths of their clients (Lynch & Hanson, 2004).

Although there is no true endpoint to cultural competence or cultural proficiency, because cultures are fluid and dynamic and each person in a culture is unique, we use the term *culturally competent* across this text to indicate a professional who has taken the steps to learn more about the cultures of their clients in an attempt to broaden their practice, demonstrate respect, and improve the overall clinical experience. *Cultural responsiveness* is used when cultural competence is put into action—for instance, when a professional makes a change in their behavior, advocates for a specific group, or acknowledges a misstep. Although we all strive for excellence, we know that in practice we may fall short. Cultural responsiveness recognizes those moments and how we react and grow from them. Perhaps consider them as moments of "stretching the soul."

HOW TO USE THIS RESOURCE

This resource is a culmination of information gathered through work done by the Multicultural Issues Board, specifically in regard to increasing one's cultural responsiveness. It is intended as a self-study course or personal workbook that will expand on the knowledge you have about the relationships between culture, communication, language, and clinical practice. It is our hope that it will challenge the ways you think about and respond to cultural issues. The target audience includes learners at any point in their professional careers—from students in training programs to experienced practitioners seeking to reflect on and enhance their cultural knowledge and improve their interactions with clients. The guided exercises are designed to help you understand the ways in which culture plays a critical role in every part of our work, and how our own individual cultures can and do influence our clinical practice. Each guided scenario is inspired by true events. Specific details and names have been removed, and some narratives have been combined in an effort to eliminate identifiable information and to add more detail to the presented case.

This resource is not a definitive authority on all populations and issues related to cultural competence; it is based on the expertise of the authors, with specific emphasis placed on clinical expertise. There may be instances in which alternative approaches or opinions may be equally as viable or culturally appropriate for the given scenario. Culture is dynamic and unique, and so the approaches to these scenarios will never have a "one size fits all" response. We encourage the reader to reflect on the presented scenarios and responses and to consider their own approach.

We hope that this tool serves as a starting point as we all continue to cultivate our clinical skills by increasing our cultural competence and responsiveness. Some situations may evoke strong emotions in the reader; this result is intentional. When confronted with discomfort, the authors encourage you to work through those feelings using the guiding questions provided and to engage in further self-reflection.

It is important to remember that the endpoint of this work is not competence or proficiency. There is never a moment when one fully achieves cultural competence. Developing cultural competence and becoming culturally responsive is an ongoing process that involves a practice of constant learning, self-reflection, and action. When cultural competence is paired with cultural humility, it encompasses a curiosity regarding the experiences of others, a desire to seek out new experiences, and a respect for the unique cultural existence of others.

Each scenario is presented in a standard format: a short prebrief, objectives, the case scenario, critical thinking and debriefing questions, a commentary, critical thinking and debriefing responses, take aways, references, and additional resources.

PREBRIEF

The prebrief includes a general overview of the concepts to be presented by the scenario and primes the reader for the topic.

OBJECTIVES

Learner objectives are provided in an effort to frame the scenario and guide the learner to focus on the main ideas. Learner objectives also serve as a tool for self-evaluation after completing the scenario exercise.

CASE SCENARIO

The scenario is presented in a narrative. Each detail mentioned in a case is important to the overall interpretation of the information and possible recommendations for approaches that follow. As you read the case, it is recommended that you take notes, underline or highlight significant passages that stand out to you, and note any emotions or reactions you may have. Be sure to note the cultural details in the scenario. These notes will help you as you complete the critical thinking and reflection questions.

CRITICAL THINKING AND DEBRIEFING QUESTIONS

After each scenario, questions are presented that challenge you to think critically and to reflect on what you have read. This section may contain additional perspectives to provide further insight on the topic. These questions help the reader debrief the scenario by providing opportunities for candid reflection and extended learning. As you read through the questions, you are encouraged to refer back to the scenario and any notes you have taken. The critical thinking questions are designed to assist you in considering how you may approach similar clinical situations in the future. The questions encourage you to engage with any emotional responses you may have and to consider the impact of any implicit or explicit cultural bias. Culture is unique to individuals and, as a result, personal. Consequently, certain scenarios may resonate deeply with a reader because of similar experiences. The cases may also elicit strong, unexpected reactions. We invite you to sit with these feelings, process them, and use the resources, commentary, and responses to the critical thinking questions to reflect on your experience.

COMMENTARY

The commentary follows the critical thinking and reflection questions. This section is critical because it provides an analysis of the information provided in the scenario. It shapes the case within the context of using cultural competence and responsiveness, and it cites useful evidence-based and best practices available in current literature. This commentary may also provide more context, research, and reflection, giving the reader additional opportunities to make notations as new thoughts arise.

CRITICAL THINKING AND DEBRIEFING RESPONSES

The answers to the critical thinking and reflection questions are included after the commentary and are separate from the questions to encourage candid evaluation. The answers expand on aspects presented in the commentary and incorporate research, best practice, and clinical expertise. They are not final, and there may be other valid approaches that are not shared.

TAKE AWAYS

The "take aways" wrap up the case and underscore the main points. This is another area where the reader can complete a self-assessment to indicate mastery of the learning objectives.

We hope that you find this resource useful and that it challenges you in many different ways. Thank you for reading.

REFERENCES

American Speech-Language Hearing Association. (n.d.). *Cultural competence.* Retrieved from https://www.asha.org/Practice-Portal/Professional-Issues/Cultural-Competence/

American Speech-Language Hearing Association. (2016a). *Code of Ethics.* Retrieved from http://www.asha.org/Code-of-Ethics/

American Speech-Language-Hearing Association. (2016b). *Scope of practice in speech-language pathology.* Retrieved from https://www.asha.org/policy/SP2016-00343/

American Speech-Language Hearing Association. (2017). *Issues in ethics: Cultural and linguistic competence.* Retrieved from http://www.asha.org/Practice/ethics/Cultural-and-Linguistic-Competence/

American Speech-Language-Hearing Association. (2018). *Scope of practice in audiology.* Retrieved from https://www.asha.org/policy/

Arora, N. (2017). Look at your blind spots: Do unconscious preconceptions shape your clinical judgment? A school-based clinician offers ways to uncover—and address—implicit bias. *The ASHA Leader, 22*(11), 6-7.

Betancourt, J., Green, A., & Carrillo, J. (2002). *Cultural competence in health care: Emerging frameworks and practical approaches.* New York, NY: The Commonwealth Fund.

Burnham, K. (2019, July 17). *5 culturally responsive teaching strategies* [Blog post]. Retrieved from https://www.northeastern.edu/graduate/blog/culturally-responsive-teaching-strategies/

Cross, T., Bazron, B., Dennis, K., & Isaacs, M. (1989). *Towards a culturally competent system of care* (Vol. 1). Washington, DC: CASSP Technical Assistance Center, Georgetown University Child Development Center.

Hook, J. N., Davis, D. E., Owen, J., Worthington, E. L., Jr., & Utsey, S. O. (2013). Cultural humility: Measuring openness to culturally diverse clients. *Journal of Counseling Psychology, 60,* 353–366.

Kohnert, K. (2008). *Language disorders in bilingual children and adults.* San Diego, CA: Plural Press.

Ladson-Billings, G. (1994). Who will teach our children? Preparing teachers to successfully teach African American students. In E. Hollins, J. King, & W. Hayman (Eds.), *Teaching diverse learners: Formulating a knowledge base for teaching diverse populations* (pp. 129-158). Albany: State University of New York Press.

Lynch, E. W., & Hanson, M. J. (2004). Family diversity, assessment, and cultural competence. In M. McLean, M. Wolery, & D. B. Bailey (Eds.), *Assessing infants and preschoolers with special needs* (3rd ed., pp. 72-74). Upper Saddle River, NJ: Pearson Education.

Mosher, D. K., Hook, J. N., Farrell, J. E., Watkins, C. E., Jr., & Davis, D. E. (2017). Cultural humility. In E. L. Worthington, Jr., D. E. Davis, & J. N. Hook (Eds.), *Handbook of humility: Theory, research, and applications* (pp. 91-104). Abingdon-on-Thames, England: Routledge/Taylor & Francis Group.

National Center for Cultural Competence. (n.d.). *Self-assessments.* Retrieved from https://nccc.georgetown.edu/assessments/

Tervalon, M., & Murray-Garcia, J. (1998). Cultural humility versus cultural competence: A critical distinction in defining physician training outcomes in multicultural education. *Journal of Health Care for the Poor and Underserved, 9,* 117-125.

ADDITIONAL RESOURCES

Battle, D. (2012). Becoming a culturally competent clinician. *Perspectives on Communication Disorders and Sciences in Culturally and Linguistically Diverse Populations, 6*(3), 19-22.

FitzJefferies, K. (2017, September). *Cultural humility: Reflection on self and practice.* Paper presented at the annual conference of the National Association for Alcoholism and Drug Abuse Counselors, Denver, CO.

Nuri-Robins, K., Lindsey, R. B., Lindsey, D., & Terrell, R. (2011). *Culturally proficient instruction* (3rd ed.). Thousand Oaks, CA: Corwin.

Roseberry-McKibbin, C. (2018). *Multicultural students with speech language needs: Practical strategies for assessment and intervention* (5th ed.). Oceanside, CA: Academic Communication Associates.

Torres, I. (2015). How to recognize your cultural competence: A group activity at the ASHA convention opened this SLP's eyes to the fluidity of her own cultural identity. And to how much that matters. *The ASHA Leader, 20*(3), 6-7.

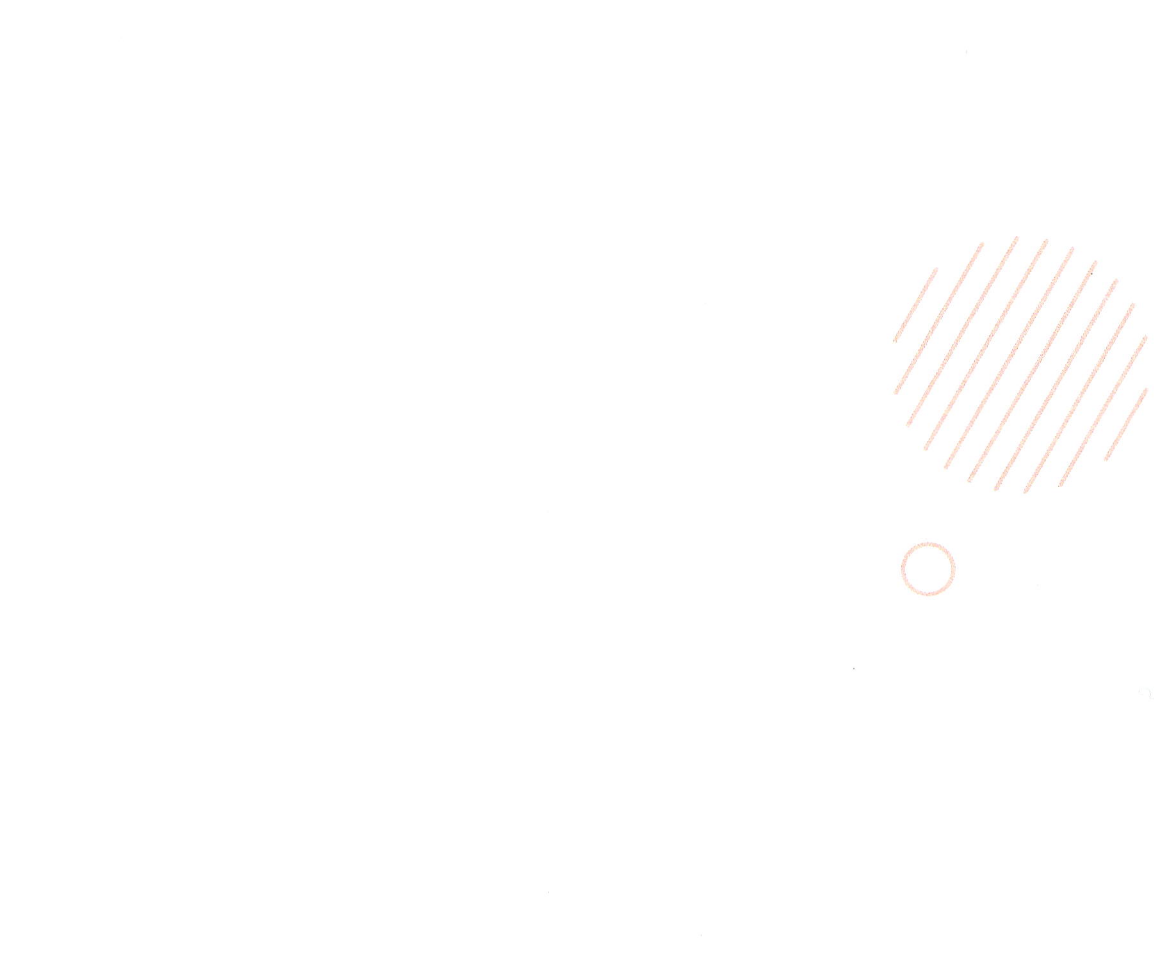

Border Trauma and Blurred Lines

— When Personal Feelings Affect Clinical Decisions

ALICIA FLEMING HAMILTON

PREBRIEF

As audiologists and speech-language pathologists (SLPs), we seek to make communication a right for all. As professionals, we have a vested interest in the welfare of our clients. This scenario focuses on the forced separation of one immigrant family and the impacts it has on their daughter. It also addresses the difficult decisions that professionals may face when working with children who are forcefully separated from their asylum-seeking parents. Immigrants and their U.S.-born children make up about 28% of the U.S. population, according to the 2019 Current Population Survey (CPS), a number which is projected to rise to about 36% by 2065 (Zong, Batalova, & Hallock, 2018). Almost 18 million children ages 0–17 years have at least one immigrant parent (Zong et al., 2018). Immigrants and refugee youth are the fastest growing group of children in the United States and are expected to make up one third of all U.S. children by 2050 (Zong et al., 2018).

notes:

OBJECTIVES

- Understand how trauma may affect overall development and place children at risk for communication disorders.
- Evaluate ethical implications when choosing whether or not to provide services.
- Ascertain the best practices when working with sequential versus simultaneous bilingual learners when there is a lack of bilingual staffing available (American Speech-Language-Hearing Association [ASHA], n.d.).

CASE SCENARIO

Shannon is a bilingual (Spanish-English) SLP who works in a large, urban school district providing services in their program for children from birth to 3 years old. Shannon is the only Spanish-speaking member of the district's early intervention interdisciplinary team, which includes an occupational therapist, an early childhood education teacher, a physical therapist, and a social worker. Recently, the social worker presented a new student referral for their team and requested assistance from Shannon.

Definitions

Simultaneous bilingualism—the acquisition of two languages at the same time, typically with both languages introduced prior to age 3

Sequential bilingualism—a second language introduced after age 3, at which time some level of proficiency has been established in the primary language, also referred to as successive bilingualism or second language acquisition

Dual language learners—individuals learning two languages simultaneously from infancy or who are learning a second language after the first language

https://www.asha.org/practice-portal/professional-issues/bilingual-service-delivery/

The referral involved Lucia, a 20-month-old girl, who was in crisis foster care. Lucia, her mother Marta, and her father Diego were from Guatemala. Their native language was K'iche', a Mesoamerican language from the Mayan language family, and they spoke Spanish as their second language. This brief description of their experience was documented in their case file:

> *Six months ago, they fled Guatemala because of the violence they were witnessing and made their way to Mexico. Lucia was just beginning to say her first words at this time. Her family arrived in Mexico 3 months later and were advised to wait their turn to complete the asylum application process for entry into the United States. Weary from their travels, Marta and Diego chose instead to cross the U.S. border independently and to request asylum from the first border patrol agent they encountered. As they attempted to cross the border, agents stopped Marta. The border agents used Spanish to explain the content of a document written in English to Marta while pointing to her daughter and then to the document to sign. Even though Marta did not fully understand the nature of the document, fearfully she signed it in the presence of the border patrol. As she signed it, Diego carried Lucia across the border and was immediately arrested and detained, with agents taking Lucia from his arms. Marta was barred from crossing the border to retrieve Lucia and was told to go back to the processing center in Mexico. The border patrol agents explained to Diego and Marta, in Spanish, that Lucia would now be placed in the U.S. foster care system until their case was seen. The family was now separated.*

Notes from her file indicated that Lucia initially cried out, saying "mama, dada, agua," as she was detained, but after a week in the detainment center, she stopped communicating verbally.

Lucia arrived at the home of her crisis foster mother, Sally, 1 month after she was separated from her parents. Sally and the early childhood interdisciplinary team's social worker had frequently worked together through the early intervention program. Sally was a married, English-speaking woman, who had two children of her own, ages 9 and 14. The team and Sally were not able to obtain information on where Lucia's father was being held, and they had no knowledge of other family members living in the United States or abroad. They were told that the form Marta signed at the border terminated her parental rights for Lucia, and they had no further contact information for Marta.

Sally reported that in the past 2 months she observed that Lucia did not talk and cried often. She ate very little, appeared lethargic, and had issues with constipation. She reported that Lucia had a flat affect and did not initiate communication or demonstrate joint attention. She reacted strongly to any physical touch, affection, and attempts to comfort her. Lucia appeared to understand everything that was said to her in Spanish and followed directions in Spanish when supplemented with gestures. She was beginning to demonstrate understanding of some directions in English. Overall, Sally described her as appearing "depressed."

The social worker brought this information back to the interdisciplinary team. After reviewing, the team had many concerns, and agreed that Lucia was a good candidate for early intervention services. They also supported intervention services in Spanish, but Shannon, the SLP, was the only bilingual team member. Shannon was concerned that Lucia may be exhibiting much more than a speech delay, and she agreed to go on a home visit to meet Lucia and learn more about her.

During the visit, the team observed Lucia sitting quietly and not interacting. After 10-15 minutes, Shannon approached her with a baby doll and asked her, in Spanish, whether she would like to play with it. Lucia made eye contact with Shannon, reached out her hand, and grabbed the doll. Shannon presented a bottle for the doll. She told Lucia that she could use the bottle to feed the baby if it was hungry. Lucia looked at Shannon, then the bottle, and back at Shannon. Lucia stretched out her hand. Shannon gave her the bottle, and Lucia "fed" the baby. Shannon continued to play with Lucia for the remainder of the visit while the social worker obtained more information for their developmental questionnaire.

After completing her clinical checklist in Spanish, Shannon concluded that Lucia's receptive language skills were age appropriate. Lucia identified common objects in Spanish, followed routine and novel directions, and answered yes-no questions by shaking her head. She demonstrated a few social smiles and joint attention. Lucia was beginning to imitate single words with Shannon. Lucia's foster mother expressed that this was the most language and interaction she had seen from Lucia since she arrived in her home. As Shannon was packing the toys to leave, Lucia hugged Shannon and would not let go. Shannon told Lucia, in Spanish, that she could keep the doll, but that Shannon had to go visit other children. Lucia began to cry as the team left.

The team reconvened after the visit to discuss service options. Shannon was torn—she knew that Lucia had experienced major trauma in her recent past, which put her at risk for future language and developmental disabilities. However, on the basis of Shannon's assessment, Lucia was currently demonstrating age-appropriate skills and did not show a need in the area of communication. If Lucia was a monolingual child, Shannon would not provide services. However, Shannon felt that because of her bilingualism, she was in a unique position to provide strategies to Lucia's caregivers that would support the maintenance of Lucia's Spanish while she learned English in her foster placement. Additionally, Shannon was disturbed by the forced separation that Lucia endured and wanted to find a way to contact Lucia's father or other family members. Shannon strongly considered reporting a language delay and bending the rules for services so that she could continue to work with and advocate for Lucia.

CRITICAL THINKING AND DEBRIEFING QUESTIONS

1. **What effect could trauma have on a child's development, including speech and language?**
2. **How do you accurately measure developmental milestones in a case like this?**
3. **What are the potential impacts and implications of participating in systems that forcibly separate families?**
4. **What are some ways to advocate for this student and family?**
5. **Are there any other ways that Shannon could support Lucia if she is not truly demonstrating a delay?**

COMMENTARY

Immigration has become a highly politicized topic in recent years. As policy enforcement changes in the United States, the increase in family separations and implications for children, the foster care system, and educational systems have become more apparent. SLPs must be cognizant of the possible cognitive, social, psychological, and physical sequalae of trauma endured by children who experience these separations (Brabeck, Lykes, & Hunter, 2014). Trauma may precipitate the development of mental and behavioral disorders, both of which are correlated to language disorders and language development (ASHA, 2018). Other research demonstrates the impact of trauma on communication, including the onset of selective mutism or acquired stuttering (Perez & Stoeckle, 2016; Wong, 2010). The conditions under which children are separated, housed, transported, and eventually placed in foster care may all contribute to the experience of trauma. ASHA has spoken out against the unnecessary and unacceptable trauma of family separation and abhorrent living conditions that these children are exposed to (ASHA, 2019).

It is essential that communication professionals attempt to understand a child's or client's experiences and approach evaluations with cultural sensitivity. This may include culturally informed interviews and assessments that capture a child's abilities in their native language. It may also include screenings for adverse childhood experiences (ACEs) and information on any exposure to trauma. Additionally, bilingual SLPs and practitioners must be prepared to share community resources with team members to support them in providing culturally appropriate referrals and interventions.

The SLP initially visited Lucia because of her foster mother's concerns about Lucia's language development. Because of her bilingual skills and clinical experience, the SLP also had a unique opportunity to advocate for Lucia by educating her team and caregivers

Expand Your Knowledge

Statement by ASHA President Shari Robertson on Immigrant Children's Living Conditions at Southern U.S. Border

June 28, 2019

(Rockville, MD) One year ago, the American Speech-Language-Hearing Association (ASHA) called upon the Trump Administration to ensure that then recently separated immigrant families were reunited in timely fashion. Today, ASHA not only renews that call, but expands it to include urging an immediate end to the horrific living conditions immigrant children in the Administration's care now find themselves having to endure.

This unacceptable situation is potentially setting them up for lifetimes of struggle. Often, traumatized children require long-term comprehensive and sustained supports, including the treatment of resulting communication disorders, in order to successfully transition into adolescence and adulthood.

As ASHA noted last year, research shows the impact of trauma on communication such as the onset of selective mutism or acquired stuttering.* Back then, family separation was trauma enough—now it is being compounded by enforced living conditions barren of basics critical to children's overall welfare and development.

"As the president of an organization that represents thousands of professionals who work daily to foster the development of children in ways that are not only healthy but also their right, we find it abhorrent that any child would be caught in terrible situations like the one happening on the southern U.S. border," ASHA President Shari Robertson, PhD, CCC-SLP said. "It must end now, before any further or irreparable damage is done to innocent children."

*See Perez, H.R., & Stoeckle (2016). Stuttering: Clinical and research update. Canadian Family Physician, 62(6), 479–484, and Wong, P. (2010). Selective mutism: A review of etiology, comorbidities, and treatment. *Psychiatry, 7*(3), 23–31

https://www.asha.org/News/2019/Statement-by-ASHA-President-Shari-Robertson-on-Immigrant-Children-s-Living-Conditions-at-Southern-U-S--Border/

about the impact that Lucia's traumatic experiences may have on her future development. Although the SLP determined that Lucia's language skills were developing appropriately given her age and language background, the SLP noticed that Lucia was exhibiting symptoms of trauma, on the basis of her own observations and those of Lucia's foster mother. The SLP knew that because of the trauma Lucia experienced as a result of forced separation from her family, Lucia was now at risk for learning and language difficulties in the future. Additionally, the SLP knew that supporting Lucia's primary language (Spanish) would be critically important in the development of her language skills and in maintaining the ability to hopefully communicate with her family sometime in the future.

Expand Your Knowledge

Adverse childhood experiences (ACEs) can have serious, long-term impacts on a child's health and well-being by contributing to high levels of toxic stress that derail healthy physical, social, emotional, and cognitive development. The original ACEs study (Felitti et al., 1998) considered 10 ACEs: Five ACEs were personal to the child (emotional, physical, and sexual abuse; and emotional and physical neglect), and five ACEs were related to other family members (witnessing domestic violence; living with someone who abused substances, was mentally ill, or was imprisoned; and absence of parent through death, divorce, or abandonment). The study was continued in later years, sometimes adding additional ACEs such as urban ACE indicators (racism, witnessing violence, living in an unsafe neighborhood, living in foster care, experiencing bullying), caregiver leaving for military deployment, or experiencing natural disasters or war (Westby, 2018).

The SLP faces a personal dilemma—according to the way professionals were assigned to students in her district's early intervention program, Lucia was not a candidate for SLP services because she did not have a demonstrated need in the area of communication. The SLP wanted to continue her involvement in Lucia's case to support her language development in Spanish and advocate for her, but she could not compromise policies on the basis of her personal feelings. Although the decision not to provide services was appropriate, the SLP may decide to help Lucia by providing education to Lucia's foster family about the importance of maintaining Lucia's home language of Spanish and encouraging the use of interpreters and playing with other Spanish-speaking children across Lucia's intervention. The SLP may also provide information on ACEs and how to mitigate some of the damaging impact of the trauma she experienced.

CRITICAL THINKING AND DEBRIEFING RESPONSES

1. **What effect could trauma have on this child's development, including speech and language?**

Research about childhood trauma indicates that children who are exposed to multiple ACEs are at risk of having more difficulty with social, emotional, and cognitive ability and that ACE exposure increases a child's likelihood of having poor health outcomes as they grow (Westby, 2018). It is important to provide intervention that targets resilience when children have experienced multiple ACEs (Westby, 2018). Westby (2018) noted that the guidelines of the Individuals With Disabilities Education Act of 1990 require that "multidisciplinary teams determine the presence of a language delay or impairment that is not the result of an environmental or economic disadvantage" (p. 3), but there is no supporting evidence for that recommendation, and in this specific case, it may not be appropriate. Another study of a cohort of urban children noted that experiencing ACEs in early childhood, especially three ACEs or more, was associated with below-average language and literacy skills in kindergarten (Jimenez, Wade, Lin, Morrow, & Reichman, 2016). This study underscored the importance of supporting optimal development among children who have experienced multiple ACEs (Jimenez et al., 2016). Finally, Jessica Goodkind of the American Psychological Association noted that family separation was "on par with beating and torture in terms of its relationship to mental health" and could be one of the driving factors that creates psychological distress (Stringer, 2018, para. 13). Research supports the idea that Lucia is likely at risk because of her prior experiences and may benefit from targeted interventions (Stringer, 2018).

2. **How do you accurately measure developmental milestones in a case like this?**

In this specific case, it would be appropriate for the SLP to research common developmental milestones in Spanish language development for children from similar backgrounds as Lucia or, at the very least, children who speak Spanish. Although Lucia could not directly be compared with students as part of the research, given her exposure to K'iche' and traumatic experiences in her asylum journey, it would provide a possible starting point to understand what a "typical" child with some of her background characteristics may be able to do. The SLP may consider completing a checklist to include ACEs and other trauma that Lucia has experienced, indicating that those experiences may have impacted her language or may put her language and other development at risk in the future. Given Lucia's age-appropriate skills during the play sample and clinical evaluation, her communication skills appear to be within age-level expectations at this time. However, if Lucia would not have engaged with Shannon during the initial evaluation, it would have been appropriate for Shannon to come back for another observation after Lucia had formed an attachment with a provider. The SLP may choose to provide some supplemental coaching or resources that can help Lucia to continue to remain on track for her development, given that her traumatic experiences and lack of native language input now put her at risk for language and learning difficulties.

3. **What are the potential impacts and implications of participating in systems that forcibly separate families?**

Personal response. Please consider the following: Professional practice dictates a call to action. A professional must reflect on how their actions may work with or against systems that are in place and weigh those actions within their own moral and ethical codes. Professionals are also encouraged to reflect on their client interactions to improve their professional practice and to increase their cultural competence in areas where they may lack information or training.

4. **What are some ways to advocate for this student and family?**

The SLP could take a variety of approaches in advocating for this family. Shannon could provide information that indicates support of a child's native language is the best practice when working on developing language skills, or she could provide strategies that monolingual clinicians or team members can use even though they do not speak a shared language with Lucia (Kohnert & Derr, 2004). Moreover, she may share data that show the positive relationships between forming genuine attachments with caregivers and positive overall development. Shannon could share Lucia's story with her local lawmakers to discuss how different policies may affect children's development in negative ways, or she could call national representatives to share this story. Shannon may also choose to support local or national charities that help children and families in similar situations. Shannon has specialized knowledge of bilingual development, typical language development, and how trauma affects the early global development of children, with persisting problems into adulthood. Sharing that information could provide a great impact on other children by teaching staff and caregivers effective strategies that can mitigate the negative effects of ACEs in their lives.

5. **Are there any other ways that Shannon could support Lucia if she is not truly demonstrating a delay?**

Shannon could advocate for an interpreter to work with Lucia's foster family to support her Spanish language development, make connections between the two languages, and lessen the impact of language loss because of her sudden exposure to English. She might also create a timeline of Lucia's family history and transition for her file to support future efforts of locating her family. Shannon could offer the team information on best practices for working with a child when you do not speak their language, including strategies that work on concepts that cross languages—for instance, working on conceptual knowledge, using picture supports, and finding phonemes shared across a language (Kohnert & Derr, 2004). The serving team, in addition to using an interpreter, could use resources in Spanish that utilize media incorporating songs and appropriate videos. Additionally, the team could choose to learn more about trauma-informed care practices and how to mitigate the long-term impact of ACEs on development.

TAKE AWAYS

- Children who have experienced a traumatic event such as forced separation from their parents may experience communication difficulties that require a multidisciplinary team to support their developmental needs.
- Self-reflection is an important aspect of any professional practice. SLPs and audiologists benefit from taking time to reflect on the populations they serve and how they may learn more about individual situations in an effort to enhance cultural competence.
- SLPs and audiologists are charged with advocating for their clients. It is important to understand how systems are constructed so that we can best advocate for our clients.

REFERENCES

American Speech-Language-Hearing Association. (n.d.). *Bilingual service delivery.* Retrieved from https://www.asha.org/practice-portal/professional-issues/bilingual-service-delivery/

American Speech-Language-Hearing Association. (2018, June 21). *ASHA urges quick reunification of separated families: Organization raises potential harm to children's communication development.* Retrieved from https://www.asha.org/News/2018/ASHA-Urges-Quick-Reunification-of-Separated-Families/

American Speech-Language-Hearing Association. (2019, June 28). *Statement by ASHA President Shari Robertson on immigrant children's living conditions at southern U.S. border.* Retrieved from https://www.asha.org/News/2019/Statement-by-ASHA-President-Shari-Robertson-on-Immigrant-Children-s-Living-Conditions-at-Southern-U-S--Border/

Brabeck, K. M., Lykes, M. B., & Hunter, C. (2014). The psychosocial impact of detention and deportation on U.S. migrant children and families. *American Journal of Orthopsychiatry, 84,* 496–505.

Felitti, V. J., Anda, R. F., Nordenberg, D., Williamson, D. F., Spitz, A. M., Edwards, V., Koss,

M. P., & Marks, J. S. (1998). Relationship of childhood abuse and household dysfunction to many of the leading causes of death in adults: The Adverse Childhood Experiences (ACE) Study. *American Journal of Preventive Medicine, 14*(4), 245–258. Retrieved from https://doi.org/10.1016/S0749-3797(98)00017-8

Individuals With Disabilities Education Act of 1990, Pub. L. 101-476, renamed the Individuals With Disabilities Education Improvement Act, codified at 20 U.S.C. §§ 1400–1482.

Jimenez, M. E., Wade, R., Lin, Y., Morrow, L. M., & Reichman, N. E. (2016). Adverse experiences in early childhood and kindergarten outcomes. *Pediatrics, 137*(2), e20151839. https://doi.org/10.1542/peds.2015-1839

Kohnert, K., & Derr, A. (2004). Language intervention with bilingual children. In B. Goldstein (Ed.), *Bilingual language development and disorders in Spanish–English speakers* (pp. 311–338). Baltimore, MD: Brookes.

Perez, H. R., & Stoeckle, J. H. (2016). Stuttering: Clinical and research update. *Canadian Family Physician, 62,* 479–484.

Stringer, H. (2018). *Psychologists respond to a mental health crisis at the border: Clinicians, researchers and advocates support families who are suffering in the wake of the family separation policy.* Retrieved from https://www.apa.org/news/apa/2018/border-family-separation

Westby, C. (2018). Adverse childhood experiences: What speech-language pathologists need to know. *Word of Mouth, 30,* 1–4. https://doi.org/10.1177/1048395018796520

Wong, P. (2010). Selective mutism: A review of etiology, comorbidities, and treatment. *Psychiatry, 7*(3), 23–31.

Zong, J., Batalova, J., & Hallock, J. (2018, February 8). *Frequently requested statistics on immigrants and immigration in the United States.* Retrieved from https://www.migrationpolicy.org/article/frequently-requested-statistics-immigrants-and immigration-united-states-7

ADDITIONAL RESOURCES

ARTICLES AND BOOKS

Evans, B. F., III, & Hass, G. A. (2018). *Forensic psychological* assessment in immigration court: A guidebook for evidence-based and ethical practice. New York, NY: Routledge.

Lieberman, A. F., & Knorr, K. (2007). The impact of trauma: A developmental framework for infancy and early childhood. *Pediatric Annals, 36,* 209–215.

McMinn, S., & Klahr, R. (2019, January 10). Where does illegal immigration mostly occur? Here's what the data tell us. *NPR.* Retrieved from https://www.npr.org/2019/01/10/683662691/where-does-illegal-immigration-mostly-occur-heres-what-the-data-tell-us

Outley, C., & Skuza, J. A. (2019). Perspectives on immigrant, refugee, and border youth. *Journal of Youth Development, 14*(2), 1–9.

Radford, J. (2019, June 17). Key findings about U.S. immigrants. *Fact Tank: News in the Numbers.* Retrieved from https://www.pewresearch.org/fact-tank/2019/06/17/key-findings-about-u-s-immigrants/

Teicher, M. H. (2018). Childhood trauma and the enduring consequences of forcibly separating children from parents at the United States border. *BMC Medicine, 16*(1), 146.

ONLINE RESOURCES

Early Childhood Technical Assistance Center: Part C Eligibility: https://ectacenter.org/topics/earlyid/partcelig.asp

Refugee Mental Health Resource Network: https://refugeementalhealthnet.org

To advocate for immigrant children and families, join the American Psychological Association's Federal Action Network: https://www.apa.org/science/about/psa/2016/07/federal-action-network

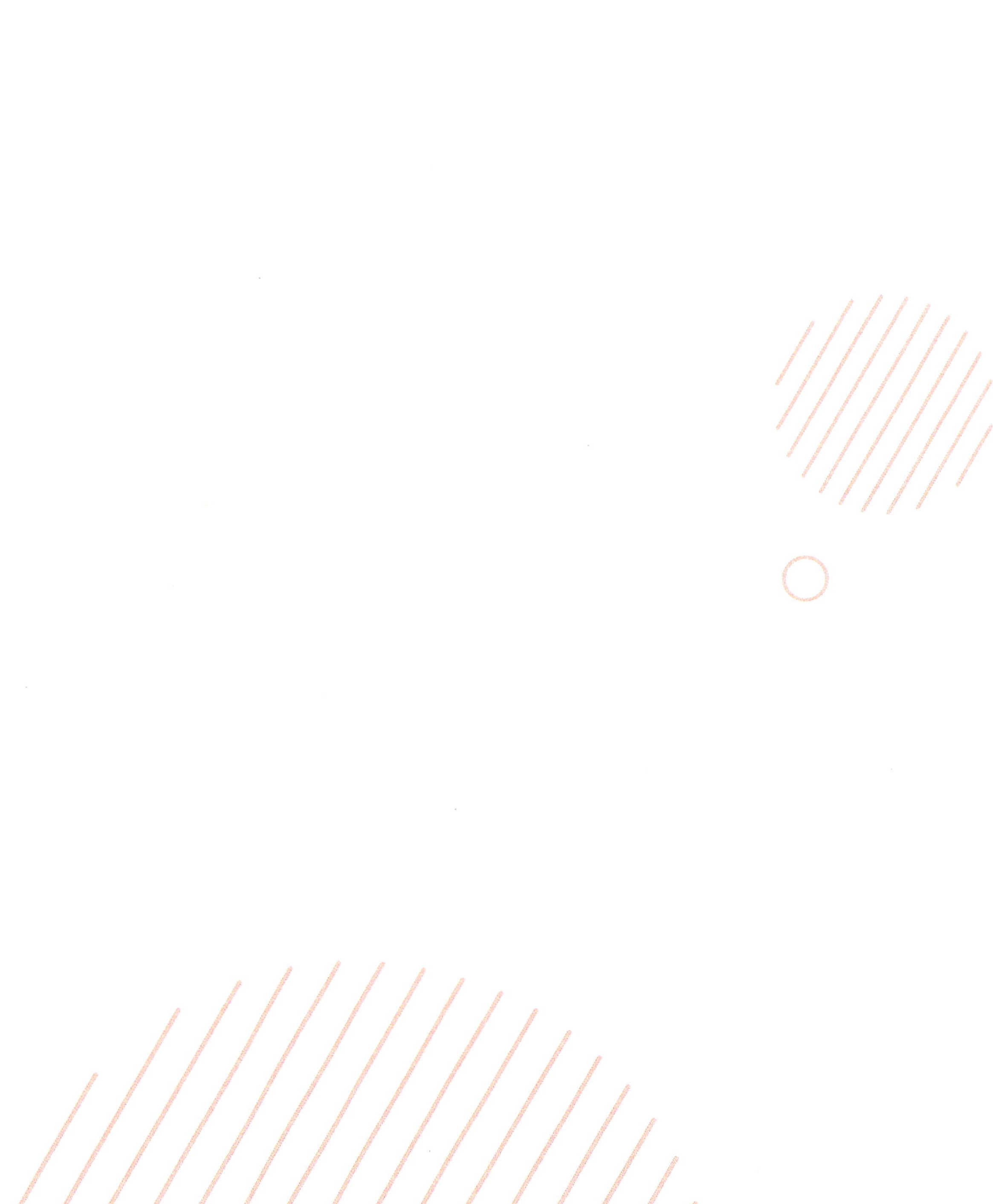

Mistaken Identity

— Reflections on Subconscious Bias and Client Deference

Alicia Fleming Hamilton

PREBRIEF

notes:

Speech-language pathologists and audiologists work with a variety of individuals who represent various cultural backgrounds. Communication sciences and disorders professionals should avoid making assumptions about clients on the basis of their appearance or other cultural practices. Researching a client's cultural background before an initial meeting may help to provide more cultural context to aid in the assessment and treatment of that client using a culturally responsive approach. As professionals, we must understand that individual differences present between and within cultures, races, and ethnic groups. Even seasoned professionals can operate under cultural assumptions and, as a result, have a cultural misstep. Each situation and client we approach are unique. As you review the following case, consider how cultural assumptions may impact the services provided to clients and their families.

As professionals, we must understand that individual differences present between and within cultures, races, and ethnic groups.

OBJECTIVES

- Identify cultural aspects of communication—style, distance, and time orientation of individuals—that may be pertinent in family and clinical interactions.
- Self-assess personal misconceptions, such as assuming that all members of cultural groups share the same appearances, beliefs, and practices.
- Identify steps to validate a client's cultural and personal traits in a situation in which power dynamics may be unequal (e.g., service delivery models or programs that are unfamiliar).

CASE SCENARIO

Lily and Anne are two White women who work for their urban district's early intervention evaluation team. Lily is an early-childhood special education teacher, able to understand and speak conversational Spanish, and Anne, a speech-language pathologist, spoke Spanish at near-native ability. They were scheduled to see a Spanish-speaking family from Guatemala regarding concerns about their 2-year-old son, Juan. Over the phone, Juan's mother, Norma, reported that her first language was Mam and that her second language was Spanish. She reported that she was also taking community education classes to learn English. Norma initially referred Juan to early childhood services because he had difficulty speaking clearly and following directions; he was also "very active." Juan's mother shared that she was pregnant, and her second baby was due in December. Lily and Anne scheduled a visit in late October, but Norma cancelled the visit. The team called back, and the visit was rescheduled for the first week of November. That visit was also cancelled. Norma gave no reasons for the cancellations. A final visit was scheduled for the first week of December. Lily explained to Norma that this would be the final attempt to meet with her and asked whether she was still interested in an evaluation. Norma affirmed her interest in an evaluation and stated that the new date and time would work. Lily requested a Spanish interpreter for herself so she could conduct a play-based observation with Juan in Spanish while Anne interviewed Norma. No Mam interpreters were available in their city.

When the team arrived at the house, a Latin American woman answered the door. She was visibly pregnant. Lily introduced herself as the teacher who called, and the interpreter relayed the introduction in Spanish. Anne introduced herself, in Spanish, as the speech-language pathologist. Once inside, the team was greeted by a 2-year-old boy who was introduced as Juan. Lily started a play-based assessment with Juan, and Anne began the interview process with the woman.

Anne asked her questions about Juan's upbringing, their family structure, language influences, and any exposure to schooling or other languages in the community. The woman noted that she felt more confident in Mam but could understand most Spanish. She reported that she spoke Mam and Spanish with Juan. She shared that she came to the United States for refuge with her toddler and left her older daughter behind. She said she was working hard on getting her daughter to the United States because Guatemala was no longer safe. Anne knew it was common for Guatemalan families to come to the United States as refugees, seeking safety from violent and unsafe conditions (Stephen, 2019).

The conversation was going well, and Anne was developing a good rapport. Anne was also visibly pregnant. As the conversation progressed the woman asked Anne how far along she was. Anne replied, "8 months," to which the woman replied, "me too." Anne was confused because she thought Juan's sibling was due in December, which would make the woman at least 9 months along, not 8. To clarify, Anne asked whether this was the woman's second child, after Juan, to which she replied in Spanish, "This is my third child, but Juan is not my son."

Anne realized that they had made a big mistake. Anne alerted Lily that the woman she was speaking with was not Juan's mother. Lily stopped playing and asked if she was speaking with Norma, and the woman replied, "No." When Lily asked whether this child was Norma's son, Juan, she replied, "yes, but Juan's mother is at the hospital. She went into labor this morning and just had her baby." After further conversation, the team found out that the woman they were speaking with was named Claudia, and she was a family friend. They learned that Norma had instructed Claudia to keep the meeting because she felt bad about the previous cancellations and was afraid Juan would not get the help he needed.

The team apologized, congratulated Claudia on her pregnancy, and asked her to pass on their congratulations to Norma. They noted they would contact Norma in a few weeks, after she had time to settle in with her new baby.

The team came back to the home to complete the evaluation, and Juan ended up qualifying for early intervention services in the areas of communication and behavior. Juan's mother, Norma, was grateful for and very involved in his home visits and the implementation of communication and behavioral strategies. Norma graciously accepted the team's apologies for their initial mistake, and the team used it as an opportunity for reflection and improvement of their home-visit practices.

CRITICAL THINKING AND DEBRIEFING QUESTIONS

1. **What is your initial reaction to this case study? Have you been in a similar situation? How would you change your response given the information above?**
2. **After reviewing the scenario, how did the team adequately address the family's needs and culture?**
3. **What were the implications of the team's inaccurate identification of the mother in this scenario? How might you have reacted?**
4. **What ethical or legal dilemmas were depicted by this case study?**
5. **What are steps teams can take to equalize the power difference that may exist as a result of cultural dissonance between families and providers?**

COMMENTARY

This scenario introduces a common home-visiting scene. A family makes a referral and is called by the evaluation or intervention team; the team then goes out to see the child. However, in this scenario, the mistakes made by the team were illustrative of physical stereotypes, cultural assumptions, and a lack of proper adherence to protocols. Although none of these mistakes were intentional, there are opportunities to learn from them and ensure they do not happen again.

One of the first mistakes made in this scenario was a lack of adherence to protocols. Generally, this early intervention team had a practice of confirming identity by asking the person present whether they are the guardian. Then the team reviews the reason for the referral and subsequent visit. If the team would have completed the appropriate introductions, shared names, and reviewed the reason for the visit, they may have avoided the entire mistake. However, the multiple missed cancellations and the federal timeline requirements to complete a birth to three referral within 45 days of receipt may have influenced the team's use of best practices (American Speech-Language-Hearing Association [ASHA], n.d.). The team also made the assumption that because this woman was pregnant, was Latina, and was at the residence that she must have been Juan's mother. Simple introductions could have prevented this entire misunderstanding.

Expand Your Knowledge

§303.310 requires that, within 45 days after the lead agency or early intervention service provider receives a referral of a child, the screening (if applicable), initial evaluation, initial assessments (of the child and family), and the initial IFSP meeting for that child must be completed (45-day timeline)." (ASHA, n.d.)

Another assumption made by the team was that Norma knew her rights to home visits and early intervention. Although the initial phone call generally explains a family's right to a screening, Norma's lack of familiarity with the U.S. system, including the right to have an interpreter, and a possible cultural practice of deference toward professionals could have affected Norma's decision to keep the visit with her approaching due date. Because of Norma's lack of knowledge regarding early intervention and the team's expertise, there may have been a power differential present that influenced Norma's actions.

It is paramount that intervention teams share protected rights and information with families, from the beginning, so that families can feel empowered and educated about the early intervention process and their rights within the process. In this scenario, specifically, we learn that Norma "felt bad" about the previous cancellations, and she may have felt as though she needed to "save face" and keep the appointment–to the extreme that she had another person stand in for her while she was giving birth. In some cultures, it is more polite to accept an appointment that one may not be able to keep than to directly decline the visit. Culturally based differences in time orientation may affect attendance and punctuality in keeping appointments (Parker et al., 2012). Parents have identified language problems, cultural differences, poverty, lack of health insurance, transportation difficulties, and long waiting times as the major access barriers to health care for Latino children. The overarching impact of poverty, including reliance on multiple agencies or systems, can affect a family's ability to prioritize other services (Flores, Abreu, Olivar, & Kastner, 1998). Norma may have felt that by cancelling a third time she was being rude, or she may have been nervous that she would not be able to complete the evaluation process because Lily told her this would be the final attempt. All of these possibilities indicate a lack of information about both the services being offered and Norma's right to these services. This lack of information, together with cultural beliefs regarding time orientation, saving face, and other identified barriers, affected Norma's ability to understand her and Juan's rights to services.

After reflection, the team realized that there may have also been a power dynamic at play in this situation. Consider that as a team sent by the public-school system, they may be viewed as an arm of the government. Many rumors are perpetuated in immigrant communities regarding accepting or declining government services and the impact that may have on future citizenship or eligibility for future programs (Rhodes et al., 2015). Specifically, families who lack information about specific details of programs available to them, or knowledge of their rights within these programs, may not realize that they can deny a visit or deny entrance to their homes. Families report that they feel obliged to follow the directions, sometimes because of a cultural deference practice and respect for educators and sometimes out of fear. Understanding the multiple factors influencing a family's decision making when accessing or accepting early intervention services can provide insight into areas that require further explanation or clarification between the serving teams and families.

The team may also consider caregiver interaction styles when deciding how to work with families that are not European American. The independent approach to caregiver interaction styles is more common in European American culture and involves independence and individual success. Another interaction style is the interdependent-collectivist style, more commonly seen in Latino and Spanish-speaking caregivers. This style emphasizes the family and the group (Greenfield, Keller, Fuligni, & Maynard, 2003). Principles of modeling, frequent repetition, and explicit teaching are consistent with interdependent caregiver interaction and may illustrate helpful suggestions for culturally compatible families and provide context for cultural expectations within this caregiver interaction style

(Guiberson & Ferris, 2019).

This scenario helps practitioners to understand the importance of following protocol, explaining processes, and understanding cultural practices when working with families, especially in their homes. Although these protocols and explanations may add more time or necessitate more visits, helping families understand their rights and responsibilities is part of our professional responsibility in providing culturally competent care.

CRITICAL THINKING AND DEBRIEFING RESPONSES

1. **What is your initial reaction to this case study? Have you been in a similar situation? How would you change your response given the information above?**

Personal reflection. Consider power dynamics you may experience when working with others who are technical experts in their fields—for example, doctors, mechanics, and electricians. Do you feel comfortable cancelling appointments? Do you understand their processes well?

2. **After reviewing the scenario, how did the team adequately address the family's needs and culture?**

Although mistakes were made during the home visit, there were some moments that addressed the family's needs and culture. Norma's ability to reschedule her evaluation multiple times demonstrated flexibility on the part of the team. The addition of an interpreter, although necessary, also demonstrated that the team knew an interpreter was essential to creating clear communication during the visit. The team also attempted to get a Mam interpreter, but none were available in the city. The teacher, Lily, also considered the need for an interpreter, recognizing that it would have been inappropriate to ask the speech-language pathologist to serve as the interpreter as well as completing her role in the visit. Finally, the team apologized for their mistakes and attempted to repair the relationship afterward.

Definition

Cultural humility is defined as the lifelong and critical self-assessment, admission of limits, and acquisition of knowledge and experience with relevant cultures of individuals one serves (ASHA, 2011).

Practitioners will not be culturally competent at all times and with all clients. In admitting their mistakes and asking the family for their input and information regarding cultural customs, the team demonstrated cultural humility. The ability to recognize mistakes, admit to them, and improve one's practice is part of learning to be a culturally responsive practitioner.

3. **What were the implications of the team's inaccurate identification of the mother in this scenario? How might you have reacted?**

The implications include violation of Health Insurance Portability and Accountability Act of 1996 (HIPAA) laws by sharing private data or information with someone who was not authorized. Additionally, the team may appear less professional or credible because of the incorrect assumptions and lack of procedural safeguards. The family may have felt offended by assumptions on the basis of their looks or by cultural generalizations, which may have led them to lose confidence in the early intervention process. Finally, the mistakes might have added more time to the process, keeping the child from getting necessary services. Personal responses may follow.

4. **What ethical or legal dilemmas were depicted by this case study?**

Several actions of the team may have had ethical or legal implications. The first instance was incorrectly identifying Juan's mother. The team made the assumption, on the basis of the woman's appearance, that she was Juan's mother, without clarifying or following established procedures. They used prior knowledge of the student's background to support generalizations about the family they were meeting. Sharing private information without consent is a violation of HIPAA laws. Because of their knowledge of Spanish, the team may have felt that they were familiar with Latin American cultural practices, giving them a false sense of cultural competence when it came to working with Norma and her family. After reflection, the team may consider how assumptions they made regarding the situation and the woman's appearance, pressures from the federal timelines, and providing services in a timely manner all affected the case in a negative way and impaired their overall judgment. Even if a professional feels familiar with a specific culture each individual adopts cultural values and practices in their own unique way.

5. **What are steps teams can take to equalize the power difference that may exist as a result of cultural dissonance between families and providers?**

When working with all clients, it is important to reflect on your own cultural practices and how those practices may relate to your client. Considering a client's familiarity with the majority culture will also provide insight into how best to explain home-visiting practices. In this scenario, the dominant European American culture is further complicated by schooling and special education requirements, setting the stage for conversations full of jargon and confusing steps.

Elements of this visit included multiple individuals, a significant amount of paperwork, and an interview that directly addressed personal questions, including those about the mother's pregnancy, health, and the place of her child's birth. For a recently immigrated family unfamiliar with this process, the steps may feel uncomfortable or even suspect. Additionally, a family may feel uneasy if a team is working for the state, as though they are being "watched" or observed by a government entity. Misunderstandings about how the special education process works or the rationale for paperwork and direct questioning may lead a family to not trust the motives of the home visit. Some immigrant families live in fear of going back to their native country or being met with violence or hostility in a new country. Although skeptical, families may also feel compelled to comply with the requests or recommendations of schools or agencies in an effort to not be seen as "difficult" or "noncompliant." Obtaining such protected information puts the team in a powerful position with the family.

Power distance is another manifestation of cultural practices. A low-power distance culture would approach students, clients and patients, and families as equals and encourage them to be part of the development of goals and objectives. In a high-power distance culture, professionals are held in high esteem, and attempts to involve families in the development of goals and therapy may cause them to question a professional's competence (Hwa-Froelich & Westby, 2003). European American practices often endorse a low-power distance culture, whereas those in Latin American may adopt a high-power distance culture. Additionally, some cultures view professionals as experts in their field, and out of respect, they do not question the expert but instead follow recommendations (Chong, 2002). Therefore, providing multiple opportunities to ask questions and clarify procedures may be met with silence because the family may feel inappropriate in challenging the "expert" or offering their own suggestions.

To understand what cultural practices and beliefs are at play, it is critical to have a skilled interpreter, a set protocol, and open communication with the client and family. Explaining processes in family-friendly ways and allowing the client and family time and space to share their culture and beliefs sends a message that they are collaborators in the process. To give families power in the decision-making process, practitioners should (a) let families know they have the right to deny a visit or entrance to their homes, (b) provide alternatives that they may have to home visits (e.g., telephone interviews or meeting at an office), and (c) inform them that they have the capacity to make choices and changes in the service delivery dynamic. Treating clients and families as equals in the planning and provision of services may help the family develop a better understanding of their own roles and participation in the process. This is cultural humility in practice and can help to facilitate a better team relationship in the long term.

TAKE AWAYS

- Even the most seasoned clinicians can make cultural mistakes. The ability to identify, admit to, and rectify those mistakes helps in demonstrating cultural humility.
- Power dynamics affect the interactions in a home visit. Partnering with families and engaging them to be informed decision makers helps to increase participation and confidence in the process.
- Protocols should be in place when working with all families to ensure equity across visits and during the provision of services.

REFERENCES

American Speech-Language-Hearing Association. (n.d.). *IDEA Part C Issue Brief: Referral timelines and requirements.* Retrieved from https://www.asha.org/Advocacy/federal/idea/IDEA-Part-C-Issue-Brief-Referral-Timelines/

American Speech-Language-Hearing Association. (2011). *Cultural competence in professional service delivery.* Rockville, MD: Author.

Chong, N. (2002). *The Latino patient: A cultural guide for health care providers.* Milton, England: Hachette UK.

Flores, G., Abreu, M., Olivar, M. A., & Kastner, B. (1998). Access barriers to health care for Latino children. *Archives of Pediatrics & Adolescent Medicine, 152,* 1119–1125.

Greenfield, P. M., Keller, H., Fuligni, A., & Maynard, A. (2003). Cultural pathways through universal development. *Annual Review of Psychology, 54,* 461–490.

Guiberson, M., & Ferris, K. P. (2019). Early language interventions for young dual language learners: A scoping review. *American Journal of Speech-Language Pathology, 28,* 945–963.

Health Insurance Portability and Accountability Act of 1996 (HIPAA), Pub. L. 104-191, 42 U.S.C. § 300gg, 29 U.S.C §§ 1181–1183, and 42 U.S.C. §§ 1320d–1320d9.

Hwa-Froelich, D., & Westby, C. (2003). Frameworks of education: Perspectives of Southeast Asian parents and Head Start staff. *Language, Speech, and Hearing Services in Schools, 34,* 299–319.

Parker, M. M., Moffet, H. H., Schillinger, D., Adler, N., Fernandez, A., Ciechanowski, P., & Karter, A. J. (2012). Ethnic differences in appointment keeping and implications for the patient centered medical home—Findings from the Diabetes Study of Northern California (DISTANCE). *Health Services Research, 47*, 572–593.

Rhodes, S. D., Mann, L., Simán, F. M., Song, E., Alonzo, J., Downs, M., . . . Reboussin, B. A. (2015). The impact of local immigration enforcement policies on the health of immigrant Hispanics/Latinos in the United States. *American Journal of Public Health, 105*, 329–337.

Stephen, L. (2019). Fleeing rural violence: Mam women seeking gendered justice in Guatemala and the U.S. *The Journal of Peasant Studies, 46*, 229–257.

ADDITIONAL RESOURCES

Cohn, D., Passel, J., & Gonzalez-Barrera, A. (2017, December 7). Rise in U.S. immigrants from El Salvador, Guatemala and Honduras outpaces growth from elsewhere: Lawful and unauthorized immigrants increase since recession. *Pew Research Center.* Retrieved from https://www.pewresearch.org/hispanic/2017/12/07/rise-in-u-s-immigrants-from-el-salvador-guatemala-and-honduras-outpaces-growth-from-elsewhere/

Global Affairs Canada. (2018, September 19). *Cultural information.* Retrieved from https://www.international.gc.ca/cil-cai/country_insights-apercus_pays/ci-ic_gt.aspx?lang=eng#cn-2

Granich, S. (2013, Fall). Culturally competent field education practice with Guatemalans. *Field Educator.* Retrieved from http://fieldeducator.simmons.edu/article/culturally-competent-field-education-practice-with-guatemalans/

Hofstede, G. (2011). Dimensionalizing cultures: The Hofstede model in context. *Online Readings in Psychology and Culture, 2*(1). https://doi.org/10.9707/2307-0919.1014

Navigating Systemic and Social Prejudice — Acknowledging Historical Trauma as a Precursor to Patient Advocacy

Wendyliza González

PREBRIEF

This scenario discusses the impact that social and systemic barriers have on access to care, education, and advocacy for underrepresented populations. It presents a situation in which a speech-language pathologist (SLP) has the opportunity to advocate for a family by providing cultural and historical context for decisions and events that were out of their control. It reminds practitioners to look at the client in a holistic manner and to remember that each client and situation are unique. The reader is encouraged to look deeper into the family structure and historical trauma present in this case to reflect on their initial reactions to the family's decisions. After reading the commentary, the reader should determine whether the context changes their perspective of the family.

notes:

OBJECTIVES

- Recognize challenges that families and children from historically underrepresented populations experience that may directly affect speech-language development and access to services.
- Understand the impact of historical trauma for specific groups of people and how that may influence their approaches to working with government agencies.
- Apply the practice of cultural humility using information from this scenario.

CASE SCENARIO

Sonia lives in a multigenerational community with her biological mother Diana, her grandmother, several cousins, and three aunts. Sonia's biological father is not involved in her life. The primary languages spoken at home are English and Ojibwe. Sonia's mother is 22 years old. She recently completed a rehabilitation stay

Expand Your Knowledge

According to the American Speech-Language-Hearing Association and the Multicultural Issues Board, underrepresented or underserved populations are those populations that "include but are not limited to individuals identified by race, ethnicity, culture, language, dialect, national origin, gender, gender identify or expression, sexual orientation, age, religion, socioeconomic status, and/or ability."

https://www.asha.org/About/governance/committees/CommitteeSmartForms/Multicultural-Issues-Board/

The theory of *historical trauma* within Native American communities was first established in 1976 by Native American social worker Maria Yellow Horse Brave Heart. The premise of this theory is that populations historically subjected to long-term, mass-trauma colonialism; slavery; war; and genocide exhibit a higher prevalence of disease even several generations after the original trauma occurred (Yellow Horse Brave Heart, 2003).

for substance abuse and is taking steps to become more independent, with her family's support. Diana works at a retail store during the day and attends night classes at the local community college four evenings a week. Because of her schedule, Diana relies heavily on her family members to take care of Sonia while she is at work or school. Diana applied for day care assistance to put Sonia into a local day care, but she was told there would not be spots available until Sonia turned 3 years old.

Just before her third birthday, while under the care of a nonfamilial babysitter, Sonia sustained multiple head and neck injuries resulting in right-sided hemiparesis; oropharyngeal dysphagia; and language, memory, speech, and cognition deficits. Before her injuries, Diana reported that Sonia was a "happy and silly" baby. She noted that she appeared to understand both Ojibwe and English and would use single words to communicate in both languages. Sonia had a "good" appetite (her favorite food was chicken nuggets) and liked to sing songs. Diana shared that Sonia's pediatrician did have concerns about her expressive language and speech skills and even suggested that a bilingual home might be "confusing" her language development. As a result, Sonia's doctor made a recommendation to get a speech and language evaluation, but Diana had found herself overwhelmed with researching speech-language pathology clinics that provided bilingual evaluation and treatment at affordable rates.

After the incident, Sonia was hospitalized. After she was stabilized, she was released to an acute care inpatient facility. Sonia received treatment from physical and occupational therapists and SLPs, and she was assigned a social services caseworker to coordinate her care. The circumstances and nature of Sonia's injuries warranted the involvement of Child Protective Services. Since initiating treatment, Sonia showed improvements in labeling objects; recognizing caregivers; and using her right hand to point, grab, and self-feed. Sonia explored various tastes and textures of food, and she used signs and gestures to communicate her basic needs, including "hurt, happy, sad, water, milk, more, no, all done, and I love you." Sonia's mother was present at the care facility every day to ensure her safety and progress. In the past, Diana and her family have witnessed other families within her community experience separation because of financial, medical, and educational circumstances. She has shared her interest with the case manager in learning about discharge care and helping Sonia communicate in her home environment. Because of the increased time commitments to care for Sonia, Diana lost her job and had to drop out of her school program. When she lost her job, Diana also lost her private insurance coverage and now depended solely on Medicaid coverage.

Because of Sonia's improvements, her discharge plan was updated to include home discharge with visits from a home nurse, an SLP, occupational and physical therapists, and a home health aide. Diana was interested in learning more about training to become Sonia's home health aide so that she could spend more time helping Sonia and decrease the financial burden on her family.

During her discharge planning conference, social services unilaterally decided that the best course of care would be to place Sonia with an experienced foster care family. This particular family frequently worked with children who had complex medical needs but was not of Native American background and had no knowledge about Ojibwe traditions. The social services worker justified their decision on the fact that Sonia's biological mother "showed a history of difficulty caring for a child with special needs" and that Diana could not provide care at a level that Sonia needed to continue to demonstrate improvements.

She also noted that the abuse happened while in her mother's care (although not under her supervision) and that given Diana's previous history of substance abuse, the potential for relapse was high because of the stress of caring for Sonia at home. Hearing these statements made Sonia's mother react strongly, and she became visibly distraught. The family was informed that the transition plan was set to occur over a period of 2 weeks. At this point, the SLP on the case requested a team meeting with the case manager, rehabilitation specialists, social services, and discharge planning to discuss and reassess Sonia's discharge plan of care.

CRITICAL THINKING AND DEBRIEFING QUESTIONS

1. **Explore obstacles that may be faced by families and children from historically underrepresented communities that may impact their speech-language development and/or access to therapy services.**
2. **How might historical trauma and/or mistrust of government agencies impact a family's willingness to participate in programming or commit to services? What can an SLP do to mitigate these perceptions and rebuild trust?**
3. **How might the team use an approach that endorses cultural humility to address the family's needs as Sonia transitions out of the rehabilitation facility? What may be the benefits of using such an approach?**

COMMENTARY

With every new client we meet, we have an opportunity to learn a new perspective on an individual's response to their culture. By approaching our clients and their families as individuals with unique cultural histories that affect their lifestyle and guide their choices, we can better collaborate with them in the assessment and treatment processes. Ensuring that we are practicing in a way that refrains from discrimination must involve the practice of self-reflection across our work. Creating time and space to review cases, celebrate positive outcomes, and analyze areas of improvement is critical in the journey of cultural competence. Analyzing cultural mishaps and reflecting on our actions and statements for instances of explicit and implicit bias help to cultivate the attitude of cultural humility across one's practice.

Practicing in a nondiscriminatory way requires constant self-reflection across all aspects of our work.

The theory of historical trauma within Native American communities was first established in 1976 by Native American social worker Maria Yellow Horse Brave Heart. The premise of this theory is that populations who are historically subjected to long-term, mass-trauma colonialism; slavery; war; and genocide exhibit a higher prevalence of disease even several generations after the original trauma occurred (Yellow Horse Brave Heart, 2003). These traumas are believed to be passed down from generation to generation and exhibit themselves in psychological and physiological behaviors, including anger, suicide, dysfunctional parenting, alcohol and drug abuse, and unemployment.

Past and present system-wide biases—including government initiatives; armed conflict; financial institutions placed to limit or strip populations of economic growth; physical displacement; and dilution or erasure of language, religion, and tradition—perpetuate the historical trauma experienced by indigenous and Native American populations (Sotero, 2006; Yellow Horse Brave Heart, Chase, Elkins, & Altschul, 2011). These experiences contribute to the narrative that those from underrepresented communities cannot trust the intentions of or be understood by people outside of their community.

Diana is a young mother who continually demonstrated her desire to improve her circumstances and become better informed about the care of her child—whether that be through attending college, completing rehabilitation services, exploring options to serve as her daughter's home health aide, or sharing her frustrations with navigating an overwhelming system when seeking services. Unfortunately, the treatment team did not "see" Diana for the person she was becoming. They did not give weight to the changes she wished to make but rather made assumptions about her intentions and parenting skills that guided their treatment of Sonia. Although the team may have felt they had Sonia's best interests in mind, by denying the historical trauma experienced by Sonia's family and subsequently silencing her mother's voice and opinions, the team has isolated Sonia and set a course of events that may negatively affect her medical, educational, personal, and emotional growth.

CRITICAL THINKING AND DEBRIEFING RESPONSES

1. **Explore obstacles that may be faced by families and children from historically underrepresented communities that may impact their speech-language development and/or access to therapy services.**

Historically underrepresented groups are defined as communities who are considered a minority, whether by ethnicity, gender, ability, or religion (Emory University, Office of Equity and Inclusion, n.d.). Typically, these groups are underrepresented in higher education and skilled career pathways as well as in literature, research, and social commentary. Repercussions of this lack of visibility within the larger community manifest in lower socioeconomic status (SES), cultural and linguistic barriers, disparities in educational history, and generalized prejudicial stereotyping.

Families with lower SES struggle with access to affordable health care options, resulting in challenges with obtaining appropriate and expedient medical services (Roseberry-McKibbin, 2001). There may be limited options for clinics and professionals in their communities, and they are faced with further obstacles when they need to find a specialist, such as a bilingual SLP. In addition, medical conditions and illnesses that go untreated can result in more health complications down the line, including conditions that directly affect the speech and language development of a growing child. Families who are financially unstable may find themselves having to choose between paying for rent, adequate child care, or food (Roseberry-McKibbin, 2001). Access to nutritional food might be a limitation for families on a strict budget.

Definition

The term **historically underrepresented groups or communities** refers to groups who have been denied access and/or who have suffered past institutional discrimination in the United States. These groups include African Americans, Asian Americans, Hispanics or Chicanos/Latinos, and Native Americans. There is an imbalance in the representation of these groups in common pursuits, including housing, education, and jobs. Other underrepresented or marginalized groups may include, but are not limited to, other ethnicities; adult learners; veterans; people with disabilities; lesbian, gay, bisexual, and transgender individuals; people from different religious groups; and people from different economic backgrounds (Emory University, Office of Equity and Inclusion, n.d.).

In addition to difficulties with meeting basic health needs, families from underrepresented communities might demonstrate educational and language gaps. Correlations between parental education, SES, and child language outcomes suggest that caregivers with lower SES may not have the resources to provide the same language enrichment or opportunities as families from more financially stable homes. Culturally, studies indicate that the overall amount of language spoken in families with lower SES is significantly lower than that spoken in higher income families, which negatively affects vocabulary, expressive language, comprehension, and educational habits in the long term (Kelly, 2010; Roseberry-McKibbon, 2001).

Families from historically underrepresented groups are often met with misinformation and social discrimination, as in the case of Diana. She was informed by a trusted pediatrician that bilingualism is detrimental for her daughter's language development, and she was later judged an inadequate caregiver by professionals who did not factor in the effects of access to care and education as well as their own personal biases with respect to Diana's underrepresented community. Diana's family support was given no weight in the decision making, and she was not consulted when decisions regarding her daughter's care were being made. Identifying and understanding these barriers is critically important when assessing, treating, and collaborating with families who come from historically marginalized communities.

2. **How might historical trauma and/or mistrust of government agencies impact a family's willingness to participate in programming or commit to services? What can an SLP do to mitigate these perceptions or rebuild trust?**

A longstanding history of being disenfranchised, alienated, and stereotyped by people in perceived positions of power can directly affect an individual's own perception of their capacity to claim and access effective and appropriate services.

In this case scenario, Diana attempted to share her story and goals with little validation from those in control of her daughter's care. In fact, little effort was made to involve Diana as an essential member of her child's treatment team. As culturally competent clinicians, we must make a commitment to acknowledging and addressing issues that affect those we work with. We must also attempt to demonstrate cultural humility by seeing our clients as experts in their own lives, sharing their values and experiences with us so that we can collaborate for the best outcomes.

As an SLP or an audiologist, your role is multitiered. The first step is to create a foundation of mutual respect and understanding with clients or families by acknowledging their language history and possible need for translation services. This can be done through ethnographic interviewing or by creating cultural ecograms. Another possibility would be using a spiritual life map (Limb & Hodge, 2007). The spiritual life map was described as a client-driven tool that allows clients to be creative, and it provides visual supports to tap into spirituality and culture, lending itself to more authentic involvements for clients in the treatment process.

After a provider has more information about the family's cultural practices and preferences, they can identify resources or specialists that are representative of Diana's background. Possible options might include multiservice clinics, Head Start programs, outreach centers servicing indigenous populations, libraries, food banks, and nonprofit organizations seeking to serve those in historically underrepresented communities. The provider can collaborate with Diana's family regarding her treatment and long-term goals. Maintaining close communication and cultivating a relationship can keep Diana involved during transitions and places the practitioner in an integral role as an advocate for the family.

With respect to Sonia's speech, language, and feeding needs, the SLP can share information with the family about early childhood development and provide information about bilingualism, which includes encouraging the family to speak their native language with Sonia, teaching indirect treatment strategies that can be generalized in the home, and locating an appropriate post-acute care provider in the community. Finally, the SLP can use their platform to confront and repair the unbal-

Definition

The **cultural ecogram** (Yasui, 2015) is an approach that can be used to facilitate the clinician-client shared understanding regarding the client's cultural, ethnic, and racial contexts and how they may affect treatment.

anced approach that this treatment facility and its case workers have taken to conduct and plan treatment for this patient and her family.

3. **How might the team use an approach that endorses cultural humility to address the family's needs as Sonia transitions out of the rehabilitation facility? What may be the benefits of using such an approach?**

As a whole, the team would benefit from reflecting on their own world views and recognize how their own cultural perspectives bring very specific experiences to the clinical team. This will allow them to embrace a culture of co-learning with colleagues and patients alike. The team has an opportunity to redefine the patient-caregiver dynamic by recognizing Diana as an expert in her own culture and as a person seeking support and advocacy from experts in their own professions. Appreciating Diana's goals and plans for her daughter and establishing a clear plan of care that echoes her voice is a tangible step toward identifying power imbalances and reflecting on behaviors that perpetuate this imbalance.

Approaching situations as a team with cultural humility involves the awareness that there may be topics and areas of conflict that cannot be truly understood because of the influence of an individual's ethnicity and life experiences. If the team desires to learn more about another culture, it may be beneficial to seek guidance from trusted cultural resources or specialists who are familiar with the Ojibwe people and their practices.

The SLP can play a crucial role in the treatment team by providing information and resources on culturally sensitive practices as a means to dispel myths about language, service delivery, and access to care for diverse families. This includes guaranteeing that translation services are available to caregivers whose primary language is not English. The SLP can function as an advocate to ensure that the caregiver's voice is heard at this meeting and to involve them in all decisions about their child's care. The clinician might take time to educate the family on topics related to language development, bilingualism, and culturally appropriate strategies to support language development in the home environment. The SLP may further provide a list of accessible clinics and support services in the family's community.

Frequent and purposeful reflection on one's biases can help to prevent damaging treatment practices caused by language barriers, preconceived judgments, close mindedness, pseudo listening, and misguided beliefs about the "best" course of care.

TAKE AWAYS

- SES is a key predictor of health, education, and language development and must be considered when reviewing a client's case history.
- Cultural competence and cultural humility require a lifetime commitment to education, self-assessment, and growth.
- Effective and comprehensive treatment stems from recognizing the patient as a dynamic, multifaceted entity—as an extension of their family, culture, and history.

REFERENCES

Emory University, Office of Equity and Inclusion. (n.d.). *Common terms: Historically underrepresented.* Retrieved from http://equityandinclusion.emory.edu/about/resources/terms.html

Kelly, D. J. (2010). Language acquisition challenges for preschoolers residing in low-SES households: Implications for speech-language pathologists and developmental researchers. *Perspectives on Language Learning and Education, 17*(2), 41-48.

Limb, G. E., & Hodge, D. R. (2007). Developing spiritual lifemaps as a culture-centered pictorial instrument for spiritual assessments with Native American clients. *Research on Social Work Practice, 17,* 296-304.

Roseberry-McKibbin, C. (2001). Serving children from the culture of poverty: Practical strategies for speech-language pathologists. *The ASHA Leader, 6*(20), 4-17.

Sotero, M. (2006). A conceptual model of historical trauma: Implications for public health practice and research. *Journal of Health Disparities Research and Practice, 1,* 93-108.

Yasui, M. (2015). The cultural ecogram: A tool for enhancing culturally anchored shared understanding in the treatment of ethnic minority families. *Journal of Ethnic and Cultural Diversity in Social Work, 24*(2), 89-108.

Yellow Horse Brave Heart, M. (2003). The historical trauma response among natives and its relationship with substance abuse: A Lakota illustration. *Journal of Psychoactive Drugs, 35,* 7-13. https://doi.org/10.1080/02791072.2003.10399988

Yellow Horse Brave Heart, M., Chase, J., Elkins, J., & Altschul, D. B. (2011). Historical trauma among Indigenous Peoples of the Americas: Concepts, research, and clinical considerations. *Journal of Psychoactive Drugs, 43,* 282-290. https://doi.org/10.1080/02791072.2011.628913

ADDITIONAL RESOURCES

About the Ojibwe Language. (n.d.). In *The Ojibwe People's Dictionary.* Retrieved from https://ojibwe.lib.umn.edu/about-ojibwe-language

American Speech-Language-Hearing Association. (2010). *Code of Ethics.* Retrieved from https://www.asha.org/Code-of-Ethics/

Hammer, C. S., Farkas, G., & Maczuga, S. (2010). The language and literacy development of Head Start children: A study using the Family and Child Experiences Survey database. *Language, Speech, and Hearing Services in Schools, 41,* 70-83.

Hyter, Y. D., Henry, J., Atchison, B., Sloane, M., Black-Pond, C., & Shangraw, K. (2003). Children affected by trauma and alcohol exposure: A profile of the Southwestern Michigan Children's Trauma Assessment Center. *The ASHA Leader, 8*(21), 6-14.

Inglebret, E., Eagle, D. B., & Pavel, D. M. (2007). American Indian stories enrich intervention. *The ASHA Leader, 12*(1), 1-27.

Leffel, K., & Suskind, D. (2013). Parent-directed approaches to enrich the early language environments of children living in poverty. *Seminars in Speech and Language, 34*(4), 267-278.

Morgan, P. L., Hammer, C. S., Farkas, G., Hillemeier, M. M., Maczuga, S., Cook, M., &

Morano, S. (2016). Who receives speech/language services by 5 years of age in the United States? *American Journal of Speech-Language Pathology, 25,* 183–199.

Multicultural Constituency Groups (MCCGs) https://www.asha.org/practice/multicultural/opportunities/constituency/

Rodríguez, B. L., Hines, R., & Montiel, M. (2009). Mexican American mothers of low and middle socioeconomic status: Communication behaviors and interactive strategies during shared book reading. *Language, Speech, and Hearing Services in Schools, 40,* 271–282.

Sotero, M. (2006). A conceptual model of historical trauma: Implications for public health practice and research. *Journal of Health Disparities Research and Practice, 1,* 93–108.

Yellow Horse Brave Heart, M., Chase, J., Elkins, J., & Altschul, D. B. (2011). Historical trauma among Indigenous Peoples of the Americas: Concepts, research, and clinical considerations. *Journal of Psychoactive Drugs, 43,* 282–290. https://doi.org/10.1080/02791072.2011.628913

Engendering Cultural Responsiveness in Clinical Practice

— Regarding Gender Identity and Expression

Ishara Ramkissoon

PREBRIEF

notes:

The relationship between a clinical educator and a student clinician is a critical component of clinical education. Clinical educators are charged with teaching specific skills, clarifying concepts, assisting with critical thinking skills, conducting performance evaluations, mentoring, and modeling professional behavior. They are involved in the clinical training, education, and supervision of audiology and speech-language pathology students (American Speech-Language-Hearing Association [ASHA], n.d.-a).

Clinical education involves developing the ability to communicate, including defining expectations and engaging in difficult conversations. Modeling appropriate communication regarding the gender identity and sexual orientation of clients as well as their caretakers can provide valuable learning opportunities for clinicians during the assessment and treatment process.

OBJECTIVES

- Identify how personal beliefs can influence perceptions and possibly impact service delivery.
- List the components of an appropriate clinical educator–student clinician relationship and identify when to take steps to report inappropriate behavior.
- Reflect on personal perceptions of outward appearances and how those perceptions may impact clinical practice.

CASE SCENARIO

Kathleho is a 3-year-old boy who came to the university clinic for a speech-language assessment. Kathleho is assigned a student clinician named Mary-Sue, who is observed by a clinical educator. Mary-Sue welcomed Kathleho and his mother into the clinic and began the assessment. Mary-Sue conducted an interview regarding Kathleho's speech and language development. Kathleho's mother stated that he recently started to put some words together, such as "big boy" and "no see," but she shared that his overall development seemed to be lagging behind his 6-year-old brother at that age. During the interview, Kathleho's mother also noted that Kathleho has not recently had a hearing

Definitions

Gender identity—An individual's sense of being male, female, both male and female, or an alternative gender. An individual who is cisgender is an individual whose gender identity is congruent with their sex assigned at birth. An individual who is transgender has a gender identity that differs from their sex assigned at birth. In English, transgender is an adjective (e.g., the correct usage would be "a transgender person") and should not be used as a noun (Bouman et al., 2017).

Gender expression—Characteristics in personality, appearance, and behavior that may be perceived as masculine, feminine, both, or neither. Gender expression may vary along the gender continuum. Gender expression may change over time and may differ depending on the environment (ASHA, n.d.-c).

Soft skills—A combination of interpersonal skills, emotional intelligence, and personal attributes. They include work ethic, professionalism, courtesy, initiative, and communication. Soft skills are generally more difficult to teach than technical skills and knowledge, and they are also challenging to measure (Shollenbarger, 2019).

test. Mary-Sue continued the assessment using standardized measures, noting significant delays in both receptive and expressive language but not reporting scores because of the influence of a possible hearing loss.

After she shared the results, Mary-Sue recommended that Kathleho receive a hearing evaluation with the audiologists in the clinic to rule out hearing loss as a contributing factor for language delay. Mary-Sue directed Kathleho and his mother toward the audiology department in the university clinic to make their appointment.

When Mary-Sue returned to the clinic, her clinical educator said, "I think Kathleho's mom is a man." Mary-Sue, caught by surprise, did not respond to the clinical educator's comment. The clinical educator repeated the comment a second time, with increased volume and emphasis on the word "man." Mary-Sue did not respond.

Kathleho came back to the clinic the following week and received his audiology results. The report indicated that threshold testing conducted in sound field with visual reinforcement audiometry revealed a severe hearing loss. Individual ear thresholds could not be obtained at this time, and the audiologist recommended further testing, such as auditory brainstem response and otoacoustic emissions testing, to confirm the behavioral report and to provide additional information.

Kathleho's mother was eager to begin treatment with speech-language therapy as well as audiological management. As they scheduled the upcoming visits, the student clinician asked Kathleho's mother whether there was any additional information the clinicians should know about the family to better tailor the therapy sessions to their needs. Kathleho's parent indicated their family uses "they/them/theirs" to refer to either parent. These were also the pronouns they wanted Kathleho to use with them. Mary-Sue noted this on Kathleho's information sheet and said goodbye to the family.

The client and family left the facility, and the student clinician and her clinical educator had a meeting to debrief the case. Once again, the topic of the parent's gender identity was raised by the clinical educator who asked Mary-Sue, "Did you think she was a man? I really couldn't tell. I'm so glad you asked about the family information, that was a great way to figure it out." The student clinician left the debrief meeting feeling confused because she did not understand how the clinical educator's comments pertained to the child's assessment or treatment, and she was unsure of the appropriateness of the comment and whether she should discuss the situation with the clinic or program director.

CRITICAL THINKING AND DEBRIEFING QUESTIONS

1. Does the gender identity of parents or guardians matter when assessing their children? Why or why not?
2. What are some approaches the student clinician could have used to address her clinical educator's inappropriate comments about the family?
3. What could have been done at the initial interview that may have addressed gender identity in a more professional way?
4. Do you consider gender identity and personal pronouns when addressing families

and clients? How could you incorporate this into your practice?

5. How might a similar situation look in your current workplace? How would you handle this conversation as it pertains to where you currently work?

COMMENTARY

This case presents a clinical situation in which a staff member's supervisor is making inappropriate comments about the clients. Part of the difficulty in this situation is that the person making inappropriate comments is the clinical educator, and the one hearing the comments is the student clinician, creating a power imbalance. Reporting inappropriate behavior of a supervisor can be daunting. The protocol for addressing inappropriate behavior, on behalf of the student clinician or the clinical educator, is best addressed before the relationship begins. This helps to clearly outline expectations for all parties.

Conversations about the gender identity of clients or family members need to be addressed in a sensitive and respectful manner when it is relevant to the provision of clinical care. Clinicians should avoid judgmental statements about gender identity because this is unprofessional and does not create a welcoming environment. Instead, clinical providers are encouraged to reflect on their professional practices to avoid any act that many be perceived as discriminatory or biased.

Gender identity can be important in a clinical setting—for example, when considering how to address families or clients, choosing clinical materials, or when working on voice therapy (ASHA, n.d.-c). Clinics benefit from policies that outline how to address clients in a sensitive and appropriate manner. Another important aspect of clinical training includes learning how to work with families and clients effectively. These skills, although less technical, are often referred to as "soft skills" and can be developed through observation and practice. Developing soft skills helps a clinician create effective relationships with clients and other clinicians. A clinician with strong soft skills also understands the importance of cultural responsiveness in clinical practice (Shollenbarger, 2019).

Approaching this situation with an attitude of cultural humility would involve asking the family what they feel is best and adapting the evaluation or treatment plans accordingly. This approach allows clinicians to support clients and families with plans that align with their wishes and beliefs. Although all practitioners have personal beliefs and values, it is important to realize how those beliefs may create a bias that affects clinical interactions and service delivery.

During the debriefing, Mary-Sue's clinical educator made the comment, "Did you think she was a man?" This comment misgendered the parent and ignored their specific request to be addressed using "they/them/theirs." When a clinician is unfamiliar with use of nonbinary pronouns, there may be a learning period with instances of error. In these situations, clinicians can use the approach of cultural humility to address the misstep, apologize, and move forward with a sincere commitment to do better. Cultural responsiveness allows clinicians to grow in their practice and to improve their interactions with all clients.

Understanding the importance of cultural responsiveness in clinical practice, establishing guidelines to address discriminatory speech and behavior, and cultivating soft skills across the staff can help all involved to provide more inclusive, culturally competent assessment and intervention.

CRITICAL THINKING AND DEBRIEFING RESPONSES

1. **Does the gender identity of parents or guardians matter when assessing their children? Why or why not?**

In this particular case study, the parent's gender identity was not a critical piece of information for the assessment of the child. However, ASHA (n.d.-c) stated,

> *It is important to know your client's name and pronouns, including whether they use more than one pronoun or set of pronouns depending on the setting or situation. Clinicians are mindful of potential barriers that influence the client's day-to-day functioning and their impact on communication. (Overview section, para. 1)*

The way in which this is addressed is important in maintaining an appropriate client-clinician relationship and in honoring the client's correct gender pronouns. When asking about gender pronouns, consider whether additional information is necessary for treatment, including sex assigned at birth, aspects about transition, or other information. Only seek what is necessary for the client's evaluation and treatment. Clients should divulge information at their own pace and comfort level, and they should be approached with sensitivity. After correct pronouns are shared, they should be used and applied throughout the treatment journey. Furthermore, gender identity information may influence what materials are selected for treatment and whether they should be considered as appropriate. Clinicians will want to be mindful of using the appropriate pronouns when referring to the child's parents.

2. **What are some approaches the student clinician could have used to address her clinical educator's inappropriate comments about the family?**

When entering into a relationship as a student clinician and clinical educator, expectations should be addressed (ASHA, n.d.-a, 2017). This can involve processes for approaching uncomfortable situations or asking questions about approaches that may be in conflict with either the clinician's or the clinical educator's training. In this case, some possible options for addressing the inappropriate comments could include the student clinician expressing her discomfort with the discussion. Or, the student clinician could have used the moment to educate, sharing something like, "The family chose not to share their gender identity with me. This may have indicated they did not feel safe discussing it or did not feel it was appropriate to do so. Because of this, I provided an opportunity later for them to share but did not directly ask." The student clinician may also approach the clinical or program director at her university to ask for further guidance in this situation. Regardless of the approach, the supervisor's behavior was not appropriate and should be documented.

Other useful resources for the clinician and the clinical educator may include ASHA's (n.d.-b) practice portal on cultural competence and the information on voice and communication services for transgender and gender diverse populations (ASHA, n.d.-c).

3. **What could have been done at the initial interview that may have addressed gender identity in a more professional way?**

Clinical practitioners are encouraged to review their policies and procedures and determine whether they are inclusive to diverse groups of people. The review should consider inclusion of a variety of gender identities. Some considerations may include asking clients which pronouns they use during intake meetings, creating a space that has a gender-neutral bathroom, and revising paperwork to allow for a variety of responses regarding gender identity and sex. The student clinician could adapt her own therapy materials to be more inclusive to gender diversity and could ask that the university clinic do the same with their treatment materials.

4. **Do you consider gender identity and personal pronouns when addressing families and clients? How could you incorporate this into your practice?**

The answer to this question is a personal response; there is no right or wrong answer. ASHA recommends looking at the entire clinical experience from the moment a client contacts the clinic, via phone or in person, to the moment they leave. Important things to consider include the following: Are the administrative staff trained in diversity and welcoming to all clients? Does the art reflect a variety of family structures and people of diverse backgrounds and beliefs? Do the forms provide opportunities for gender diverse people to note their preferences? Are gender neutral bathrooms available? These questions may serve as a starting point.

5. **How might a similar situation look in your current workplace? How would you handle this conversation as it pertains to where you currently work?**

The answer to this question involves personal reflection. While contemplating your response, consider the following: Who makes recommendations for and changes to the training and environmental setup in your work place? What is the protocol for addressing cultural missteps or asking for enhanced cultural competence training for staff? Do you feel comfortable addressing inappropriate comments? Is there a process for doing so?

TAKE AWAYS

- Clinics providing services to a wide range of populations, including gender diverse individuals, may consider reviewing their policies and procedures to determine whether there are clear statements of inclusiveness and nondiscrimination to guide clinicians in their interactions.
- Gender diverse families may or may not self-identify during interactions with communication professionals. Clinicians should avoid asking or speculating about the gender identity of the client or any of the family members.
- Cultural humility is a valuable concept to use as guiding principle in our interactions with diverse populations as we seek to partner with families to create the best therapeutic outcomes.

REFERENCES

American Speech-Language-Hearing Association. (n.d.-a). *Clinical education and supervision.* Retrieved from https://www.asha.org/PRPSpecificTopic.aspx?folderid=8589942113§ion=References

American Speech-Language-Hearing Association. (n.d.-b). *Cultural competence.* Retrieved from https://www.asha.org/Practice-Portal/Professional-Issues/Cultural-Competence/

American Speech-Language-Hearing Association. (n.d.-c). *Voice and communication services for transgender and gender diverse populations.* Retrieved from https://www.asha.org/PRPSpecificTopic.aspx?folderid=8589944119§ion=Key_Issues

American Speech-Language-Hearing Association. (2017). *Issues in ethics: Supervision of student clinicians.* Retrieved from https://www.asha.org/Practice/ethics/Supervision-of-Student-Clinicians/

Bouman, W. P., Schwend, A. S., Motmans, J., Smiley, A., Safer, J. D., Deutsch, M. B., ... & Winter, S. (2017). Language and trans health. *International Journal of Transgenderism, 18*(1), 1–6. Retrieved from https://doi.org/10.1080/15532739.2016.1262127

Shollenbarger, A. (2019, May 28). The importance of soft skills for professional success [Blog post]. *ASHA Leader Live.* Retrieved from https://blog.asha.org/2019/05/28/the-importance-of-soft-skills-for-professional-success/

ADDITIONAL RESOURCES

Rogers, M., & Nunez, L. (2013). From my perspective: How do we make interprofessional collaboration happen? *The ASHA Leader, 18*(6), 7–8.

Listening to the Silence

— Second Language Acquisition and Preventing Misdiagnosis

Jean Franco Rivera Pérez and Ishara Ramkissoon

PREBRIEF

Audiologists and speech-language pathologists are trained to recognize and understand how cultural and linguistic variables can affect every part of their practice from structure of language to a client's communication style. A strong understanding of the multiple ways in which learning a second language can affect a client's native language and communication is critical to provide effective and culturally appropriate audiology and speech-language pathology services in this population.

OBJECTIVES

- Review personal knowledge regarding the stages of second language acquisition and development.
- Self-assess possible assumptions regarding second language learning and use related to clients who speak a different language.
- Identify differences between the "silent period" of second language acquisition and selective mutism.

CASE SCENARIO

Pierre is a 4-year-old boy who came to the United States from the Democratic Republic of the Congo as a refugee with his family. He has been enrolled in Head Start, a program that helps promote school readiness in young children of low-income families, for 2 months. He participates in an English-only instruction program with his teacher, Sarah, a monolingual English speaker from the United States. Two weeks into the school year, Sarah completed paperwork for all children in her classroom. On Pierre's form, she mentioned concerns about him not engaging with other kids in the classroom, and she noted that he appeared "excessively" shy. She also said he did not speak to the teachers or children in the classroom and that he liked to observe the children from a distance.

Pierre's background information, obtained from his parents with the support of an interpreter, indicated that his home language is French and that he is currently exposed to English in his Head Start classroom. The form noted that his exposure to English has been less than 4 months. When the teacher contacted Pierre's parents to share her concerns

notes:

Definitions

Nonverbal period or silent period—A 3- to 6-month period in which children do not seem to be talking; this has been described as a normal part of second language acquisition. In this stage, students are learning the second language, listening and gaining comprehension, and they produce little output. The child will respond in his or her first language, which has been described as a typical stage of second language acquisition (Roseberry-McKibbin, 2014).

Selective mutism—A childhood anxiety disorder that is characterized by a child's inability to speak and communicate effectively in select social situations; there is no response in either language (Richard, 2011). It appears to affect females more than males (Cunningham, McHolm, Boyle, & Patel, 2004), and prevalence is very high in immigrant children who are learning a second language (Preston, 2014).

about his language skills, they said that he does not speak much at home, but they are not concerned. His parents described him as a "laid back" kid who doesn't "fuss much." His family members at home and nearby neighbors speak French only.

Pierre was scheduled for a hearing screening at Head Start as part of a program-wide screening initiative. The hearing screening was conducted by an audiology graduate student with a French interpreter. Pierre's parents were also present. The graduate student gave Pierre the instructions "raise your hand when you hear a beep" in English, his second language. When Pierre did not respond, the interpreter provided the same instructions in French. Pierre did not respond to the 35-dB familiarization tone. The graduate student proceeded to increase the stimulus to 50 dB and to provide directions with the interpreter, but Pierre still did not respond to the tone. After multiple presentations of the stimulus tone at 30 dB and 50 dB, Pierre remained unresponsive to the tones. The graduate student indicated that Pierre's "lack of response" led to him failing the hearing screening, and she recommended a follow-up audiological evaluation. She also referred Pierre for a speech and language assessment because she suspected a possible language disorder because of Pierre's lack of response and lack of any verbal communication during the screening. When a speech-language pathologist contacted the graduate student to ask the rationale for the referral, the student commented that "Pierre couldn't even raise his hand for the screening; all these foreign children I tested were dumb!"

When she returned to the clinic, the graduate clinician shared her frustrations with her clinical educator. She shared that she was upset that none of the children would respond to her prompts and that Pierre, specifically, seemed to ignore everything she asked him to do. She didn't understand why they had to spend so much time reviewing his intake questionnaire and playing with him if he didn't even cooperate. She asked whether they could make sure all the students were "cognitively appropriate" the next time she conducted screenings. After she shared this information, her clinical educator asked her whether she could provide more details about Pierre's language history or his educational exposure during his time in the refugee camp. The student admitted that she did not probe further about his language use at home, and she did not know that he had previously been in a refugee camp.

After this admission, the clinical educator explained that Pierre's behavior could have been the result of a variety of factors. The first important piece was to note that he had only been enrolled in Head Start for 2 months, and it was likely his first formal schooling experience in English only. His intake information noted that he had been exposed to English for 4 months. Before that, Pierre spent time as a refugee and moved around frequently. The clinical educator explained that Pierre may be in the early phases of second language development, sometimes called the nonverbal or silent period (Tabors, 1997). During this period, children focus on listening and comprehension of the new language. Children in this stage may appear very quiet, speaking little. Sudden English-only immersion in young children, without having previous exposure to the language, may be a stressful process that can lead to a nonverbal or silent stage, lasting a few weeks or, in some preschool children, up to a year (Tabors, 1997). However, children in the silent period are expected to continue to respond in their home language and familiar communication environments.

The clinical educator also noted that it can be common for children to experience trauma as a result of displacement or traumatic exposure in refugee camps. She went on to inform her student that children who experience trauma may appear to ignore or refuse to respond. Rarely, students may exhibit characteristics of selective mutism as an avoidance reaction to trauma (McInnes & Manassis, 2005; Wong, 2010). Some signs that supported this were that Pierre did not respond verbally in either language per observations and per his parents' report. The graduate student was surprised to hear this because she was not aware that the characteristics of selective mutism could impact behavioral responses in hearing tests. The clinical educator then described alternative hearing screening methods that did not require a behavioral response from the listener. Finally, the clinical educator addressed the inappropriate comment made by the audiology clinician to the speech-language pathologist. The clinical educator suggested that the student complete additional cultural competence training, specifically addressing her knowledge and beliefs about refugee children and their families.

CRITICAL THINKING AND DEBRIEFING QUESTIONS

1. **How could the audiology graduate student have made the child feel more comfortable during the hearing screening?**
2. **What missteps did the graduate student clinician take? What did the clinician do well?**
3. **Compare and contrast the silent period with selective mutism. What differentiates the two?**
4. **What other steps can be taken to address the lack of cultural empathy on the part of the student clinician?**

COMMENTARY

This scenario touches on a variety of situations that may arise across clinical settings. The first major theme was completing testing on a student who was not familiar with English. Although the audiologist had an interpreter present, it was likely Pierre's first experience completing a hearing screening. Pierre's parents, who were present during the screening, may have served as a more informative resource in this case providing information on Pierre's communication development across setting. The audiology student appeared to have limited experience completing hearing screenings on young children and lacked cultural competence skills, as referenced by her prejudicial comments.

While discussing language development, the topic of selective mutism was addressed, in contrast to the typical stages of second language development. Being instantly immersed in an English-only environment without any home language support may be a deeply traumatic event for many dual language learners and a frustrating experience for school personnel (Combs, Evans, Fletcher, Parra, & Jiménez, 2005). When children are suddenly plunged into a classroom with a language of instruction that they do not know, their communication habits may change. Students in this situation have been described as being more observational and in a stage known as the "silent period," where they are reluctant to speak because they are still acquiring the new language (Tabors, 1997). Although many experts and scholars believe that the silent period is a normal stage of second language acquisition, there is little empirical evidence of this stage (for discussion, see Roberts, 2014). However, this information is valuable for educational and health professionals in understanding rationale for specific behaviors of children learning a new language. Moreover, these professionals should also be proactive by providing rich activities to engage children who may be demonstrating characteristics of the silent period. Selective mutism should not be confused with the silent period because selective mutism typically presents across both languages, in unfamiliar settings, and lasts longer than the silent period (Toppelberg, Tabors, Coggins, Lum, & Burger, 2005).

Selective mutism is defined as a childhood anxiety disorder that is characterized by a child's inability to speak and communicate effectively in select social situations; there is no response in either language (Richard, 2011). In this scenario, Pierre exhibited some characteristics that were consistent with selective mutism. They included the following: Pierre's preference to observe peers and adults from a distance, his lack of engagement in the classroom, limited verbal responses, and "excessive shyness." Reviewing Pierre's behavior at school, in the community, and at home can provide more context about his language skills and whether he is demonstrating difficulties in all settings, or just in particular ones. Considering Pierre's prior experience of trauma as a result of his experiences in fleeing one country to move to another, as well as Pierre's immersion in a new language setting, Pierre would be considered at risk for selective mutism (McInnes & Manassis, 2005). Although bilingualism does not cause selective mutism, some research indicates that there is a higher incidence of selective mutism in bilingual immigrant populations (Toppelberg et al., 2005).

When assessing bilingual children who do not appear to speak or who are hesitant to participate, it is important to consider all contributing factors in their case history. For Pierre, it was critical to understand his prior experience of trauma as a refugee, the length of time he had been in the United States, the social expectations in his home regarding verbal communication, his lack of familiarity with the screening task, or other unknown factors. The American Speech-Language-Hearing Association's (ASHA's) practice portal provides considerations in the role and responsibilities to serve children with selective mutism (ASHA, n.d.-b). In such cases, alternative hearing screening may be used, such as otoacoustic emission testing (ASHA, n.d.-a).

Finally, the student's use of unprofessional language related to her client is a violation of ASHA's (2016) *Code of Ethics* (Principle of Ethics IV, Section D: Individuals shall not engage in any form of conduct that adversely reflects on the professions or on the individual's fitness to serve people professionally). Although the *Code of Ethics* applies to those who hold the clinical certificate of competence or may be applying for it, the student should still view the *Code of Ethics* as a professional guide for practice.

Under the Principle of Ethics IV, the speech-language pathologist (who received the referral) has a responsibility to report this violation, and the clinical collaborator has an ethical responsibility to instruct the clinician on their error and resolve the situation. Additionally, the student's reference to the client's race and pejorative language could be viewed as discriminatory. This student's supervisor has the responsibility to ensure that the student understands the gravity of her errors and receives additional instruction in cultural competence. Specific subjects may include stages of second language acquisition or typical bilingual development, modifications to assessments, implicit bias training, and ethics.

CRITICAL THINKING AND DEBRIEFING RESPONSES

1. **How could the audiology graduate student have made the child feel more comfortable during the hearing screening?**

Several things could have been done to make the child comfortable and to improve the reliability of the screening test:

a. Research and review the client's file before testing. In this case, that would include learning basic information about the refugee population, Pierre's home, his primary languages, history, newborn hearing screening results, and pertinent medical data and other vital background information.

b. If known, research the history and characteristics of refugee groups, including population, history, and practices.

c. Establish rapport briefly before beginning the test—for example, introduce yourself, show a toy, and engage with the child. Consider toys that are familiar to the child, including items that are culturally representative (e.g., pictures, foods).

d. When providing instructions, confirm that the child understands the task; look for verbal or nonverbal acknowledgment of the task—that is, raise hand when tone is heard. Consider playing a game first to ensure that the child understands the process.

e. Use the child's first language via an interpreter to instruct if no response to the second language. Directly address the child, and not the interpreter, when giving directions. Use gestures when appropriate.

Consider doing a play-based assessment that can turn the task into a game or complete an otoacoustic emission test.

2. **What missteps did the graduate student clinician take? What did the clinician do well?**

Missteps include the following:

a. Not confirming that the child understood the task;

b. Failing to do a quick check for auditory response to loud environmental noise—for example, clap hands loudly behind the child or use a noisemaker to produce loud tone/noise to check for startle response; and

c. Using judgmental language and name calling to explain Pierre's lack of response.

The clinician did the following things well:

a. Alternating decibel levels,

b. Referring to a speech-language pathologist, and

c. Openly sharing her impressions with her clinical educator.

3. **Compare and contrast the silent period with selective mutism. What differentiates the two?**

Generally, language acquisition can be classified into the following stages: preproduction, early production, speech emergence, intermediate fluency, and advanced fluency (e.g., Krashen & Terrell, 1983; Tabors, 1997). Although most individuals will follow this trajectory, language development is unique to each person. For example, a student like Pierre may spend more time in the preproduction phase given variables such as his personality, time in the immersive culture (United States), and peer group (English speaking). Other individuals, such as adults who are traveling to a foreign country, may move quickly out of preproduction into the early production and speech emergence stages when trying to learn and master a second language. Language fluency may remain variable in all languages, across settings.

Selective mutism is a childhood anxiety disorder. The characteristics in identifying selective mutism include the inability to speak and communicate effectively in social settings. A child may communicate well at home but refuse to communicate at school. The ways in which selective mutism manifest may vary in degree—one child may never talk outside their home, whereas another may whisper or speak to certain people in social settings. When forced to communicate in a setting where they are not comfortable, people with selective mutism may choose to gesture or nod, or they may have more severe emotional reactions, including tantrums, running away, or crying.

A child who appears nonverbal, uses gestures to communicate, and appears very anxious in social settings outside of the home should be monitored by staff and parents. Obtaining a thorough speech and language history of communication interactions at home along with skilled observations across the day are important pieces in obtaining information to differentiate between second language acquisition, selective mutism, and possible language disorder.

4. **What other steps can be taken to address the lack of cultural empathy on the part of the student clinician?**

The clinical educator could assign the student a project to help increase cultural competence in the topics of second language acquisition, experiences of refugees, and other activities that can increase her cultural knowledge and sensitivity. Additionally, learning about the process of second language acquisition may provide further insight on the cognitive demands and stages that occur when attempting mastery of another language. Depending on her program and its rules and requirements, she may also be subject to some sort of discipline because of her insensitive and inappropriate comments about a client. Although students are not technically held to ASHA's (2016) *Code of Ethics,* they should consider it as a guidepost for their training and future professional practice.

TAKE AWAYS

- Knowledge of the process of second language acquisition can help clinicians interpret observed patterns of responses or limited spontaneous communication in dual language learners when compared with children with language disorders.
- Children who experience trauma, including those who have a history of being refugees, may be at higher risk for developing language disorders and, in some cases, selective mutism.
- Alternative hearing assessments are available to support the evaluation of clients with limited or developing English-language abilities.

REFERENCES

American Speech-Language-Hearing Association. (n.d.-a). *Childhood hearing screening.* Retrieved from https://www.asha.org/PRPSpecificTopic.aspx?folderid=8589935406§ion=Key_Issues

American Speech-Language-Hearing Association. (n.d.-b). *Selective mutism.* Retrieved from https://www.asha.org/PRPSpecificTopic.aspx?folderid=8589942812§ion=Signs_and_Symptoms

American Speech-Language-Hearing Association. (2016). *Code of Ethics.* Retrieved from https://www.asha.org/Code-of-Ethics/

Combs, M. C., Evans, C., Fletcher, T., Parra, E., & Jiménez, A. (2005). Bilingualism for the children: Implementing a dual-language program in an English-only state. *Educational Policy, 19,* 701–728. https://doi.org/10.1177/0895904805278063

Cunningham, C. E., McHolm, A., Boyle, M. H., & Patel, S. (2004). Behavioral and emotional adjustment, family functioning, academic performance, and social relationships in children with selective mutism. *Journal of Child Psychology and Psychiatry, 45,* 1363–1372. https://doi.org/10.1111/j.1469-7610.2004.00327.x

Krashen, S. D., & Terrell, T. D. (1983). *The natural approach: Language acquisition in the classroom.* London, England: Alemany Press.

McInnes, A., & Manassis, K. (2005). When silence is not golden: An integrated approach to selective mutism. *Seminars in Speech and Language, 26*(3), 201–210.

Preston, K. (2014). When a child goes silent. *The ASHA Leader, 19*(11), 34–38.

Richard, G. J. (2011). *The source for selective mutism.* East Moline, IL: LinguiSystems.

Roberts, T. A. (2014). Not so silent after all: Examination and analysis of the silent stage in childhood second language acquisition. *Early Childhood Research Quarterly, 29*(1), 22–40. https://doi.org/10.1016/j.ecresq.2013.09.001

Roseberry-McKibbin, C. (2014). *Multicultural students with special language needs: Practical strategies for assessment and intervention* (4th ed.). Oceanside, CA: Academic Communication Associates.

Tabors, P. O. (1997). *One child, two languages: A guide for preschool educators of children learning English as a second language.* Baltimore, MD: Brookes.

Toppelberg, C. O., Tabors, P., Coggins, A., Lum, K., & Burger, C. (2005). Differential diagnosis of selective mutism in bilingual children. *Journal of the American Academy of Child and Adolescent Psychiatry, 44,* 592–595.

Wong, P. (2010). Selective mutism: A review of etiology, comorbidities, and treatment. *Psychiatry, 7*(3), 23–31.

ADDITIONAL RESOURCES

ARTICLES AND BOOKS

Elizur, Y., & Perednik, R. (2003). Prevalence and description of selective mutism in immigrant and native families: A controlled study. *Journal of the American Academy of Child and Adolescent Psychiatry, 42*, 1451–1459. https://doi.org/10.1097/00004583-200312000-00012

Goldstein, B. (2000). *Resource guide on cultural and linguistic diversity.* San Diego, CA: Singular Publishing Group.

Hungerford, S., Edwards, J., & Lantosca, A. (2003, November). *A socio-communication intervention model for selective mutism.* Seminar presented at the American Speech-Language-Hearing Association Convention, Chicago, IL. Retrieved from http://www.speech-languagepathologist.org/archives/chat/SLP/files/ASHA2003HandoutRe_formatted.doc

Kohnert, K., Yim, D., Nett, K., Kan, P. F., & Duran, L. (2005). Intervention with linguistically diverse preschool children. *Language, Speech, and Hearing Services in Schools, 36*, 251–263. https://doi.org/10.1044/0161-1461(2005/025)

Lavie, L. (2014). Under the Iron Dome: As bombs interrupt fittings, an Israeli audiologist hustles her elderly patients to the shelter–And prays for peace. *The ASHA Leader, 19*(9), 72.

Mayo, L. H., Florentine, M., & Buus, S. (1997). Age of second-language acquisition and perception of speech in noise. *Journal of Speech, Language, and Hearing Research, 40*, 686–693. https://doi.org/10.1044/jslhr.4003.686

Schum, R. L. (2002). Selective mutism: An integrated approach. *The ASHA Leader, 7*(17), 4–6. https://doi.org/10.1044/leader.FTR1.07172002.4

ONLINE RESOURCES

American Speech-Language-Hearing Association's *Code of Ethics*: https://www.asha.org/Code-of-Ethics/

Selective mutism: https://www.asha.org/PRPSpecificTopic.aspx?folderid=8589942812§ion=Overview

When Collaboration Meets Contrasting Beliefs — Navigating Autism Spectrum Disorder Treatment Within Cultural Expectations

Ivan Campos, Puja Goel, Dorian Lee-Wilkerson, Alicia Fleming Hamilton, and Wendyliza González

PREBRIEF

This scenario discusses cultural beliefs surrounding autism spectrum disorder (ASD) and how it affects a Chinese family in the United States. It provides a perspective regarding the way a family's traditional Chinese beliefs surrounding disability and gender can influence their choices for service delivery. It also illustrates the importance of involving all family members in the decision-making process. Finally, it highlights evidence-based, best practices for treatment and how they may work in harmony with complementary and alternative medicine (CAM) practices.

notes:

OBJECTIVES

- Identify beliefs and perceptions surrounding autism and disability that may exist in the Chinese community.
- Understand complementary approaches to treatment, such as CAM, that may be considered in conjunction with evidence-based approaches.
- Explore decision-making processes for parents of children with autism, including approaches to selecting interventions.

CASE SCENARIO

Bo Zhao is a 4-year-old boy whose family speaks Mandarin Chinese. Bo is nonverbal and has recently been diagnosed with ASD by his pediatrician. Bo has a twin sister, Chen, who is typically developing. The children live with their mother, father, and grandmother. Their mother and grandmother care for them in the home. Bo does not attend preschool or day care. Bo's family moved to the United States for his father's job and have been there for 2 years. Mr. Zhao works for an international business, and the family lives a modest, middle-class life. The family hopes to move back to China in 5–10 years after Mr. Zhao's work contract is over.

Bo's medical history is unremarkable. His parents were surprised when they learned that they were having twins. As the children grew, the parents reported that Bo appeared to lag behind his sister, Chen, in all developmental milestones and described Chen as a "helper" who pushed Bo in his learning. When Bo at-

Definitions

Complementary and alternative medicine (CAM)—A broad domain of healing resources that encompasses all health systems, modalities, and practices and their accompanying theories and beliefs, other than those intrinsic to the politically dominant health system of a particular society or culture in a given historical period.

Speech-generating devices (SGDs)—Defined by the Centers for Medicare and Medicaid Services (n.d.) as "durable medical equipment that provides an individual who has a severe speech impairment with the ability to meet his or her functional speaking needs" (I. Proposed Decision, Speech Generating Devices section, para. 2).

tended his yearly medical checkup at 3 years old, his pediatrician shared concerns that Bo was not yet using words and did not appear to socially engage with anyone but his sister. The pediatrician suspected that Bo may have ASD and referred him for an early childhood evaluation. Bo was diagnosed with ASD shortly after his third birthday. The family reported that when they heard his diagnosis, they were shocked and confused.

Bo demonstrated behaviors typically associated with ASD, including arm-flapping, difficulty with joint attention, being easily agitated, and having a strong preference for playing with small action figures. Initially, his grandmother shared that she was disappointed that Bo was the twin with a disability and said it would have been "much better if it were his twin sister, Chen." The parents expressed that when he was diagnosed, they felt as though "the sky was falling down." After the diagnosis was briefly explained, the family appeared more hopeful about Bo's prognosis and agreed to start therapy. The diagnosing speech-language pathologist (SLP) shared information with Bo's parents about Child Find: a legal mandate under the Individuals With Disabilities Education Act of 1990. Child Find offered the parents the option of having the school evaluate Bo to identify possible educational disabilities and to provide needed services, should he qualify. Bo's parents were appreciative of the information but declined this option. The family, instead, chose to seek home-based services through a local private practice.

Bo was offered an English-speaking SLP paired with an interpreter. However, the family wanted to find a bilingual, Mandarin-speaking clinician. They used a database from their state speech-language-hearing association and found an SLP who, although not fully fluent, knew conversational phrases in Mandarin Chinese and was familiar with Chinese cultural practices. When the clinician asked whether her abilities would meet the family's needs, the family reported yes, that they felt more comfortable having someone who "understood their culture" providing services for Bo. He received private speech-language pathology services for 1 hour, twice a week, in the home.

Over the past year Bo demonstrated gains in his communication skills, including the ability to point to desired objects, make a choice between two objects or pictures, and tolerate hand-over-hand assistance. Bo learned to use some gestures to communicate, including pointing; clapping; and the signs for no, yes, and water/drink. Bo used primitive vocalizations (grunting, squealing, screeching) and exaggerated facial expressions to initiate communication.

The treating SLP recently introduced a picture-based communication system with extensive research supporting its positive outcomes in developing verbal communication (Flippin, Reszka, & Watson, 2010). The picture-based system was used to observe Bo's responses. With this system, Bo was successful at pointing to a desired object in a field of two. This particular strategy helped to decrease his frustration when trying to communicate with his family and his SLP. Initial picture-based trials were successful during therapy. As a result, the SLP scheduled a consultation with a speech-generating device (SGD) company to trial digital devices for presentation of pictures.

When the SLP shared this news with the family, they became very upset. The family did not like the idea of using a computer to talk for their son. They expected Bo to catch up to his sister and speak like her after a few years of therapy. They shared that previous doctors and therapists had told them that this was possible. The strongest opponent to the use of the SGD was Bo's grandmother, who warned that if he used a device to speak like this in public, he would bring dishonor on their family. She believed that Bo's autism was a punishment for the misbehavior of an ancestor. As the only male child, it was incredibly important to the family that Bo learn to communicate verbally, and they shared they did not want to send him to school with typically developing children until he could speak "normally." The SLP listened respectfully to the family's opinions. She restated their statements and asked whether they may be interested in taking the SGD home, "just for a trial." The family agreed reluctantly. When they returned for a follow-up visit, the device was still in the box, unopened. The SLP politely asked how the device trials went, and Mrs. Zhao shared that they would be suspending speech therapy for the moment to pursue other treatments including acupuncture and medicinal herbs. Bo and his sister would be staying home so his mother could teach them.

CRITICAL THINKING AND DEBRIEFING QUESTIONS

1. **In what ways can an SLP support a family's cultural beliefs regarding their child's care?**
2. **How can the SLP work with this family to address the cultural conflicts that occurred?**
3. **What resources can the SLP provide to demonstrate how SGDs can support Bo in his communication?**
4. **What are ways that evidence-based practice and CAM or other holistic approaches can complement each other during treatment?**

COMMENTARY

According to recent Centers for Disease Control and Prevention data, about one in every 59 children has been identified with ASD (Baio et al., 2018). As awareness of autism increases, it is likely that the identification of children with autism will also increase. Over the years, early identification of autism has seen a dramatic increase, with some countries identifying cases relatively recently, such as in China where the first cases of autism were not diagnosed until 1982. Programs providing autism services to children and their families in China were not available until the 1990s. Although awareness about autism in China is growing, families with children who have developmental disabilities (autism included) continue to report the need for more support, professional help, and information about how to raise their children (S. Y. Wong et al., 2004).

Understanding cultural practices and views regarding Chinese beliefs about developmental disabilities, especially autism, is critical in working with the Zhao family. Their cultural background influences the way they view autism and the impact they feel it may have on their lives and Bo's success in life. In this case, Bo's family was candid about their feelings of disappointment especially that Bo, their male child, was diagnosed with ASD. Historically, China has enforced a family planning policy that restricted the size of families to one or two children per couple, with male children more highly prized. This policy was revised in 2013 to allow parents who were only children to have a second child (Bloomberg News, 2020). It can also be common for Chinese families to believe that disabilities are caused by fate. Understanding cultural beliefs and views surrounding disability provides a strong foundation for a treating clinician when working with all families.

Family involvement is critical when working with students who have communication disorders, and research has indicated that quality educator-parent collaboration is necessary to establish effective educational programs for students with disabilities, including ASD (Fish, 2008). A collaborative approach to decision making would have involved the SLP making the decisions with the family (Smith, Summers, Mueller, Carillo, & Villaneda, 2018) instead of for them, as occurred in this scenario. This approach may have resulted in a more effective treatment plan that combined traditional and nontraditional clinical methods and demonstrated respect and value for the family's treatment desires. Some families may use alternative and holistic medicine as a primary approach to treat illness and disorder. Other families may use it as a supplement to other European American methods. Bo's family made the decision to use alternative and holistic medicine as a primary intervention for ASD when they became dissatisfied with the progress Bo was making with traditional speech therapy. Starting the therapy process in a collaborative way may have allowed the SLP and the family to have a more productive conversation regarding their concerns about Bo's progress and may have included opportunities to review treatment options and timelines that could better align with the family's expectations of Bo developing verbal language. It may also have provided an opportunity to consider ways that CAM could complement the evidence-based interventions provided by the SLP.

Understanding cultural beliefs and views surrounding disability provides a strong foundation for clinicians when working with all families.

Collaborative decision making also considers the communication styles and language competencies of family members. It is possible that the parents and grandmother did not fully understand Bo's diagnosis and prognosis as explained by the pediatrician. Through collaboration, the SLP can assist families in understanding medical terms and technical concepts associated with diagnosing disorders and prognoses; the SLP can also help the family determine therapy approaches that use bilingual materials, interpreters, or both. This understanding can also provide for a better cultural foundation in working with the family.

The family may have been disappointed that their SLP did not directly align with their cultural beliefs, even though they had sought out a Mandarin-speaking clinician. Although the SLP was Chinese, her individual culture appeared to align more with standard European American values and practices. Discussing cultural beliefs and values before starting services could have shed light on this difference in expectations.

CRITICAL THINKING AND DEBRIEFING RESPONSES

1. **In what ways can an SLP support a family's cultural beliefs regarding their child's care?**

First, SLPs can research a client's culture before meeting with them to have an idea of general practices. If an SLP does not know a client's cultural background before the meeting, they can conduct a thorough interview and case history to provide more in-depth cultural information from the client. The client in this scenario noted that they hoped to return to China within the next 5–10 years. This information may have been an indication that the family valued their Chinese heritage and language even though they did not openly discuss their desire. The family also rejected the offer of an English-speaking clinician paired with an interpreter and chose a Mandarin-speaking SLP. By choosing a Mandarin-speaking SLP, the family may have been indirectly indicating that the knowledge of, respect for, and integration of the family's cultural practices were important for effective intervention.

A study on the decision-making processes of parents who had children with ASD and how they chose interventions was completed by Finke, Drager, and Serpentine (2015); they noted that parents considered a variety of sources when making their intervention decisions for their children, including professional recommendations and anecdotal information from other parents through support groups or online, weighing each piece of evidence equally. This study also highlighted the need to have a collaborative decision-making process for parents because they felt solely responsible for the intervention decisions for their children. It may be helpful to demonstrate processes that can help families objectively assess information using evidence-based practices to help parents increase confidence in the decisions they make.

Given this information, the SLP may have avoided some possible conflicts by engaging the family in collaborative decision making. For most children, and Bo specifically, home is where most of their communication will occur. For that reason, it is paramount that his family supports his treatment plan and is involved in its design. If a family does not agree with a treatment approach, it is up to the treatment team and family to decide on another approach based on available evidence and the child's needs. The SLP should always strive to address potential conflicts by considering the family's and client's needs and preferences.

2. **How can the SLP work with this family to address the cultural conflicts that occurred?**

In this situation, the SLP could take several steps to address the cultural conflicts. The SLP could research and review literature that discusses traditional Chinese views of illness and disorder. These resources may include articles that discuss traditional Chinese views of ASD and the history of its treatment. The SLP may ask the family to share information with her about their cultural practices and beliefs in an attempt to integrate their traditions and practices into the therapy session.

For instance, in many Chinese families, it is common to place great value and deference to the opinion of elders (Battle, 2012). Traditionally in Chinese families, the decision maker is the father, whereas the mother is charged with the responsibility for care and education. In Bo's case, the decision makers were his parents and grandmother, as a respected elder. Additionally, his mother may have felt shame because of his disability (Richmond, 2011). Understanding the cultural dynamics at play could help the SLP when presenting diagnoses and prognosis, including information about programs available in the United States and possibly meeting with other families they could connect with. The shame that Bo's mother may feel has also been illustrated with families in China who do not send their children to school for fear of "losing face" if they attend school with "normal" children (Liu, 2003).

3. **What resources can the SLP provide to demonstrate how SGDs can support Bo in his communication?**

Although Bo's family rejected the idea of using an SGD, research overwhelmingly points to the use of SGDs as beneficial for nonverbal children. Kasari et al. (2014) demonstrated that intervention for minimally verbal, school-age children with ASD that included the use of an SGD improved their spontaneous output of novel utterances when compared with interventions that did not use SGDs. Drager, Light, and McNaughton (2010) demonstrated that augmentative and alternative communication (AAC) use can lead to increases in receptive vocabulary in young children. Providing this research to the family could help them to be informed decision makers in the care of their child. The SLP could also share that using an SGD does not affect the motivation to use natural speech, and when therapy focuses on natural speech in conjunction with AAC use it can facilitate the production of natural speech (Millar, Light, & Schlosser, 2006).

To encourage maintenance of the home culture and language, the SLP may refer to research that cites specific considerations for programming an SGD in Chinese (Oxley & Ma, 2020). Smith and colleagues (2018) confirmed that the home language should be supported either directly or indirectly through intervention. This can be done through the use of a bilingual clinician or interpreter or by training caregivers through collaboration. These multicultural and multilingual approaches help to ensure the best treatment options for children who speak multiple languages. Providing the family with evidence that children with ASD who are bilingual are more flexible thinkers and that using the device can promote verbal bilingual output may provide the family with additional hope. Helping parents and families understand that total communication (spoken, gestured, or through a device) is the goal may also help bridge the gap between the family's ideas about treatment, ways to increase Bo's communication skills, and the SLP's ideas.

4. **What are ways that evidence-based practice and CAM or other holistic approaches can complement each other during treatment?**

In Bo's scenario, CAM is important to the family and something they have chosen as an alternative to the treatment practices selected by the SLP. A study in China demonstrated that 47% of parents of children diagnosed with ASD wanted to use both CAM and Western medicine (V. C. N. Wong, 2009). A review of multiple CAM treatments (Brondino et al., 2015) indicated that there was no conclusive evidence for the efficacy of CAM therapies in ASD. The authors suggested that all practitioners encourage patients and their families to discuss the safety and efficacy of all CAMs. CAMs can be used to augment conventional treatment but not as a replacement. A family may choose to use massage to reduce anxiety and enhance positive responses to behavioral and educational treatments. If interested, families should be advised to try one CAM at a time and consistently monitor any clinical changes or adverse responses.

In this scenario, the SLP may have asked more about the CAM treatments Bo was receiving and could have suggested a meeting with his healers to integrate their work into the speech sessions. The SLP can help to create a nonjudgmental environment and discuss with families the advantages and disadvantages of using CAM on the basis of empirical evidence. The SLP could use picture boards or program the SGD device with words for herbs, food, or other CAM that acknowledge this practice. It is important when working with all families to provide opportunities for them to share their cultural practices and beliefs at the onset and throughout intervention. This collaborative approach emphasizes the partnership when executing treatment and can lead to positive clinical outcomes.

TAKE AWAYS

- Clinicians should be aware of the many ways culture influences a family's decision-making process and develop collaborate and flexible plans that are congruent with a family's cultural practices.
- Recognizing alternative medicine in therapy approaches can result in positive and productive therapist-client relationships.
- Sharing information about families' and clients' use of CAM with members of the

interprofessional team improves intervention processes and clinical outcomes.

REFERENCES

Baio, J., Wiggins, L., Christensen, D. L., Maenner, M. J., Daniels, J., Warren, Z., . . . Dowling, N.F. (2018). Prevalence of autism spectrum disorder among children aged 8 years—Autism and Developmental Disabilities Monitoring Network, 11 sites, United States, 2014. *Morbidity and Mortality Weekly Report: Surveillance Summaries, 67*(6), 1-23.

Battle, D. (2012). Becoming a culturally competent clinician. *Perspectives on Communication Disorders and Sciences in Culturally and Linguistically Diverse Populations, 6*(3), 19-22.

Bloomberg News. (2020, January 22). China's two-child policy. *The Washington Post.* Retrieved from https://www.washingtonpost.com/business/energy/chinas-two-child-policy/2020/01/22/a1bd70e2-3cfc-11ea-afe2-090eb37b60b1_story.html

Brondino, N., Fusar-Poli, L., Rocchetti, M., Provenzani, U., Barale, F., & Politi, P. (2015). Complementary and alternative therapies for autism spectrum disorder. *Evidence-Based Complementary and Alternative Medicine, 2015,* 258589.

Centers for Medicare and Medicaid Services. (n.d.). *Speech generating devices.* Retrieved from https://www.cms.gov/medicare-coverage-database/details/medicare-coverage-document-details.aspx?MCDId=26

Drager, K. D. R., Light, J., & McNaughton, D. (2010). Effects of AAC interventions on communication and language for young children with complex communication needs. *Journal of Pediatric Rehabilitation Medicine: An Interdisciplinary Approach, 3,* 303-310.

Finke, E., Drager, K., & Serpentine, E. C. (2015). "It's not humanly possible to do everything": Perspectives on intervention decision-making processes of parents of children with autism spectrum disorders. *Perspectives on Language Learning and Education, 22*(1), 13-21.

Fish, W. W. (2008). The IEP meeting: Perceptions of parents of students who receive special education services. *Preventing School Failure, 53,* 8-14.

Flippin, M., Reszka, S., & Watson, L. R. (2010). Effectiveness of the Picture Exchange Communication System (PECS) on communication and speech for children with autism spectrum disorders: A meta-analysis. *American Journal of Speech-Language Pathology, 19,* 178-195.

Individuals With Disabilities Education Act of 1990, Pub. L. 101-476, renamed the Individuals With Disabilities Education Improvement Act, codified at 20 U.S.C. §§ 1400-1482.

Kasari, C., Kaiser, A., Goods, K., Nietfeld, J., Mathy, P., Landa, R., . . . Almirall, D. (2014). Communication interventions for minimally verbal children with autism: A sequential multiple assignment randomized trial. *Journal of the American Academy of Child and Adolescent Psychiatry, 53,* 635-646.

Liu, L. M. (2003). Shequ qingjing yu chengxiang ruozhi ertong jiaoyu moshi de chayi: Dui Beijing shi ruozhi ertong anli de fenxi [Community circumstances and the difference between educational models for urban and rural children with mental retardation: An analysis of children with mental retardation in Beijing]. *Shehui Xue Yanjiu, 1,* 95-101.

Millar, D. C., Light, J. C., & Schlosser, R. W. (2006). The impact of augmentative and alternative communication intervention on the speech production of individuals with developmental disabilities: A research review. *Journal of Speech, Language, and Hearing Research, 49*(2), 248-264. https://doi.org/10.1044/1092-4388(2006/021)

Oxley, J., & Ma, Y. (2020). Considerations for Chinese text input methods in the design of speech generating devices: A tutorial. *Clinical Linguistics & Phonetics, 34,* 366-387. https://doi.org/10.1080/02699206.2019.1652934

Richmond, A. S. (2011). Autism spectrum disorder: A global perspective. *Perspectives on Global Issues in Communication Sciences and Related Disorders, 1*(2), 39-46.

Smith, V., Summers, C., Mueller, V., Carillo, A., & Villaneda, G. (2018). Evidence-based clinical decision making for bilingual children with autism spectrum disorders: A guide for clinicians. *Perspectives of the ASHA Special Interest Groups, 3*(14), 19-27.

Wong, S. Y., Wong, T. K. S., Martinson, I., Lai, A. C., Chen, W. J., & He, Y. S. (2004). Needs of Chinese parents of children with developmental disability. *Journal of Learning Disabilities, 8,* 141-158.

Wong, V. C. N. (2009). Use of complementary and alternative medicine (CAM) in autism spectrum disorder (ASD): Comparison of Chinese and Western culture (Part A). *Journal of Autism and Developmental Disorders, 39,* 454-463. https://doi.org/10.1007/s10803-008-0644-9

ADDITIONAL RESOURCES

AUTISM IN CHINA

McCabe, H., Wu, S. X., & Zhang, G. J. (2005). Experiences with autism in the People's Republic of China: Viewing social change through one family's story. *The Journal of International Special Needs Education, 8,* 11-18.

McCabe Hobart, H. (2008). Autism and family in the People's Republic of China: Learning from parents' perspectives. *Research & Practice for Persons With Severe Disabilities, 33*(1-2), 37-47.

Richmond, A. S. (2011). Autism spectrum disorder: A global perspective. *Perspectives on Global Issues in Communication Sciences and Related Disorders, 1*(2), 39-46.

BILINGUAL AUGMENTATIVE ALTERNATIVE COMMUNICATION (AAC) APPS: PORTLAND STATE UNIVERSITY

https://sites.google.com/pdx.edu/multicsd/adult/other-toolstopics-for-slps/bilingual-aac-apps

PRACTICE PORTAL ON AUGMENTATIVE ALTERNATIVE COMMUNICATION (AAC)

https://www.asha.org/PRPSpecificTopic.aspx?folderid=8589942773§ion=Key_Issues#AAC_Myths_and_Realities

SPEECH-GENERATING DEVICES

An, S., Feng, X., Dai, Y., Bo, H., Wang, X., Li, M., . . . Wei, L. (2017). Development and evaluation of a speech-generating AAC mobile app for minimally verbal children with autism spectrum disorder in Mainland China. *Molecular Autism, 8,* 52. https://doi.org/10.1186/s13229-017-0165-5

Centers for Medicare and Medicaid Services. (n.d.). *Speech generating devices.* Retrieved from https://www.cms.gov/medicare-coverage-database/details/medicare-coverage-document-details.aspx?MCDId=26

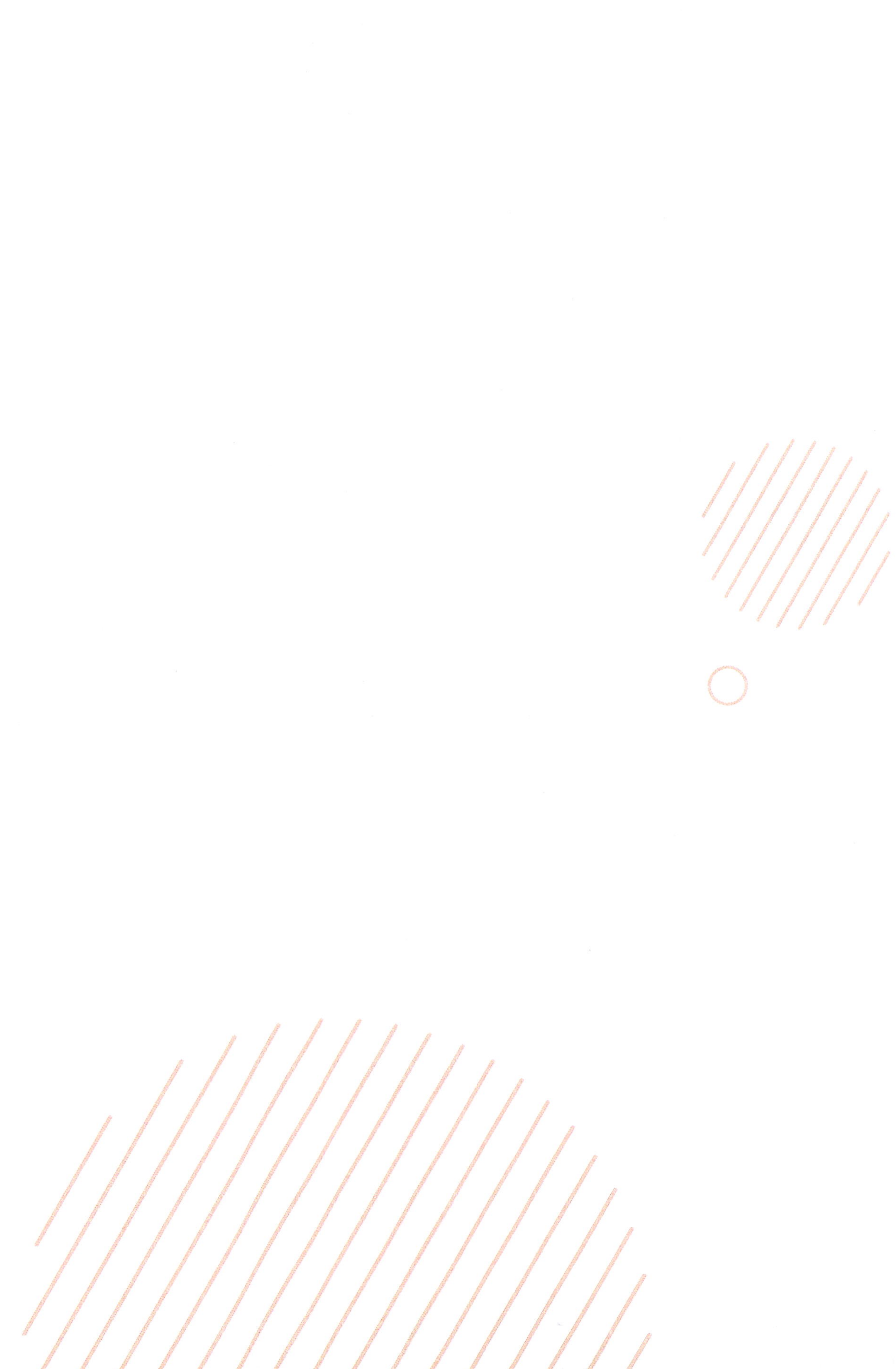

Assimilation and Language Assumptions — Why English Isn't "Better"

Alicia Fleming Hamilton and Carmen Ana Ramos-Pizarro

PREBRIEF

notes:

U.S. Census Bureau (2018) data indicate that 23% of children in the United States speak a language other than English at home. Although parents of dual language learners (DLLs) may likely recognize the value of their children learning English, communities may vary in their knowledge about the value of maintaining their native language and culture. Cultural assimilation may contribute to the practice of adopting all aspects of a new culture without regard for the benefit of the home culture. This case highlights how a speech-language pathologist (SLP) worked with a family to adjust expectations and priorities.

OBJECTIVES

- Explain best practices related to communicating results from speech-language testing to parents of DLL students.
- Summarize the main advantages of bilingualism in cognitive and linguistic development.
- Differentiate between cultural liaison, interpreter, and translator.

CASE SCENARIO

Catherine is an SLP who works with the early childhood team at a suburban school. The team received a referral from a teacher in one of their early childhood classrooms, for a 4-year-old girl named Fairuza. Fairuza recently moved to the United States with her family from Iran. Fairuza's parents were both doctors in Iran, and Fairuza's mother, Dr. Ghasemi, was currently working as a doctor in the United States. The family speaks both Farsi (Persian) and English in their home. As part of her intake into the new school, Fairuza completed early childhood screening. She passed all areas of development, except communication. When her parents received the results they were not surprised because they also had communication concerns when they observed their daughter play with the English-speaking children in their neighborhood. They noticed that Fairuza rarely initiated play with other children, seemed to go along with whatever game they chose, and rarely protested when the children played something she did not like. At home in Farsi, Fairuza was able to tell stories, ask for what she wanted, and protest when she was unhappy.

After an explanation about early childhood screening and Fairuza's performance, her parents requested a full communication evaluation. They were concerned that if she had difficulty with her communication, Fairuza would face challenges in her academic achievement. The SLP met with the family and completed a full evaluation of Fairuza's language and articulation skills in Farsi and English, with the help of a Farsi interpreter. After testing, the SLP concluded that Fairuza's communication skills were within normal limits, including her articulation skills, when tested in English and Farsi.

When the team met with Fairuza's family to share results, her father was furious. He shared that he pulled Fairuza out of a local preschool where they spoke Farsi only because he did not want her to become "confused" learning two languages. He felt that she would be most successful if she advanced in English. He insisted that she needed to improve her English skills and that the smaller ratios and specialized service in the special education classes they told him about, along with being among English speaking peers, would help her accomplish that. Catherine, the SLP, noted that because Fairuza's language skills were within normal limits for her age and gender in her home language, and because they were still within the low end of the normal range for English speakers, she did not have a disability and did not qualify for special education services. She clarified that to be diagnosed with a language disorder, Fairuza would have needed to exhibit deficits in her home language and any other language she used. Fairuza's parents were still concerned. They did not understand why their daughter failed the communication screening and appeared to lag behind in learning English but did not qualify for extra help. Catherine shared that Fairuza had age-appropriate skills in Farsi, and the things they noticed on the screener were likely common occurrences for students who were learning a second language.

After the parents acknowledged the results, they were at a loss about how to proceed. Catherine recommended and strongly encouraged Fairuza's father to reenroll her in her Farsi preschool because it would continue to strengthen both of her languages. Catherine explained the importance of continuing with Farsi for both language development and cultural benefits. When Fairuza's father heard this explanation, his demeanor changed. He spent the next 30 minutes asking Catherine about language learning and bilingualism. When he left, he asked Catherine to forward him more information to share with his community about the benefits of speaking multiple languages.

CRITICAL THINKING AND DEBRIEFING QUESTIONS

1. Did the SLP provide an appropriate recommendation to the family regarding continuing Fairuza's education in Farsi school?
2. Is it the SLP's role to provide counseling to these parents if the results of the assessment showed that there was no communication problem?
3. In this case, the SLP was not fluent in Farsi and had to rely on the use of an interpreter. What are the implications of using a nonprofessional interpreter during speech-language evaluations? What alternatives are there when there is no one who speaks the native language?
4. What are the social and cultural benefits of maintaining a native language?
5. How would you respond if a parent insisted on having their child speak English only?

COMMENTARY

DLLs frequently have different levels of mastery of both their native language and English. The Ghasemi family wanted Fairuza to be fluent in English. These desires may stem from family preferences or perceptions regarding cultural assimilation. In this case, the SLP maintained professionalism by sharing resources about bilingual language development and native language preservation with the family. The SLP could have explained earlier in the process, and in more detail, the differences between typical bilingual language development and characteristics of disordered language (Hoff & Core, 2015). This information may have given the family better context for the special education evaluation from the beginning.

A foundational understanding of bilingual language development and its benefits may have provided the family with the background knowledge to better interpret the results of the language tests. Bilingual advantages have been reported for executive function (Bialystok, Craik, Klein, & Viswanathan, 2004), metalinguistic awareness (Cummins, 1978), phonetic perception (Antoniou, Liang, Ettlinger, & Wong, 2015), cognitive flexibility (Adi-Japha, Berberich-Artzi, & Libnawi, 2010), creative thinking (Lee & Kim, 2011), and even delay in the onset of symptoms of dementia (Bialystok, Craik, & Freedman, 2007).

Bilingual advantages have been reported for executive function (Bialystok, Craik, Klein, & Viswanathan, 2004), metalinguistic awareness (Cummins, 1978), phonetic perception (Antoniou, Liang, Ettlinger, & Wong, 2015), cognitive flexibility (Adi-Japha, Berberich-Artzi, & Libnawi, 2010), creative thinking (Lee & Kim, 2011), and even delay in the onset of symptoms of dementia (Bialystok, Craik, & Freedman, 2007).

Some public school systems may have close to 30% of students who speak one or more of 155 languages other than English at home (New York City Department of Education, n.d.). SLPs have a responsibility to provide valid assessments in languages in which they are not fluent. The use of interpreters is a reality that most SLPs will face at some point in their careers. The American Speech-Language-Hearing Association (ASHA) has provided a clear map to guide practitioners on how to select the best qualified interpreter, how to provide instructions on their role, and how to ensure that the person strives to extend their role from a strictly linguistic broker to being a cultural interpreter, ensuring that relevant aspects of the family's culture are interpreted and decoded for the clinician.

Multiple contributing factors—including a lack of consistent teacher training regarding typical bilingual development, a lack of administrative support when providing necessary resources to teachers and students who speak multiple languages, and a lack of a centralized methodology or curriculum in bilingual teaching—may impact the number of DLL students referred to special education services for assessment. SLPs armed with knowledge about what is typical bilingual development and what is disordered bilingual development will be able to advocate for the use of classroom strategies that foster use of the native language as a strategy to facilitate language learning and to provide appropriate, equitable identifi-

Definitions

Cultural broker—person knowledgeable about the client's/patient's culture and/or speech-language community. The broker passes cultural/community-related information between the client and the clinician in order to optimize services.

Linguistic broker—a person knowledgeable about the client's/patient's speech community or communication environment who can provide valuable information about language and sociolinguistic norms in the client's/patient's speech community and communication environment.

An informant or broker can provide

- grammaticality judgments, indicating whether the client's/patient's language and phonetic production are consistent with the norms of that speech community or communication environment;
- information on the language socialization patterns (i.e., use of language in socially appropriate ways based on the culture) of that speech community or communication environment; and
- information on other areas of language, including semantics and pragmatics (ASHA, n.d.).

The ASHA website has more information at https://www.asha.org/PRPSpecificTopic.aspx?folderid=8589935334§ion=Key_Issues

cation of students who truly need special education support.

CRITICAL THINKING AND DEBRIEFING RESPONSES

1. **Did the SLP provide an appropriate recommendation to the family regarding continuing Fairuza's education in Farsi school?**

Multiple bodies of research indicate that bilingualism—especially when maintaining the home, or native, language—is critical for a student to develop their highest level of language proficiency in both languages. Research also shows that discouraging a family's use of their native language can cause adverse effects on the overall language development, but it also impacts their cultural learning and social communication within their community (Barac, Bialystok, Castro, & Sanchez, 2014; Moore, Pérez-Méndez, & Boerger, 2006). It is not an appropriate recommendation to discourage use of a native language. When this is suggested, there is evidence that developing only one of a child's languages can cause irreversible negative effects on children's development (Moore et al., 2006).

2. **Is it the SLP's role to provide counseling to these parents if the results of the assessment showed that there was no communication problem?**

Yes. When an SLP is providing an assessment that is accurate and authentic, it is critical to describe each task, its validity, and discuss the student's performance. SLPs must take time to explain the difference between errors that are developmentally appropriate and errors that indicate a disorder. Parents may become confused when told their child has made an error; as a result, SLPs should take care to review qualification criteria so that parents have a solid understanding of their child's performance. Comprehensive service delivery can involve two categories of counseling: information counseling and personal adjustment counseling (Flasher & Fogle, 2012). Informational counseling is also called client and family-caregiver education, and it involves discussing the nature of a disorder, possible treatment approaches and techniques, prognosis, and material and community resources. Personal adjustment counseling involves the feelings, emotions, thoughts, and beliefs expressed by clients as part of the information exchange with the SLP or audiologist (Flasher & Fogle, 2012). In this case, the SLP is providing both, which are within her scope and are an important skill to help families as they learn about results and possible treatment options.

3. **In this case, the SLP was not fluent in Farsi and had to rely on the use of an interpreter. What are the implications of using a nonprofessional interpreter during speech-language evaluations? What alternatives are there when there is no one who speaks the native language?**

Best practice involves using a professional interpreter to complete an assessment in a client's native language. An SLP should set aside time before and after the evaluation to brief the interpreter and to review the testing and discuss results. Ideally, sessions can be videotaped to refer to later in case there are differing opinions regarding performance or whether there is confusion regarding a task. When a professional interpreter or bilingual SLP is not available, the next best approach would be to use a bilingual assistant, bilingual staff from an outside discipline, or a cultural liaison (listed in order of preference on the basis of training) and to provide appropriate time to explain the testing protocol and expectations. At times, when there is no one else available, a family member may be used, but clinicians should only turn to family members as a last resort and not as a result of organizational factors (e.g., improper funding or poor planning). It is important to consider that family members may be less reliable and may have their own biases or conflicts of interests given the outcome of the results (ASHA, n.d.).

4. **What are the social and cultural benefits of maintaining a native language?**

The social and cultural benefits of maintaining a native language include literacy and academic knowledge; the continuation of family storytelling; and the ability to connect with others in the community, to carry on traditions, and to establish a strong cultural identity. Caregivers may find it easier to communicate in their native language, leading to more opportunities to share language about emotions and feelings that can deepen the child-caregiver relationship. This is why it is critical that early intervention providers approach bilingualism in a positive way. When a child's home language is not developed, they are at risk for language loss (Hoff, Rumiche, Burridge, Ribot, & Welsh, 2014). When a child loses their home language, they also lose their cultural identify, values, and beliefs (Moore et al., 2006).

5. **How would you respond if a parent insisted on having their child speak English only?**

There are many excellent resources at the end of this scenario that tout the benefits of maintaining native language and the benefits of bilingualism for children. An SLP could select appropriate resources, on the basis of their interactions with the family and clinical judgment. They may also offer themselves as a resource and provide contact information in the event that questions or concerns arise in the future. However, the final decision will always lie with the client or, in this case, the client's parents.

TAKE AWAYS

- Bilingual families are not all alike. They present with differing expectations for screening and evaluation processes as well as different levels of understanding of these systems. Because these systems may be unfamiliar, it is paramount for SLPs to create systems that clearly and accurately describe processes and present possible outcomes from the beginning. This transparency can help to avoid difficult situations after completion of the evaluation.
- Just because someone is bilingual does not mean they are an expert in the field of bilingualism. In reality, they may have little knowledge of evidence base for the benefits of bilingualism and what is "typical" in bilingual development. SLPs have rigorous training and are experts in atypical and typical language development. Often SLPs undergo additional, specialized training regarding bilingualism and its development.

REFERENCES

Adi-Japha, E., Berberich-Artzi, J., & Libnawi, A. (2010). Cognitive flexibility in drawings of bilingual children. *Child Development, 81,* 1356-1366.

American Speech-Language-Hearing Association. (n.d.). *Collaborating with interpreters.* Retrieved from https://www.asha.org/PRPSpecificTopic.aspx?folderid=8589935334§ion=Key_Issues

Antoniou, M., Liang, E., Ettlinger, M., & Wong, P. C. (2015). The bilingual advantage in phonetic learning. *Bilingualism: Language and Cognition, 18,* 683-695.

Barac, R., Bialystok, E., Castro, D. C., & Sanchez, M. (2014). The cognitive development of young dual language learners: A critical review. *Early Childhood Research Quarterly, 29,* 699–714.

Bialystok, E., Craik, F. I., & Freedman, M. (2007). Bilingualism as a protection against the onset of symptoms of dementia. *Neuropsychologia, 45,* 459–464.

Bialystok, E., Craik, F. I., Klein, R., & Viswanathan, M. (2004). Bilingualism, aging, and cognitive control: Evidence from the Simon task. *Psychology and Aging, 19,* 290–303.

Cummins, J. (1978). Bilingualism and the development of metalinguistic awareness. *Journal of Cross-Cultural Psychology, 9,* 131–149.

Flasher, L. V., & Fogle, P. T. (2012). *Counseling skills for speech-language pathologists and audiologists.* Clifton Park, NY: Thomson Delmar Learning.

Hoff, E., & Core, C. (2015). What clinicians need to know about bilingual development. *Seminars in Speech and Language, 36*(2), 89–99.

Hoff, E., Rumiche, R., Burridge, A., Ribot, K. M., & Welsh, S. N. (2014). Expressive vocabulary development in children from bilingual and monolingual homes: A longitudinal study from two to four years. *Early Childhood Research Quarterly, 29,* 433–444. https://doi.org/10.1016/j.ecresq.2014.04.012

Lee, H., & Kim, K. H. (2011). Can speaking more languages enhance your creativity? Relationship between bilingualism and creative potential among Korean American students with multicultural link. *Personality and Individual Differences, 50,* 1186–1190.

Moore, S. M., Pérez-Méndez, C., & Boerger, K. (2006). Meeting the needs of culturally and linguistically diverse families in early language and literacy intervention. In L. Justice (Ed.), *Clinical approaches to emergent literacy intervention* (pp. 29–70). San Diego, CA: Plural Press.

New York City Department of Education. (n.d.). *English language learners demographics report for the 2016–2017 school year.* Retrieved from https://infohub.nyced.org/reports/academics/ELL-demographic-report

U.S. Census Bureau. (2018). *American Community Survey (ACS): 2018 data release.* Retrieved from https://www.census.gov/programs-surveys/acs

ADDITIONAL RESOURCES

ARTICLES

Campbell-Wilson, F. (2002). Middle Eastern and Arab American cultures. In D. E. Battle (Ed.), *Communication disorders in multicultural populations* (pp. 113–134). Boston, MA: Butterworth-Heinemann.

Cardenas, J. (1993, September). Current problems in bilingual education: Part II. *Intercultural Development Research Association (IDRA) Newsletter.* Retrieved from https://www.idra.org/resource-center/current-problems-in-bilingual-education-part-ii/

Chan, K. (2016, December 2). These are the most powerful languages in the world. *World Economic Forum.* Retrieved from https://www.weforum.org/agenda/2016/12/these-are-the-most-powerful-languages-in-the-world/

Diamond, J. (2010, October 15). The benefits of multilingualism. *Science, 330,* 332–333.

Giambo, D. A., & Szecsi, T. (2015). Promoting and maintaining bilingualism and biliteracy:

Cognitive and biliteracy benefits and strategies for monolingual teachers. *The Open Communication Journal, 9,* 56–60.

Huang, A. J., Siyambalapitiya, S., & Cornwell, P. (2019). Speech pathologists and professional interpreters managing culturally and linguistically diverse adults with communication disorders: A systematic review. *International Journal of Language & Communication Disorders, 54,* 689–704.

Hwa-Froelich, D. A., & Westby, C. E. (2003). Frameworks of education: Perspectives of Southeast Asian parents and Head Start staff. *Language, Speech, and Hearing Services in Schools, 34,* 299–319.

Lee, H., & Kim, K. H. (2011). Can speaking more languages enhance your creativity? Relationship between bilingualism and creative potential among Korean American students with multicultural link. *Personality and Individual Differences, 50,* 1186–1190.

Namazi, M. (2014). Cultural and linguistic considerations: The case of Persian. *Perspectives on Communication Disorders and Sciences in Culturally and Linguistically Diverse (CLD) Populations, 21*(3), 88–95.

Poarch, G. J., & Bialystok, E. (2015). Bilingualism as a model for multitasking. *Developmental Review, 35,* 113–124.

Santhanam, S. P., Gilbert, C. L., & Parveen, S. (2019). Speech-language pathologists' use of language interpreters with linguistically diverse clients: A nationwide survey study. *Communication Disorders Quarterly, 40*(3), 131–141.

WETA. (n.d.). *Raising bilingual kids.* Retrieved from https://www.colorincolorado.org/raising-bilingual-kids

Zarifian, T., Modarresi, Y., Tehrani, L. G., Kazemi, M. D., Salavati, M., Sadeghi, A., & Shahshahani, S. (2017). Persian articulation assessment for children aged 3–6 years: A validation study. *Iranian Journal of Pediatrics, 27*(4), e8217.

ENGLISH LANGUAGE LEARNERS

New York City Department of Education. (n.d.). *English language learners demographics report for the 2016–2017 school year.* Retrieved from https://infohub.nyced.org/reports/academics/ELL-demographic-report

GUIDELINES ON USING INTERPRETERS

American Speech-Language-Hearing Association. (2015). *Collaborating with interpreters.* Retrieved from https://www.asha.org/PRPSpecificTopic.aspx?folderid=8589935334§ion=Key_Issues

IRAN

Wahlstrom, A. (2007). *Iran.* Retrieved from Portland State University website: https://sites.google.com/pdx.edu/multicsd/international-cultures/iran?authuser=0

PUBLIC LAWS

Individuals With Disabilities Education Act of 1990, Pub. L. 101-476, renamed the Individuals With Disabilities Education Improvement Act, codified at 20 U.S.C. §§ 1400–1482.

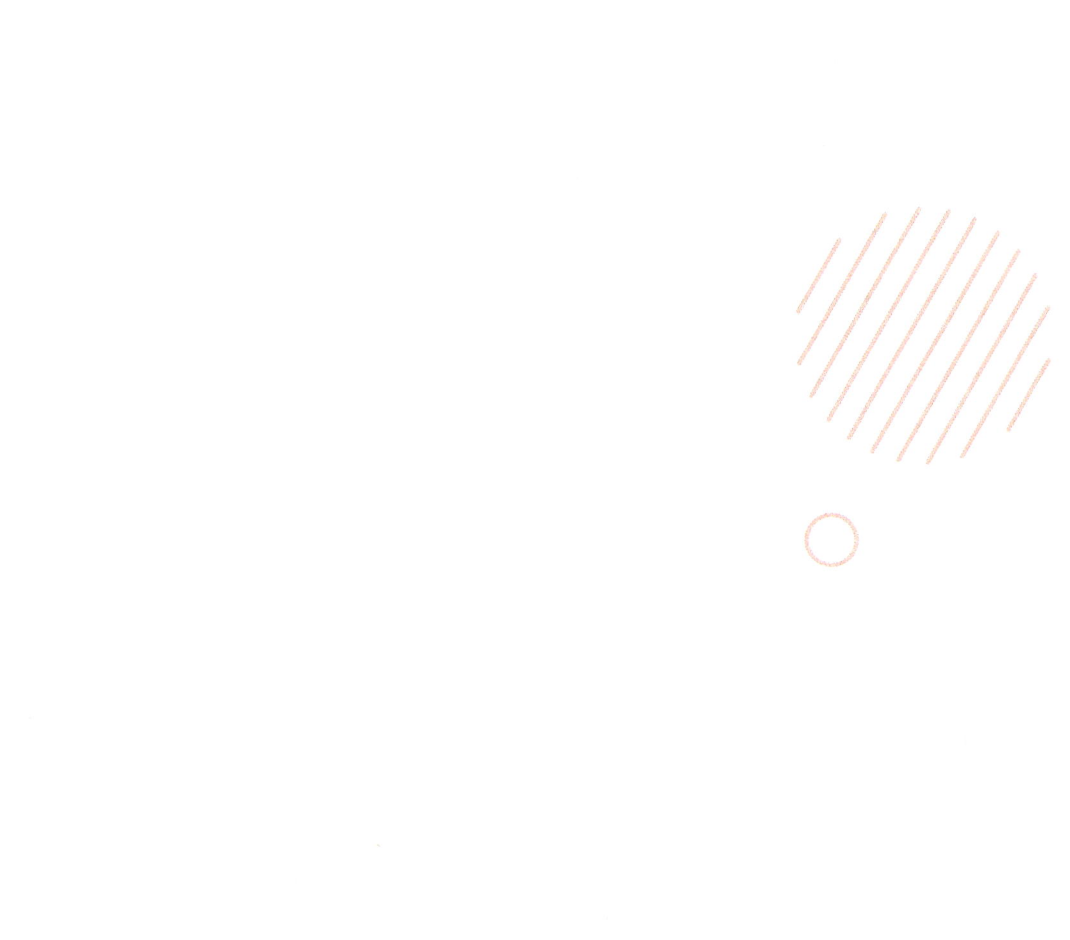

Every Child Is Unique

— Overrepresentation of Linguistically Diverse Students in Special Education

Ivan Campos, Alicia Fleming Hamilton, and Wendyliza González

notes:

PREBRIEF

It can be difficult to accurately assess non-native speakers of English. Some data suggest that children who are exposed to more than one language are often overrepresented in special education (DeMatthews, Edwards, & Nelson, 2014; Sullivan, 2011). This information illustrates the difficulty speech-language pathologists (SLPs) may experience when accurately assessing dual language learners (DLLs). This scenario presents one example of the consequences of inappropriate referrals, testing, and educational placements and illustrates strategies that address these issues.

OBJECTIVES

- Select appropriate assessment strategies to use when evaluating children who are DLLs.
- Define the responsibilities of the SLP as part of the assessment team when completing a bilingual assessment.
- Cite current resources that present evidence-based practice for evaluations in this population.

CASE SCENARIO

José is a 5-year-old bilingual (Spanish-English) preschooler in an English special education classroom with a special education label of speech-language impairment. José is exposed to Spanish at home and speaks it with his parents and siblings. His parents have no concerns about his Spanish language skills.

José was initially evaluated and qualified for early intervention services at 2 years old. The team reported that José demonstrated a delay in the area of communication on the basis of English-only assessments conducted by the early intervention team. José received home-based services for a year, in English. When José turned 3 years old, he was evaluated again by the district evaluation team to determine whether he was eligible for Part B special education services under the Individuals With Disabilities Education Improvement Act of 2004 (IDEA). Once again, all assessments were conducted in English language only. José earned English receptive language standard scores, which demonstrated low average skills when compared with monolingual English peers. His English expressive language standard scores indicated significantly low and impaired skills. Developmental scores in the areas of cognition, communication, adaptive behavior, and physical skills—obtained through parent interview with the support of a Spanish interpreter—reflected standard scores in the low 90s, the broad average range. The information from the most recent parent interview was almost identical to José's initial evaluation when his parents noted they had no concerns about his language skills. José scored in the high 70s, or moderately below average, in the area of social emotional development often tied to communication skills. Using the social emotional and expressive language scores, the team determined that José was eligible for special education services in the area of developmental delay, with a secondary diagnosis of speech and language impairment. The team wrote an individualized education plan (IEP) with goals in the area of communication.

José was placed in a special education classroom with six children who had a variety of special education diagnoses. The classroom had one licensed teacher and two paraprofessionals. Instruction was in English only. José spent a portion of his day "mainstreamed" or in the regular education preschool classroom for specific classes such as art, science, and gym. Additionally, José received weekly speech and language services to work on his goals that included using the correct present progressive tense and learning prepositions in English. José spent almost a year and a half in this classroom setting.

As José's team planned his transition to kindergarten, his SLP recommended that they reassess his skills to determine whether he still needed special education services. His general education preschool teacher, who collaborates with the special education teacher, reported that José was doing well in her classroom and did not think he needed to be in the restrictive special education only classroom. She observed José successfully communicating his wants, needs, and opinions with her and other students in the classroom. However, his special education teacher noted that José is slow to respond to her and that he makes some grammatical errors while speaking. She reported that José does not yet speak English "well enough" to be in the mainstream class full time.

José's current reassessment for special education was conducted in English and Spanish, to consider the languages used both at home and at school. José is now 5 years old. A Spanish interpreter was used to interview José's parents. José earned English receptive language standard scores in the low 90s and English expressive language standard scores in the high 70s (very low average), with the majority of his errors noted in morphosyntax. On bilingual English-Spanish measures that accept responses in either language, José's scores were in the average range. When José's narrative retell task was compared with bilingual Spanish-English speakers on a standardized measure, his scores were within the typical range (Squires et al., 2014). Additional narrative measures were attempted in Spanish; however, José only responded in English, despite prompting. After reviewing the data, the IEP team determined that José was not eligible for special education services and instead they recommended that he be placed in a general education setting with DLL support services in his classroom.

The IEP team noted that this case was the fifth student within a year who was inappropriately diagnosed receiving special education services. The lack of assessment in José's native language provided inaccurate information for his initial evaluations. The team is frustrated that bilingual-multicultural students of diverse linguistic backgrounds are being identified as qualifying for special education services, when later evaluations indicate they are typically developing.

CRITICAL THINKING AND DEBRIEFING QUESTIONS

1. **After reviewing the assessment process for José's Part B assessment (right before he turned 3 years old), what could have been done differently?**
2. **As part of an assessment team, how would you approach a colleague who was reporting scores and testing bilingual children using monolingual English tests?**
3. **What other alternative language testing measures might be included in a team toolbox when evaluating a DLL student?**
4. **Given that José responded mostly in English during his final evaluation, would it be appropriate to report standard scores? Why or why not?**

COMMENTARY

Many standardized tests that are used to determine eligibility for speech and language services in the school setting are normed on monolingual English speakers. Administering these tests to a non-native English speaker, or to a child who speaks multiple languages, may result in inaccurate information about the child's skills. In cases like José's, his initial assessments compared his skills with students who spoke English as their first language, immediately placing him at a disadvantage. His team did not include conceptual scoring to measure his abilities in both English and Spanish (e.g., Bedore, Peña, García, & Cortez, 2005) and did not use an interpreter to determine José's skills in Spanish only. Although the team had information that José's parents were not concerned about his language skills, they appeared to dismiss his parents' perceptions of his abilities. Finally, reporting standard scores when the student being assessed is not represented in the norming sample illustrates an incomplete understanding of speech-language assessment development and use, which will yield incorrect results.

Definition

Conceptual scoring—where responses are accepted in either language and credited on a single-word test—has been demonstrated to mitigate some of the documented differences in vocabulary scores between monolingual and bilingual children (Bedore, et al., 2005).

Per the IDEA, federal law requires that part of an initial assessment be conducted with an interpreter present. This can include testing that uses parts of standardized assessments with modifications, the parent interview, or other SLP-created measures. In José's case, there are standardized assessments available in Spanish that may be given with the help of a bilingual SLP or trained interpreter. If the protocol in the manual is followed, standard scores can accurately be reported. Alternative approaches could include dynamic assessment or response to intervention approaches, especially given that José has been in a classroom and evaluators as well as teachers have daily access to him there. Measuring José's progress regarding his ability to learn and retain new skills could provide additional data to help indicate whether his learning or language abilities are disordered. Alternative assessment approaches consider the multiple languages a student may be exposed to, the degree of acculturation they are experiencing, and both their strengths and needs as a learner. At a time when DLLs in Grades 6–12 are 3.5 times more likely to qualify for special education (Tankard Carnok & Silva, 2019), and children who are referred to child study teams have greater than a 50% chance of being identified as disabled, clinicians must be mindful of the overidentification of DLLs and ensure that children are receiving accurate and appropriate diagnoses (Schon, Shaftel, & Markham, 2008).

As noted in the scenario, this district team is observing a pattern of evaluation practices that are inappropriate and providing scores that may not be indicative of a student's true abilities. It would be prudent for the team to approach both evaluation teams to discuss best practices in evaluations, including using alternative evaluation measures, using a bilingual SLP, and discussing alternative staffing ideas or evaluation approaches with an administrator. The team may consider scheduling in-service activities focused on special education professionals that highlight best practices when evaluating students who speak more than one language. They may look at staffing to allocate bilingual staff in better ways and keep more robust data on English learners in special education to see whether changing evaluation practices produces more accurate assessments and diagnoses.

Team education may be especially critical in this case, given the attitudes conveyed by the special education teacher. Note that she recommended José should remain in the special education classroom because he did not yet "speak English well enough" to be in the mainstream class full time. A lack of proficiency in a second language is not a disability and does not support placement in a restrictive, special education classroom. If this belief is the foundation of the teacher's instruction, cultural competence training should be addressed, including what typical bilingual language development looks like to give the teacher a better understanding of "normal" versus disordered language use.

A lack of proficiency in a second language does not constitute a reason for a special education diagnosis or placement in a special education classroom.

The school SLP may provide information to colleagues regarding the stages of second language acquisition and what typical dual language learning may look like in a student versus disordered language learning. SLPs have a unique understanding of typical and disordered language development that is vital when working with students who are multilingual. It is especially important to convey this information to classroom teachers and service providers who are providing instruction and treatment to students in special education. Accurate assessment and diagnoses, as well as appropriate identification and intervention methods, should be the goal for district special education teams.

It is the responsibility of all speech-language professionals to ensure services are provided in a manner that yields accurate and reliable results. Clinicians, their evaluation teams, and their supervisors can work together to ensure that all activities reflect this best practice.

CRITICAL THINKING AND DEBRIEFING RESPONSES

1. **After reviewing the assessment process for José's Part B assessment (right before he turned 3 years old), what could have been done differently?**

José's home and primary language was Spanish when he was first referred for special education, but his initial assessment was done in English. Best practice is to evaluate in a child's native language. If a child has a true language disorder, deficits will present in all languages the child uses (Gutiérrez-Clellan & Simon-Cereijido, 2009). José's assessments should have been conducted in both English and Spanish because these are the languages he is exposed to. Additionally, the assessment team should have adopted a more thorough set of protocols for bilingual or multicultural assessments. This could have included the use of narrative and dynamic assessments, observations, and possible criterion-based measures (Goldstein, 2000). José's last evaluation used narrative retell tasks, standardized testing that allowed conceptual scoring (see Anaya, Peña, & Bedore, 2018), and a more robust assessment of his skills in both Spanish and English. His final evaluation also incorporated an interpreter throughout the assessment process. Although an interpreter was used for his Part B evaluation, José was still given tests in English only, and the team reported those scores. However, it is not appropriate to report scores if the student being tested is not represented in the norming sample. In José's case, he is a bilingual student, and the tests that he was given were normed on monolingual, English-only speakers. The team may have also considered using a bilingual SLP for José's initial testing.

2. **As part of an assessment team, how would you approach a colleague who was reporting scores and testing bilingual children using monolingual English tests?**

In this situation, it would be appropriate to address the colleague and probe more deeply into their evaluation practices. Perhaps the colleague was instructed incorrectly or was not aware of alternative testing options. Approaching the colleague with helpful information or examples of alternative practices could be another way of sharing information about best practices. If a colleague is not receptive to peer-to-peer feedback, it may be appropriate to involve a supervisor or principal. If a colleague continues their prior testing practices after multiple opportunities for feedback and coaching with peers and supervisors, and continues to appear unreceptive, it may be appropriate to talk to the ethics board or initiate a complaint.

3. **What other alternative language testing measures might be included in a team toolbox when evaluating a DLL student?**

Possible bilingual language testing measures (Kohnert, 2013) include the following:

- A comprehensive parent or family interview to obtain complete and detailed information about language exposure, use, and level of fluency;
- Clinical observations;
- Administration of bilingual assessment with a trained, bilingual SLP;
- Appropriate use of an interpreter or translator during testing, using recommendations in testing manuals;
- Spontaneous language samples in all languages spoken by the student;
- Portions of standardized assessments that may provide descriptive information about the student's language skills, without reporting scores;
- Narrative assessment of morphosyntactic variation in all languages spoken by the student; and
- Evaluation of learning potential such as dynamic assessment tasks involving a test, teach, and retest approach.

4. **Given that José responded mostly in English during his final evaluation, would it be appropriate to report standard scores? Why or why not?**

Reporting scores for an assessment that was normed on monolingual, English speakers is not appropriate and is not considered best practice. Although José appears to speak English fluently, his foundational exposure to language and his home language were Spanish, which keeps him separate from appropriate comparison with the norming group (American Speech-Language-Hearing Association, n.d.).

TAKE AWAYS

- Best practice in evaluations is including assessment in all languages that a client uses or is exposed to.
- Reporting a bilingual client's assessment scores from evaluations normed on monolingual, English speakers is not appropriate and is not considered best practice.
- SLPs have an obligation to advocate for the use of appropriate testing practices within their own teams, special education teams, and across their districts to ensure accurate identification of students who are multilingual.

REFERENCES

American Speech-Language-Hearing Association. (n.d.). *IDEA Part B Issue Brief: Culturally and linguistically diverse students.* Retrieved from https://www.asha.org/Advocacy/federal/idea/IDEA-Part-B-Issue-Brief-Culturally-and-Linguistically-Diverse-Students/

Anaya, J. B., Peña, E. D., & Bedore, L. M. (2018). Conceptual scoring and classification accuracy of vocabulary testing in bilingual children. *Language, Speech, and Hearing Services in Schools*, *49*(1), 85–97.

Bedore, L. M., Peña, E. D., García, M., & Cortez, C. (2005). Conceptual versus monolingual scoring. *Language, Speech, and Hearing Services in Schools, 36,* 188–200.

DeMatthews, D. E., Edwards, B., & Nelson, T. E. (2014). Identification problems: US special education eligibility for English language learners. *International Journal of Education Research, 68,* 27–34.

Goldstein, B. (2000). *Cultural and linguistic diversity resource guide for speech-language pathologists.* San Diego, CA: Singular.

Gutiérrez-Clellan, V., & Simon-Cereijido, G. (2009). Using language sampling in clinical assessments with bilingual children: Challenges and future directions. *Seminars in Speech and Language,* 30, 234–245.

Individuals With Disabilities Education Improvement Act of 2004, Pub. L. 108-446, 20 U.S.C. §§ 1400-1482.

Kohnert, K. (2013). *Language disorders in bilingual children and adults.* San Diego, CA: Plural Publishing.

Schon, J., Shaftel, J., & Markham, P. (2008). Contemporary issues in the assessment of culturally and linguistically diverse learners. *Journal of Applied School Psychology, 24,* 163–189.

Squires, K. E., Lugo-Neris, M. J., Peña, E. D., Bedore, L. M., Bohman, T. M., & Gillam, R. B. (2014). Story retelling by bilingual children with language impairments and typically developing controls. *International Journal of Language & Communication Disorders,* *49*(1), 60–74.

Sullivan, A. (2011). Disproportionality in special education identification and placement of English language learners. *Exceptional Children, 77*(3), 317–334.

Tankard Carnock, J., & Silva, E. (2019, July 30). *English learners with disabilities: Shining a light on dual-identified students.* Retrieved from https://www.newamerica.org/

education-policy/reports/english-learners-disabilities-shining-light-dual-identified-students/

ADDITIONAL RESOURCES

ARTICLES AND BOOKS

American Speech-Language-Hearing Association. (n.d.). *Bilingual service delivery.* Retrieved from https://www.asha.org/PRPSpecificTopic.aspx?folderid=8589935225§ion=Key_Issues

American Speech-Language-Hearing Association. (2008). *Roles and responsibilities of speech-language pathologists in early intervention: Technical report.* Retrieved from https://www.asha.org/policy/tr2008-00290/

Aud, S., Fox, M. A., & KewalRamani, A. (2010, July). *Status and trends in the education of racial and ethnic groups* (NCES 2010-015). Retrieved from https://nces.ed.gov/pubs2010/2010015.pdf

Fernandez, N., & Inserra, A. (2013). Disproportionate classification of ESL students in U.S. special education. *TESL-EJ, 17*(2). Retrieved from http://www.tesl-ej.org/wordpress/issues/volume17/ej66/ej66a1/

Gutiérrez-Clellen, V. F., & Peña, E. (2001). Dynamic assessment of diverse children: A tutorial. *Language, Speech, and Hearing Services in Schools, 32,* 212–224.

Harry, B., & Klingner, J. (2006). *Why are so many minority students in special education? Understanding race and disability in schools.* New York, NY: Teachers College Press.

Lazewnik, R., Creaghead, N., Combs, S., & Raisor-Becker, L. (2010). Perspectives on preparing graduate students to provide services to diverse populations in schools. *Perspectives on School-Based Issues, 11*(2), 33–39.

Osborne, A. G., Jr., & Dimattia, P. (1994). The IDEA's least restrictive environment mandate: Legal implications. *Exceptional Children, 61*(1), 6-14.

Pretti-Frontczak, K., & Bricker, D. (2000). Enhancing the quality of individualized education plan (IEP) goals and objectives. *Journal of Early Intervention, 23*(2), 92-105.

Smith, V., Summers, C., Mueller, V., Carillo, A., & Villaneda, G. (2018). Evidence-based clinical decision making for bilingual children with autism spectrum disorders: A guide for clinicians. *Perspectives of the ASHA Special Interest Groups, 3*(14), 19–27.

TIER 1 INTERVENTIONS

https://www.pbisworld.com/tier-1/

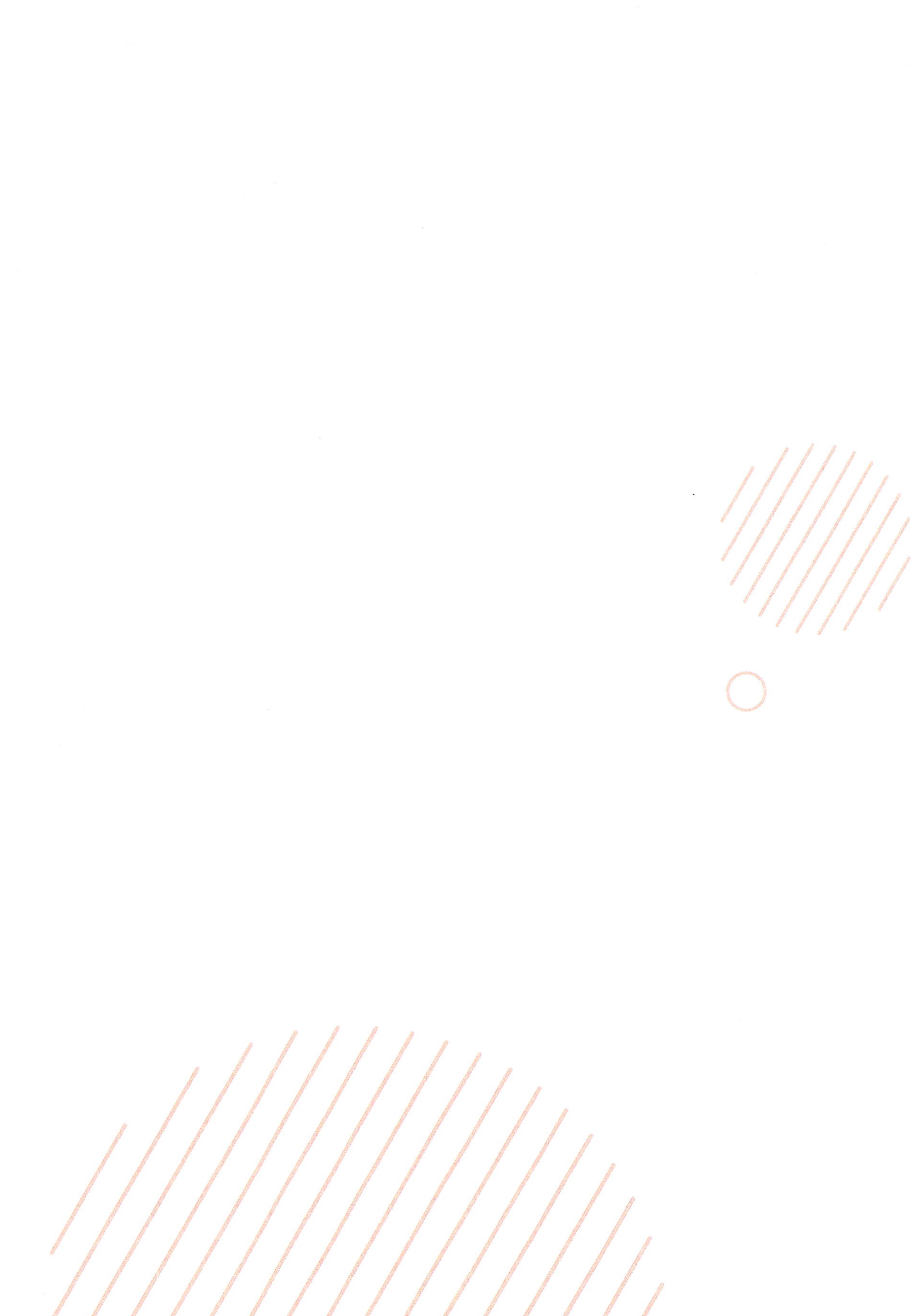

Conflicts in Culture

— When the Special Education Process Has Unintended Consequences

ALICIA FLEMING HAMILTON AND CARMEN ANA RAMOS-PIZARRO

notes:

PREBRIEF

This scenario discusses the importance of understanding how disabilities are viewed across cultures and the impact that a diagnosis may have on an individual and their entire family. In the United States, federal law dictates regulations for initial eligibility for special education services in a school setting (Individuals With Disabilities Education Improvement Act [IDEA], 2004). These laws include requirements for the qualification and treatment of speech and language disorders. Practices for identification and provision of services for disabilities vary across cultures. This scenario illustrates the importance of explaining the special education practices and systems of the United States to families.

OBJECTIVES

- List appropriate options for conducting an articulation assessment in a language in which you are unfamiliar.
- Compare the perception of "disability" across different cultures and regions—specifically, Pakistan and the United States.
- Reflect on the importance of accurately describing the U.S. special education process to families who may not be familiar with its rules and regulations.

CASE SCENARIO

Laila is a 5-year-old girl who recently completed early childhood screening through her local school district. Laila's family is of Pakistani descent, but Laila was born in the United States. Laila's family speaks Urdu and English at home. Laila passed all areas of her early childhood screening except the area of articulation/intelligibility. Laila's parents agreed with the results of her performance and reported understanding Laila less than 50% of the time when she speaks in either English or Urdu.

Laila's family met with a speech-language pathologist (SLP) named Ms. Gardner. Ms. Gardner completed an assessment to rule out a possible articulation disorder. Although the family declined the need for an interpreter during the interview, stating they could communicate in English fluently, Ms. Gardner indicated that she would need an interpreter present to assist her as she completed the Urdu portion of the articulation testing. She explained that this was a requirement of federal law when assessing children for special education services (IDEA, 2004).

The SLP used a standardized English articulation assessment, but she did not report scores. She also recorded a language sample and had Laila's parents complete an intelligibility rating scale for her in English to identify any sound productions errors. Ms. Gardner, who had never worked with clients from Pakistan, developed an informal articulation inventory of Urdu phonemes she found during her research of online resources. She used this list to create an inventory in which Laila could imitate the sounds in words with an interpreter present. During the assessment, the interpreter stated that Laila made mistakes on a variety of words. Ms. Gardner and the interpreter reviewed the sound-specific errors. Afterward, the SLP debriefed with the interpreter, who reported that Laila's speech was very difficult to understand for a child of her age and that her difficulties did not appear to be related to her Urdu accent. Assessment findings confirmed that Laila was presenting with an articulation disorder in both English and Urdu. Laila's parents were present for the entire evaluation and agreed with all findings.

The special education team met to review the evaluation results and to develop Laila's initial individualized education plan (IEP). Laila's parents and the Urdu interpreter were present during this meeting. Recommendations for intervention were provided by the team. Ms. Gardner explained that Laila now qualified for special education services, and with their input, an IEP would be developed to work on the sounds she produced in error and to learn strategies for speaking more clearly. At the mention of special education, Laila's mother began to weep. The SLP offered reassurance to the parents that services would positively impact their daughter's outcomes and gave Laila's mother some time to process the information. Ms. Gardner asked the parents to sign the documents and with their signature indicate that they understood and agreed with all recommendations provided.

At that point, Laila's parents turned to the interpreter and spoke animatedly for a few moments before indicating that they were refusing to sign the paperwork. The father expressed in English, before leaving, that although they were thankful for her time, they were no longer interested in SLP services. The SLP was confused by the parents' decision because they had participated in all other parts of the process without issue.

Ms. Gardner turned to debrief and thank the interpreter for her time and service. The interpreter explained that in Pakistani culture, girls are promised to be married from a young age. She related that although Laila's parents had lived in the United States for a number of years, they still wanted to arrange for their daughter to be married and settled before she was 15 years old. Now that Laila had been diagnosed with an articulation problem, the parents felt that their community would see Laila as having a "disability" and therefore would not be a desirable marriage candidate.

CRITICAL THINKING AND DEBRIEFING QUESTIONS

1. **What are some alternative treatment options the family could seek out that do not include "special education" services to address Laila's needs?**
2. **How would you respond to a situation in which a family was in agreement that their child was exhibiting a disorder, but they did not want to adopt the special education label to receive services?**

3. Have you ever reported results to a family or client and had to navigate strong emotional reactions? How did you help the family or client work through the results? After reflection, is there anything you would do differently in the future?
4. Are there any other tools that Ms. Gardner could have used to assess Laila?
5. If Laila's family was interested in treatment, what goals would you focus on for her articulation errors?

COMMENTARY

Understanding a client's cultural backgrounds provides practitioners with a broader understanding of how a family may receive the assessment and diagnosis of a speech or language disability. In Pakistan, like in many other cultures, there is great stigma and discrimination associated with a diagnosis of disability. A study by the Economist Intelligence Unit (2014) illustrates that marriage prospects are different for women with disabilities because they are seen as "caretakers of a household" and their disability makes it more difficult to find a partner. This perception that women with disabilities have difficulty serving as caretakes of a household may be due to a lack of educational opportunities for people with disabilities in this culture. Special education schools in Pakistan are often centered in urban areas, and the fees make them accessible to wealthy families only. Views that disability is associated with a lack of opportunity become reinforced when there is not ample educational support for those with special educational needs. The results can be that people with disabilities lack proper education, sometimes ending up in impoverished situations.

Although Laila's parents have lived in the United States for many years, their active participation in the local Pakistani community and adherence to cultural customs may indicate their preference toward upholding traditional Pakistani views and not adopting the cultural practices and views of the United States. Their experience of disability and how it impacted people in Pakistan caused great distress to them when considering their daughter's future. A disability diagnosis would have made a significant impact in the family's cultural practice of planning for her arranged marriage.

Ms. Gardner, after identifying the rationale for the parent's rejection of services, could have contacted them to provide details about the typically positive outcomes through therapeutic treatment of articulation disorders. She could have asked the interpreter whether it would be appropriate to disclose the information about arranged marriage and cultural beliefs surrounding disability. If the interpreter said yes, the SLP could have called the family and asked to meet again with a culturally sensitive social worker or community liaison in an attempt to build a bridge between the two cultures and provide Laila's parents with more information about available resources to help Laila that are more aligned with their desire to not include special education services, including private therapy options.

Ms. Gardner, in spite of not having experience with the assessment of Urdu articulation disorders, excelled in finding alternative assessments using available resources. The development of an inventory of sounds and the use of elicitation of sounds in error were appropriate ways to explore the child's sound production in Urdu. This strategy may be implemented, in conjunction with an interpreter, with any language that an SLP is evaluating in which they are not fluent.

The use of interpreters provides another opportunity to not only assist with the child's assessment but also to create a window into the family's cultural background that would not be available otherwise. The Urdu interpreter became a valuable cultural broker by providing background on the parents' perception of disability and, after brief instruction and training from the SLP, actively participating in the assessment and the judgment of the level of speech intelligibility of the child. The SLP could have gone even further by meeting with the interpreter before this meeting to have a better context before the assessment. The SLP could have also scheduled a separate meeting to debrief with the interpreter in an attempt to gain more information about how families in this culture view special education and ways that she may present the information in a more culturally sensitive way.

Although the decision related to an arranged early marriage for Laila may seem foreign to mainstream culture in the United States, professionals must remain focused on the purpose of the evaluation, which is identifying the presence or absence of a disorder and, when applicable, seeking services for a child who may be demonstrating a disability. Additional cultural beliefs surrounding the cause of a disability should be explored with the family. Perceptions of disability being caused by "evil eye," stress to the mother while pregnant, or a sense of fatalism that it is in "God's hands" may all contribute to a family's reactions to a diagnosis of an articulation or other language or learning disorder (Kilshaw, Al Raisi, & Alshaban, 2015).

CRITICAL THINKING AND DEBRIEFING RESPONSES

1. **What are some alternative treatment options the family could seek out that do not include "special education" services to address Laila's needs?**

If the family is able, they may choose to receive services through a private clinic or a local independent contractor. This would require payment and may not be covered by their school district because of funding constraints. However, if the family thought this was an option that could help them address Laila's speech issues and not experience cultural stigma through a special education label, it might be an appropriate alternative.

2. **How would you respond to a situation in which a family was in agreement that their child was exhibiting a disorder, but they did not want to adopt the special education label to receive services?**

We must remember that the family's and client's preferences are paramount. Ultimately, the decision of whether to receive therapy belongs to the parents. If they choose to decline services, that should be properly documented. A practitioner could provide information regarding attitudes of peers toward children with articulation disorders and how they are viewed negatively when compared with peers without speech sound errors (Crowe-Hall, 1991). They may also provide the parents with information on behaviors to watch for if Laila's speech production decreases and steps to take if or when this occurs. This information may be useful to the parents if they see changes in Laila because of her speech difficulties and decide to pursue treatment at a later date.

3. **Have you ever reported results to a family or client and had to navigate strong emotional reactions? How did you help the family or client work through the results? After reflection, is there anything you would do differently in the future?**

Personal response. Some ideas for this SLP would include researching Pakistani practices and perceptions regarding disability. This may have impacted the way the SLP presented the information. Another suggestion may have included laying out the special education process at the first meeting with family-friendly materials and visuals or consulting a cultural broker earlier in the process.

4. **Are there any other tools that Ms. Gardner could have used to assess Laila?**

The tools that Ms. Gardner used—including an intelligibility rating scale for parents, standardized assessments (without reporting scores), and language samples in both English and Urdu—were appropriate choices in this situation. Parent and interpreter reports added valuable information for her evaluation. Using available phonemic inventories and devising an imitative articulation assessment was another appropriate way of measuring Laila's articulation abilities in her native language. Ms. Gardner could have added a more robust parent interview in the beginning of the evaluation to address cultural beliefs and practices, including how the special education process may be received by this family and viewed through their cultural perspective.

5. **If Laila's family was interested in treatment, what goals would you focus on for her articulation errors?**

A common approach that is well supported in the research literature is to create a list of the phonemes that are in error/developmentally appropriate in both languages. In this case, there would be a list of phonemes in error in Urdu and English. The SLP would then target the shared phonemes between the two languages, with the idea that the improvements would impact the other phonemes specific to Urdu or English (Kohnert & Derr, 2004).

TAKE AWAYS

- When assessing articulation, it is vital to assess all languages a child uses or is exposed to.
- When determining a "difference versus disorder," one must consider phonemes present in a native language and understand that the influence of the native language's phonemes on the second language is not necessarily a sign of a disorder.
- Discussing cultural views and traditions as well as identifying clear expectations are essential when beginning the assessment process. Providing full, clear explanations of what will happen, including possible evaluation outcomes, may help a family understand and address information that may challenge their cultural views.
- Interpreters provide rich contributions to culturally sensitive assessments and treatment services when they work in coordination with SLPs.
- SLPs can develop novel strategies for the assessment of articulation or language abilities when working with clients who speak a language in which they are not fluent.

REFERENCES

Crowe-Hall, B. (1991). Attitudes of fourth and sixth graders toward peers with mild articulation disorders. *Language, Speech, and Hearing Services in Schools, 22,* 334-340.

Economist Intelligence Unit. (2014, August). *Moving from the margins: Mainstreaming persons with disabilities in Pakistan.* Retrieved from https://www.britishcouncil.pk/sites/default/files/moving_from_the_margins_final.pdf

Individuals With Disabilities Education Improvement Act of 2004, Pub. L. 108-446, 20

U.S.C. §§ 1400-1482.

Kilshaw, S., Al Raisi, T., & Alshaban, F. (2015). Arranging marriage; negotiating risk: Genetics and society in Qatar. *Anthropology & Medicine, 22*(2), 98-113.

Kohnert, K., & Derr, A. (2004). Language intervention with bilingual children. In B. Goldstein (Ed.), *Bilingual language development and disorders in Spanish-English speakers* (pp. 311-338). Baltimore, MD: Brookes.

ADDITIONAL RESOURCES

ARTICLES AND BOOKS

Baldizón, F., Rutherford-Blowes, D., O'Neal, M., Powers, A., & Rashiti, L. (n.d.). *Alternative methods of assessment for English language learners (ELL) pamphlet.* Retrieved from http://www.ctspeechhearing.org/media/files/alternative_methods_of_assessment_for_english_language_learners_(ell)_pamphlet.pdf

British Council. (n.d.). *Global skills spotlight–Promoting effective skills frameworks for disabled peoples' economic empowerment.* Retrieved from https://www.britishcouncil.org/education/skills-employability/opportunities-updates/promoting-skills-frameworks-disabled-peoples-economic-empowerment

Girls Not Brides. (n.d.). *Pakistan.* Retrieved from https://www.girlsnotbrides.org/child-marriage/pakistan/

Johnson, R. (2019, January 11). *How the U.S. immigration system encourages child marriages.* Retrieved from https://www.hsgac.senate.gov/imo/media/doc/Child%20Marriage%20staff%20report%201%209%202019%20EMBARGOED.pdf

McLeod, S., & Goldstein, B. (Eds.). (2012). *Multilingual aspects of speech sound disorders in children* (Vol. 6). Tonawanda, NY: Multilingual Matters.

McLeod, S., Harrison, L. J., & McCormack, J. (2012). *Intelligibility in Context Scale.* Retrieved from http://www.csu.edu.au/research/multilingual-speech/ics

Riaz, S. (2013). Shariah perspective on marriage contract and practice in contemporary Muslim societies. *International Journal of Social Science and Humanity, 3*(3), 263-267.

URDU INFORMATION SHEET FOR PARENTS

Nottinghamshire Healthcare. (n.d.). *Urdu information sheets.* Retrieved from https://www.nottinghamshirehealthcare.nhs.uk/childrens-slt-resources

Representation and Race in Foster Care — Including and Informing All Parties

Wendyliza González and Alicia Fleming Hamilton

notes:

PREBRIEF

Children are sometimes placed in foster care as a result of challenging family situations. When this happens, a legal decision is made to separate them from their biological parents. Foster parents are appointed and may also serve as advocates for these children. Research indicates that African American, Native American, and Latino children are overrepresented in the child welfare system and foster care in reported cases of child maltreatment compared with their percentages in the population at large, which can have lasting impacts on their development (U.S. Department of Health and Human Services, Administration for Children and Families, Children's Bureau, 2013).

When a child in foster care is referred for special education services, it can be difficult to know who the legal decision maker is for the child and how to proceed within the confines of the law. This case depicts a scenario in which biological parents and foster parents do not agree on the child's educational placement. It highlights the role of the speech-language pathologist (SLP) and educational team. It also touches on issues of race and placement in special education services.

OBJECTIVES

- Distinguish key behaviors associated with emotional trauma, abuse, and neglect in children.
- Appraise special management issues when completing the assessment of a child in foster care.
- Increase awareness of the disproportionate number of African American children in foster care and identify processes to support these families in the educational environment as they seek reunification.

CASE SCENARIO

Ben is a 5-year, 10-month-old, English-speaking, African American, male student currently enrolled in a general education kindergarten coteaching classroom (with both special education and general education students) in a large metropolitan area. Ben has two younger brothers (4 years old and 3 months old), and all three siblings are currently in foster care. His foster family is White. Ben's biological mother and father are staying in a homeless shelter, where they receive family education, drug counseling, and rehabilitation services with the goal of regaining custody of Ben and his younger brothers. Ben's biological parents maintain limited contact with him but have requested to stay up to date on all medical and educational concerns regarding their children. Ben's foster parents disclosed to his teacher that he has experienced significant trauma after witnessing violence while under their care. They also noted that Ben did not have any formal education before starting kindergarten because of frequent moves. Ben receives at-risk counseling with the school guidance counselor in a small group setting of two students and has a 1:1 crisis paraprofessional assigned to him to support his learning.

Definition

Paraprofessional—also known as an instructional assistant—is a certified aide in a school community who is often assigned to, and responsible for, specialized or concentrated assistance for students with special needs.

Ben was referred for a special education assessment and services in kindergarten when his teacher noted that he did not respond to questions, would not identify academic concepts, and frequently threw tantrums and had "outbursts." His teacher reported that Ben's outward behavior and emotional affect vary with the degree of his dysregulation. When he is calm, he tends to be more passive, and when he is excited or upset, he tends to exhibit tantrums and outbursts. Ben has difficulty responding to auditory stimuli; does not visually engage with people, pictures, or objects; and often speaks unintelligibly to himself during self-directed play. Ben has difficulty with transitions and often becomes limp, lies on the floor, and refuses to stand up when asked to change activities. At least once per day, Ben will scream or moan jargon words, run around the room, climb on furniture, or lay in the middle of a group of students engaged in an activity.

The school district's assessment team described their evaluation as "challenging" because of Ben's unresponsiveness to questions and testing stimuli. Behaviors described in their report were consistent with those previously identified by Ben's teacher. They concluded that Ben met the criteria for developmental delay and emotional behavioral disorder. The team felt that emotional behavioral disorder was the more appropriate diagnosis of the two, given Ben's dysregulation. To best meet Ben's needs, the team recommended that he be placed in a more restrictive learning environment, sometimes called self-contained, that consisted of 12 students with special needs individualized education programs (IEPs), one special education teacher, and two support professionals. The teacher shared that this classroom had two other African American boys, whereas the general education classroom did not. The school psychologist was not in agreement with the diagnosis of emotional behavioral disorder and felt that developmental delay was a more appropriate diagnosis for Ben, explaining that the team did not factor in Ben's traumatic childhood experiences as part of his behavior, in addition to his lack of exposure to early learning experiences. She also asked why it mattered whether there were other African American students in the classroom, when this should be a decision based on what is best for Ben.

Ben's foster parents were invited to attend the results meeting in person and supported the team's recommendation. Ben's foster mother explained that she has frequently felt overwhelmed by his behavior, and she was certain that he would benefit from "as much support as he can get." Ben's biological parents participated via conference call. When Ben's biological parents heard the results, they rejected the diagnosis and the team's placement recommendation. They believed a less restrictive classroom environment would be a better match for Ben, and they wanted him to be exposed to typically developing peer models. They shared that they didn't want him to be seen as "different" and that they would like him in a classroom that has "normal" kids.

At this point, the meeting was at an impasse because neither set of parents (biological and foster) could agree on Ben's educational needs and academic placement. Additionally, according to the laws of the state Ben lived in, his biological parents had final say, legally. Both Ben's SLP and classroom teacher thought that Ben's biological parents didn't really understand the benefit of the smaller classroom setting. The SLP, who supported the team's recommendations, suggested that Ben's case be referred to the director of special education and the district's legal counsel for further guidance on who could make the final decision.

CRITICAL THINKING AND DEBRIEFING QUESTIONS

1. **How might perceptions of race and upbringing impact educational labels and service delivery methods?**
2. **Who should ultimately make decisions related to Ben's placement?**
3. **What professionals should be involved in Ben's treatment plan? Are there any other resources that should follow him?**
4. **How can team members maintain communication with Ben's biological parents to ensure a smooth future transition?**
5. **What symptoms are Ben exhibiting that may be a result of the trauma he experienced?**

COMMENTARY

Fostering can provide needed stability for children whose parents are unable or unwilling to provide custody and care because of a variety of circumstances. The American Bar Association has noted that the rights of foster parents vary by state and, in some cases, may be limited (Barve, 2017). Although biological parents may be separated from their children because of incarceration, homelessness, emergencies, or other circumstances, they may retain their parental rights, affording them continued participation in their child's educational decision making. In this case, the team invited Ben's foster parents to his IEP meeting in an attempt to be inclusive and involved because they were currently caring for Ben, even though they may not have had legal entitlements to participate or a legal say in his final placement.

Ben's biological parents' decision regarding his placement may have been based on a variety of factors. It could have included previous experiences with special education, their personal interpretation of "disability" and how it may impact their son's educational career, or experience with the stigma of having a "label." Ben's family is African American, and they may have been offended by the mention of placing Ben in a classroom with the rationale that it contained other African American students. Ben's parents may also have had hesitations about placing Ben in a classroom that is separated from general education, adding another layer of separation from his classmates, when he is already separated from his family. Any questions or misunderstandings about placement should be discussed thoroughly so that Ben's parents and foster family fully understand what will happen when he initiates services. The SLP may have resources to present to the families, including visuals and evidence to illustrate the benefits of both placements.

With the biological parents' authorization, on the basis of the laws of their state of residence, partnerships may be created with foster parents that could benefit Ben. These partnerships might include home visiting as well as the implementation of strategies at home and at school that can help to manage Ben's outbursts and difficulty regulating himself. These interventions may be used in conjunction with Ben's placement in the general education classroom. The SLP could present visuals or other supports to help Ben communicate more clearly, in an aim to decrease his level of frustration. In this situation, the SLP and the special education team have an opportunity to model strategies that may be helpful for Ben, so that both sets of his guardians can implement them. These strategies can help to ensure that Ben and his family are interacting with strategies that enrich their home environment and reinforce skills and strategies that Ben is working on at home.

In the United States, 57% of children in foster care between 0 and 5 years old experience a language delay (Krier, Green, & Kruger, 2018).

In the United States, 57% of children in foster care between 0 and 5 years old experience a language delay (Krier, Green, & Kruger, 2018). Additionally, trauma related to neglect or abuse has been cited among environmental factors that may negatively impact a child's language development. Other data show that when children were controlled for measures of weight and height ratio, sensorimotor function, memory, and executive function, children in foster care were shorter for their age; had smaller head circumferences; and had poorer visual-spatial, language, and cognitive functioning (Pears & Fisher, 2005). Finally, when controlling for other variables (child, caregiver, household, and abuse characteristics), African American children had 44% higher odds of foster care placement when compared with White children (Knott & Donovan, 2010, p. 683).

These data could provide additional insight for the special education team and may help them when discussing placement options or having further conversations with Ben's biological and foster parents. Specifically, they may reconsider the diagnosis of emotional behavioral disorder and agree to try supporting Ben in the general education classroom. The team may provide resources for rich language strategies to use at home, either with Ben's foster family or when his is reunified with his biological parents. The team may also research interventions helpful to students who experience trauma, including being flexible; providing positive reinforcement; knowing and understanding possible behavioral triggers or aversions; creating a trusting environment for a student; choosing high-interest materials with the opportunities for many choices throughout an activity; planning predictable interventions; and fostering self-love, worthiness, and respect (White, 2019).

CRITICAL THINKING AND DEBRIEFING RESPONSES

1. **How do perceptions of race and upbringing impact educational labels and service delivery methods?**

Learning about a client's cultural background can provide a basic foundation for working with diverse clients. In this scenario, Ben is an African American child whose parents do not currently have custody of him. Ben was diagnosed with special education needs, but his biological parents appear to be resistant to putting him in a "special classroom" or with kids who aren't "normal." Additionally, the educational team tried to make the case that it would be better for Ben's placement in a self-contained classroom because other African American children were also in the class. Although the teacher may have intended her comment to imply that Ben may feel more comfortable with students who looked like him, the comment was not appropriate, and the parents, as well as the school psychologist, did not find it valid. Historical trends indicate that special education diagnoses generally assigned to European American children tend to carry fewer socially restrictive stigmas than those given to African American children (Reid & Knight, 2006). African American children who exhibit social or behavioral concerns are more likely to be designated as emotionally disturbed than their European American counterparts who receive a diagnosis of learning disabled (Gold & Richards, 2012).

Expand Your Knowledge

Historical trends indicate that special education diagnoses generally assigned to European American children tend to carry fewer socially restrictive stigmas than those given to African American children (Reid & Knight, 2006). African American children who exhibit social or behavioral concerns are more likely to be designated as emotionally disturbed than their European American counterparts who receive a diagnosis of learning disabled (Gold & Richards, 2012).

Implicit bias refers to attitudes or stereotypes that can unconsciously affect our understanding of others and our actions and decisions in daily life (Arora, 2017). Clinicians are also encouraged to reflect on the possible impact of implicit bias in their practice. It is important for all professionals to explore the ways in which their culture—including values, beliefs, and practices—can create bias and impact their interpretation of other cultures and people.

2. **Who should ultimately make decisions related to Ben's placement?**

In this scenario, on the basis of the state where Ben was located, his biological parents are the legal decision makers for his education, unless their rights have been legally terminated. Although Ben is in foster care, his biological parents continue to have legal rights to decisions regarding his education, and their ultimate goal is to be reunified with him and his biological siblings. It is important to be aware of the laws that apply to biological and foster parents in the state where you work because they may influence your approaches when working with families who have children in foster care. It is also important to reflect on your own responses to a situation, which may reveal a personal bias you have toward the decisions of either the foster or biological family.

Definition

Implicit bias refers to attitudes or stereotypes that can unconsciously affect our understanding of others and our actions and decisions in daily life (Arora, 2017).

3. **What professionals should be involved in Ben's treatment plan? Are there any other resources that should follow him?**

Those who are already involved should remain: the SLP, special education teacher, general education teacher, social worker, school psychologist, counselor, 1:1 crisis paraprofessional, foster parents, and biological parents. It would be important to also communicate with Ben's foster care case manager to ensure that information was given to the appropriate stakeholders in Ben's life and education. It would also be important to communicate with a doctor to monitor Ben's mental diagnoses and coordinate care as he grows older.

4. **How can team members maintain communication with Ben's biological parents to ensure a smooth future transition?**

Team members must be familiar with the guardianship laws for their state. Custody and decision-making capacity vary depending on the laws of your specific state. After a firm understanding of these laws and the rights of parent and guardians under the law are established, it becomes critical that the case manager maintain communication with all parties who are legally permitted to be part of the case. In this scenario, the team invited Ben's parents and foster parents to the meetings. Special education team should be sensitive to the difficulties that a family may be experiencing while separated.

5. **What symptoms are Ben exhibiting that may be a result of the trauma he experienced?**

Current research notes that children who are exposed to trauma or in foster care have a higher likelihood of presenting with speech and language disorders. Trauma exposure creates physiologic changes in children's brains that can result in cognitive, physical, emotional, and social delays (Westby, 2018). Specifically, children may be in a state of constant stress response, making it more challenging for them to pay attention, process new information, or retain information. Some of these children may have sensory processing difficulties, difficulty responding to social skills, and more negative or aggressive peer interactions. These children may also distrust adults. Trauma-informed treatment and policies can alleviate retraumatization of students and aim to help children effectively learn coping strategies for daily living.

TAKE AWAYS

- The role, responsibilities, and rights of foster parents and biological parents should be clearly established ahead of evaluation planning or other due process meetings because these vary by state.
- Research indicates that children in foster care are likely to have been exposed to trauma, and children who are exposed to trauma are at risk for developing speech and language disorders. Information about a student's living situation is critical for providing informed, effective intervention.

REFERENCES

Arora, N. (2017). Look at your blind spots: Do unconscious preconceptions shape your clinical judgment? A school-based clinician offers ways to uncover–and address–implicit bias. *The ASHA Leader, 22*(11), 6-7.

Barve, S. (2017). Special education advocacy: A guide for attorneys. *Child Law Practice Today, 36,* 147.

Gold, M. E., & Richards, H. (2012). To label or not to label: The special education question for African Americans. *Educational Foundations, 26,* 143-156.

Knott, T., & Donovan, K. (2010). Disproportionate representation of African-American children in foster care: Secondary analysis of the National Child Abuse and Neglect Data System, 2005. *Children and Youth Services Review, 32*(5), 679-684. http://dx.doi.org/10.1016/j.childyouth.2010.01.003

Krier, J. C., Green, T. D., & Kruger, A. (2018). Youths in foster care with language delays: Prevalence, causes, and interventions. *Psychology in the Schools, 55,* 523-538. https://doi.org/10.1002/pits.22129

Pears, K. C., & Fisher, P. A. (2005). Emotion understanding and theory of mind among maltreated children in foster care: Evidence of deficits. *Development and Psychopathology, 17*(1), 47-65. https://doi.org/10.1017/s0954579405050030

Reid, D. K., & Knight, M. G. (2006). Disability justifies exclusion of minority students: A critical history grounded in disability studies. *Educational Researcher, 35*(6), 18-23.

U.S. Department of Health and Human Services, Administration for Children and Families, Children's Bureau. (2013, December 17). *Child maltreatment 2012.* Retrieved from https://www.acf.hhs.gov/cb/resource/child-maltreatment-2012

Westby, C. (2018). Adverse childhood experiences: What speech-language pathologists need to know. *Word of Mouth, 30,* 1–4 . https://doi.org/10.1177/1048395018796520

White, C. (2019, July 10). Strategies for working with students who've experienced trauma. *Leader Live.* Retrieved from https://blog.asha.org/2019/07/10/strategies-for-working-with-students-whove-experienced-trauma/

ADDITIONAL RESOURCES

Amster, B. J. (1999). Speech and language development of young children in the child welfare system. In J. A. Silver, B. J. Amster, & T. Haecker (Eds.), *Young children and foster care: A guide for professionals* (pp. 117–138). Baltimore, MD: Brookes.

Arora, N. (2019). Look at your blind spots. *The ASHA Leader, 22*(11), 6–7. https://doi.org/10.1044/leader.FMP.22112017.6

Centers for Disease Control and Prevention. (n.d.). *Violence prevention: Adverse childhood experiences.* Retrieved from https://www.cdc.gov/violenceprevention/childabuseandneglect/acestudy/index.html

Henry, J., Sloane, M., & Black-Pond, C. (2007). Neurobiology and neurodevelopmental impact of childhood traumatic stress and prenatal alcohol exposure. *Language, Speech, and Hearing Services in Schools, 38,* 99–108. https://doi.org/10.1044/0161-1461(2007/010)

Hwa-Froelich, D. (2012). Childhood maltreatment and communication development. *Perspectives on School-Based Issues, 12*(2), 43–53. https://doi.org/10.1044/sbi13.2.43

Hyter, Y. D., & Way, I. (2007). Epilogue: Understanding children who have been affected by maltreatment and prenatal alcohol exposure: Future directions. *Language, Speech, and Hearing Services in Schools, 38,* 157–159. https://doi.org/10.1044/0161-1461(2007/016)

Kaufman, T. (n.d.). *Foster care, special education, and learning and thinking differences: What you need to know.* Retrieved from https://www.understood.org/en/school-learning/your-childs-rights/basics-about-childs-rights/foster-care-special-education-and-learning-and-attention-issues-what-you-need-to-know

Lum, J. A. G., Powell, M., Timms, L., & Snow, P. (2015). A meta-analysis of cross-sectional studies investigating language in maltreated children. *Journal of Speech, Language, and Hearing Research, 58,* 961–976. https://doi.org/10.1044/2015_JSLHR-L-14-0056

McInerney, M., & McKlindon, A. (n.d.). *Unlocking the door to learning: Trauma-informed classrooms and transformational schools.* Retrieved from https://www.elc-pa.org/wp-content/uploads/2015/06/Trauma-Informed-in-Schools-Classrooms-FINAL-December2014-2.pdf

Welc, J. B. (2010, November 10). *Understanding the impact of abuse and neglect on speech and language development.* Lecture presented at the American Speech-Language-Hearing Association Annual Convention, Philadelphia, PA.

Westby, C. E. (2007). Child maltreatment: A global issue. *Language, Speech, and Hearing Services in Schools, 38,* 140–148. https://doi.org/10.1044/0161-1461(2007/014)

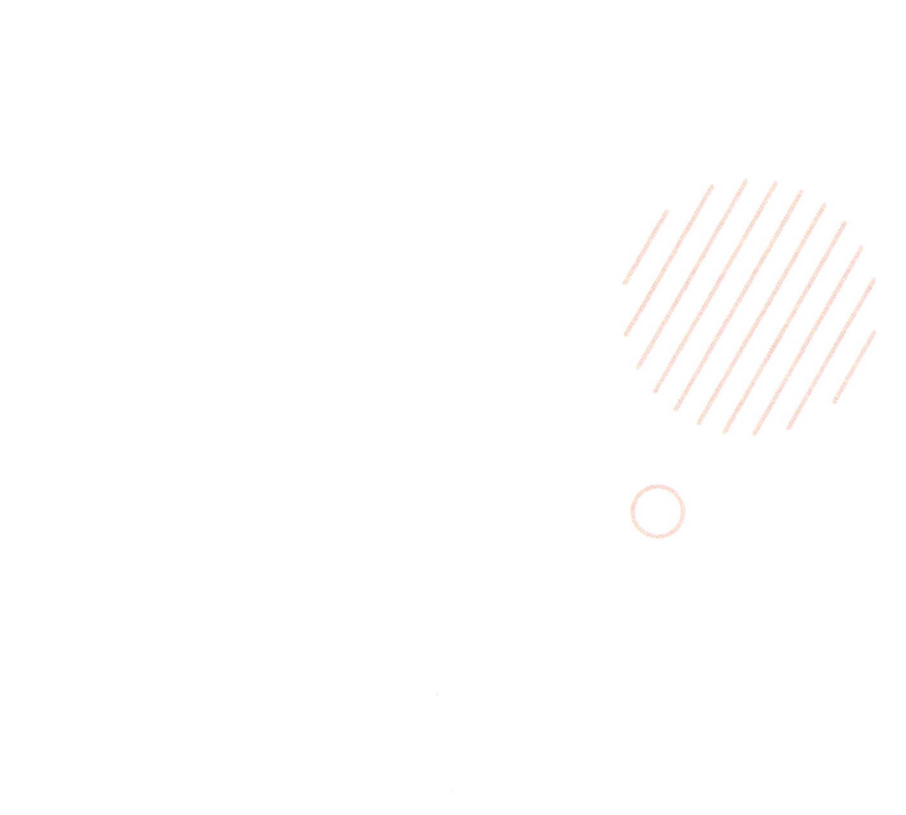

You Can't Judge a Book by Its Cover — Misconceptions About Cultural Knowledge Based on Physical Appearances

Wendyliza González and Alicia Fleming Hamilton

notes:

PREBRIEF

This scenario reviews the dynamics between a clinical educator and a student clinician. It highlights cultural differences in how power is perceived and how disagreements are approached. The scenario shows the importance of a thorough case history and family interview when working with all families, especially those who may use multiple languages. All of these factors will play a role in choosing the best assessment practices for this family.

OBJECTIVES

- Describe the importance of a home language questionnaire or ethnographic interview with clients and families when completing a clinical assessment.
- Explain when it is appropriate to report standard scores and when it is not, and provide alternative assessment procedures available to students who are not represented within the norming sample.
- Review important resources available for families and community members that reinforce the importance of bilingual language development for all children.
- Consider ways to approach cultural differences between clinicians and clinical educators.

CASE SCENARIO

Mary is a second-year speech-language pathology graduate student of Korean descent, in her fifth clinical rotation at a pediatric, center-based school. Mary is completing the bilingual emphasis track at her university, and she is under the supervision of a senior therapist, Joana. Joana is a White, monolingual English speaker and has 7 years of post-graduate experience. Mary's grandparents speak Korean, but Mary only knows a few phrases and terms in Korean; English is her native and primary language. Her family is proud of their Korean heritage and participates in Korean cultural events throughout the year.

Joana and Mary are assigned a new case. Their new client, Sue, is a 6-year-old bilingual English- and Korean-speaking female presenting with speech sound errors and a possible language disorder. Before initiating a family interview, Joana asked the family whether they required an interpreter, but the family politely declined. Joana reassured the family that Mary, her graduate student clinician, "is Korean too" and would be able to help with any interpretation, if something is confusing.

During the brief family interview focusing on the child's exposure to other languages, Mary learned that Sue has been diagnosed by a psychologist with a learning disability. No information was elicited on the student's strengths or alternative ways of communication, and the interview focused only on verbal communication. The family also shared that they speak English and Korean equally at home. Sue's father said he worries that speaking both languages to Sue has been detrimental to her speech and language development. The pediatrician and the psychologist who diagnosed Sue with a learning disability told the family that it's "harder for children with disabilities to learn two languages, which may explain why Sue is lagging behind other students her age." After sharing this information with Mary and Joana, Sue's father specifically asked whether they should stop speaking Korean to Sue. Joana advised the father that, on the basis of her experience and training, Sue's family should "stick" to one language (English) at home. At the conclusion of the interview, Mary asked her clinical educator whether they should continue asking more questions about communication, including where they communicate, who they communicate with, and what areas they would like to focus on. Joana dismissed her request saying, "The interview is just something we have to check off. The evaluation data will tell us everything we need to know."

Mary recalled from her training program that exposure to multiple languages during development is not linked to the development of a language disorder and does not make it harder for children to communicate. In fact, being bilingual is beneficial for children with disabilities because it provides them with the ability to communicate in multiple contexts and also encourages flexible thinking. Mary did not feel comfortable providing this information during the interview because she would have felt like she was disrespecting her clinical educator by contradicting her in front of the client. However, Mary was confident in her knowledge that growing up bilingual is an asset for multicultural children with disabilities because it can help the children maintain communication with their families, caregivers, and community as well as at school.

Joana completed the evaluation in English only, using evaluations normed on English speakers and criterion-referenced tests. She reported all scores in the final report. Although Mary is not a fluent speaker of Korean, her knowledge of typical and disordered language in bilingual children was at odds with her clinical educator's choice of evaluation tools that did not accurately measure Sue's total language abilities. Mary's Korean heritage has instilled in her a great respect for authority, including educators and professionals. Although she didn't agree with Joana, she felt as though asking why these assessments were chosen and disputing Joana's advice to "stick to one language" might be viewed as a challenge to Joana's authority.

CRITICAL THINKING AND DEBRIEFING QUESTIONS

1. **Have you received reports that have reported scores for children who are not represented in a norming sample? Or reports for dual language learner students that include reported scores when the test was not normed on bilinguals? How might you approach the clinician who reported the scores?**

2. What are appropriate ways of disagreeing or presenting contradictory information with a clinical educator or professor?
3. What are some resources with information regarding appropriate components of culturally competent supervision?
4. The student clinician and client have the same cultural background but different language histories. What difficulties may this present?
5. What are benefits of using an ethnographic interview in place of a traditional interview?

COMMENTARY

An essential part of a thorough speech and language assessment is obtaining information about languages and dialects that a client may be exposed to and in what contexts those languages are used. This information can be obtained by using a thorough ethnographic interview that includes questions about different settings and language exposure in those settings. Ethnographic interviews aim to get an understanding of the functional use of language for a client—including the social situations they are in and how they perceive and understand those situations. Evaluators can also complete setting observations in the home, school, or community as well as provide surveys to families and teachers on language exposure for the child. Although Mary asked during the initial assessment meeting whether the family needed an interpreter, that question should have been asked before meeting a family in person, so that if an interpreter is needed, they can be present at the initial meeting. If a family is offered interpreter services but it is clear that there is no interpreter available, the offer can feel disingenuous and the family may feel obligated to say "no."

After completing a thorough interview, the clinician could seek out culturally and linguistically appropriate assessment tools. These tools may include portions of standardized assessments (without reporting scores), criterion-referenced measures, language samples in the home language, observations in natural contexts and school settings, and parent reports (Duran, 2017). Clinicians may also consider response-to-intervention information or dynamic assessment tasks, which are types of descriptive measures of a client's abilities (American Speech-Language-Hearing Association [ASHA], n.d.). These two approaches involve measuring a skill, teaching the skill if necessary, providing intervention, and then measuring the skill again to see whether it was learned. Other assessments may include universal screening instruments available in the targeted language. The clinician can also review trusted resources to research developmental and phonological norms for particular cultures, in this case Korean speakers.

After completing a thorough interview, the clinician could seek out culturally and linguistically appropriate assessment tools. These tools may include portions of standardized assessments (without reporting scores), criterion-referenced measures, language samples in the home language, observations in natural contexts and school settings, and parent reports (Duran, 2017).

Reporting scores for an assessment that was normed on monolingual English speakers is not appropriate and is not considered a best practice (Anaya, Pena, & Bedore, 2016). Because Sue is not represented in the norming or standardization sample of the assessments given, a descriptive analysis of her performance is the most appropriate way of reporting results. Mary is within her rights to speak up and ask for clarification regarding her clinical educator's decision. If her clinical educator is not receptive to this, another option would be for Mary to speak to her academic clinical educator or program director about the discrepancy between what she is being taught in her training program and what she is observing in the community. Other assessment techniques for this student could include gathering information from her school performance, family interview, dynamic assessment, response to intervention, or criterion-referenced measures (Anaya et al. 2016).

When Mary's clinical educator was asked by Sue's parents whether she should continue learning both languages, the clinical educator provided information that was not rooted in evidence. When a clinician is unsure regarding a current practice or recommendation, the best course of action is to answer honestly and research the answer to provide to clients at a later date. In this case, the clinical educator provided information that was not based on current research, and she did not cite any research at all in her statement. Studies show that students, especially those with disabilities, can benefit from being exposed to two or more languages (e.g., Restrepo, Morgan, & Thompson, 2013). Additionally, a 2009 meta-analysis of bilingual language development indicated that bilingualism does not cause delays in language development (Kohnert & Medina, 2009). This exposure keeps them connected to their caregivers and communities, provides them with rich language input, and increases the ability to have flexible thinking skills. Additionally, principles from family-centered practices in early intervention can be useful in supporting culturally and linguistically diverse families (Peredo, 2016). Additionally, when professionals or families decide to develop only one of a child's functional languages, there are irreversible negative effects on children's development (Moore & Pérez-Méndez, 2006). Children who are still in the early developmental stages of language acquisition are susceptible to language loss (Hoff, Rumiche, Burridge, Ribot, & Welsh, 2014).

Studies show that students, especially those with disabilities, can benefit from being exposed to two or more languages (e.g., Restrepo, Morgan, & Thompson, 2013).

There were multiple instances in this case study in which Mary's clinical educator made comments that were culturally insensitive. Her comment about Mary being Korean and therefore being able to"interpret" was both culturally insensitive and incorrect. She implied that all people of a certain culture must know the language, which we discovered is not the case for Mary. This scenario illustrated Mary's cultural upbringing and cultural values of respect and deference toward authority figures. These cultural beliefs and practices should have been reviewed at the onset of the clinical practicum so that the clinical educator and student clinician can create explicit approaches to conflict resolution that are amenable for all involved. Requirements for clinical supervision include the demonstration of cultural competence as well as the ability to have difficult conversations (ASHA, 2008). Mary may want to approach her clinical educator again with the comments and suggest a debriefing to discuss how they were not appropriate given her culture and the setting. She may also seek input from a trusted professor or her clinical placement director.

CRITICAL THINKING AND DEBRIEFING RESPONSES

1. **Have you received reports that have reported scores for children who are not represented in a norming sample? Or reports for dual language learner students that include reported scores when the test was not normed on bilinguals? How could you approach the clinician who reported the scores?**

Personal response. If you have received reports that have reported scores for a population that does not fit the profile of your client, reflect on ways to reach out professionally to the examiner in an effort to understand their evaluation process and why they used those specific assessments. Building a bridge of communication might help to create a learning moment for all parties involved.

2. **What are appropriate ways of disagreeing or presenting contradictory information with a clinical educator or professor?**

Clinical educators and clinicians are guided by the *Code of Ethics* (ASHA, 2016). The ASHA *Code of Ethics* guides all practitioners to provide culturally competent services and to share accurate information. In this situation, Mary could write down the things she overhead and schedule a meeting with her clinical educator to clarify the intent. The clinical educator would have an opportunity to discuss the comments outside of the treatment area and without the client present. Giving opportunities to provide further context for specific assessment decisions in a separate setting may provide beneficial learning opportunities for both Mary and her clinical educator. It also gives Mary's clinical educator the opportunity to explain her rationale, if she was misunderstood.

3. **What are some resources with information regarding appropriate components of culturally competent supervision?**

ASHA's practice portal has information on clinical education and supervision as well as information on providing culturally competent services. Another suggestion would be to create a clinical contract for supervision that is agreed on by both the clinician and clinical educator before the practicum begins. If these contracts do not mention approaches to conflict mediation and the use of culturally competent practices, it may be valuable to contact the clinic director in a graduate program to discuss the addition of these important items or suggest their addition before the onset of the practicum during the initial clinical educator-student clinician meeting.

The ASHA Code of Ethics *guides all practitioners to provide culturally competent services and to share accurate information.*

4. **The student clinician and client have the same cultural background but different language histories. What difficulties may this present?**

Remember that each individual is a unique person within their cultural background. In this case, Mary was Korean and had limited knowledge of the language, but she described herself as a monolingual, English speaker. Although Mary may have understood many aspects of Korean culture that put Sue's family at ease, she noted that she was in no way able to interpret or assess Sue's Korean, because Korean was not a functional language for her. This serves as a reminder that assumptions about individuals because of how they appear or because of their cultural background can prove to be inaccurate.

5. **What are benefits of using an ethnographic interview in place of a traditional interview?**

There are many benefits to using an ethnographic interview with all clients. Ethnographic interviews are considered a culturally responsive and family-centered way to learn about a client within a flexible framework. They can be used with clients and families across disorders and ages (Westby, 1990, 2009). Ethnographic interviews use open-ended questions and exact rephrasing of client's answers to come to a better understanding of exactly how the communication issues impact the client's life. They also give clients more ownership in the treatment experience by using their exact words and goals to shape treatment.

TAKE AWAYS

- It is critical to know the languages and dialects that the patient has been exposed to so that culturally and linguistically appropriate assessment materials and tools can be provided.
- Research suggests that using two languages with children with language impairment is beneficial for communication at home (Kay-Raining Bird et al., 2005).
- Consider adopting ethnographic interview as part of your assessment process. This type of interviewing can provide incredible insight into a family's communication needs and how to focus treatment.
- Both clinicians and clinical educators are guided by ASHA's (2016) *Code of Ethics* to maintain current knowledge regarding the most appropriate evaluation and treatment practices and to continue to improve cultural competence across one's practice.
- Children in early intervention are capable of learning two languages, and intervention should address both of their linguistic systems (Kohnert & Derr, 2012).

REFERENCES

American Speech-Language-Hearing Association. (n.d.). *Response to intervention (RTI).* Retrieved from https://www.asha.org/SLP/schools/prof-consult/RtoI/

American Speech-Language-Hearing Association. (2008). *Clinical supervision in speech-language pathology.* Retrieved from https://www.asha.org/content.aspx?id=10737450495

American Speech-Language-Hearing Association. (2016). *Code of Ethics.* Retrieved from https://www.asha.org/Code-of-Ethics/

Anaya, J. B., Pena, E. D., & Bedore, L. M. (2016). Where Spanish and English Come Together: a two dimensional bilingual approach to clinical decision making. *Perspectives, 1*(14), 3–16. https://doi.org/10.1044/persp1.SIG14.3

Duran, L. (2017, October). *Emerging solutions to serving dual language learners in multitiered systems of support.* Paper presented at the 33rd Annual International Conference of the Division for Early Childhood, Portland, OR.

Hoff, E., Rumiche, R., Burridge, A., Ribot, K. M., & Welsh, S. N. (2014). Expressive vocabulary development in children from bilingual and monolingual homes: A longitudinal study from two to four years. *Early Childhood Research Quarterly,* 29, 433–444. https://doi.org/10.1016/j.ecresq.2014.04.012

Kay-Raining Bird, E., Cleave, P., Trudeau, N., Thordardottir, E., Sutton, A., & Thorpe, A. (2005). The language abilities of bilingual children with Down syndrome. *American Journal of Speech-Language Pathology, 14,* 187–199.

Kohnert, K., & Derr, A. (2012). Language intervention with bilingual children. In B. Goldstein (Ed.), *Bilingual language development and disorders in Spanish-English speakers* (pp. 311–338). Baltimore, MD: Brookes.

Kohnert, K., & Medina, A. (2009). Bilingual children and communication disorders: A 30-year research retrospective. *Seminars in Speech and Language, 30*(4), 219–233. https://doi.org/10.1055/s-0029-1241721

Moore, S., & Pérez-Méndez, C. (2006). Working with linguistically diverse families in early intervention: Misconceptions and missed opportunities. *Seminars in Speech and Language, 27,* 187–198. https://doi.org/10.1055/s-2006-948229

Peredo, T. N. (2016). Supporting culturally and linguistically diverse families in early intervention. *Perspectives of the ASHA Special Interest Groups, 1*(1), 154–167.

Restrepo, M. A., Morgan, G. P., & Thompson, M. S. (2013). The efficacy of a vocabulary intervention for dual-language learners with language impairment. *Journal of Speech, Language, and Hearing Research, 56,* 748–765.

Westby, C. E. (1990). Ethnographic interviewing: Asking the right questions to the right people in the right ways. *Journal of Childhood Communication Disorders,* 13, 101–111. https://doi.org/10.1177/152574019001300111

Westby, C. (2009). Considerations in working successfully with culturally/linguistically diverse families in assessment and intervention of communication disorders. *Seminars in Speech and Language,* 30, 279–289. https://doi.org/10.1055/s-0029-1241725

ADDITIONAL RESOURCES

American Speech-Language-Hearing Association. (n.d.-a). *Clinical education and supervision.* Retrieved from https://www.asha.org/practice-portal/professional-issues/clinical-education-and-supervision/

American Speech-Language-Hearing Association. (n.d.-b). *Response to intervention (RTI).* Retrieved from https://www.asha.org/SLP/schools/prof-consult/RtoI/

American Speech-Language-Hearing Association. (2008). *Clinical supervision in speech-language pathology.* Retrieved from https://www.asha.org/content.aspx?id=10737450495

American Speech-Language-Hearing Association. (2017a). *Issues in ethics: Cultural and linguistic competence.* Retrieved from https://www.asha.org/Practice/ethics/Cultural-and-Linguistic-Competence/

American Speech-Language-Hearing Association. (2017b). *Issues in ethics: Responsibilities of individuals who mentor clinical fellows in speech-language pathology.* Retrieved from https://www.asha.org/Practice/ethics/Responsibilities-of-Individuals-Who-Mentor-Clinical-Fellows-in-Speech-Language-Pathology/

Anaya, J. B., Pena, E. D., & Bedore, L. M. (2016). Where Spanish and English Come Together: a two dimensional bilingual approach to clinical decision making. *Perspectives, 1*(14), 3–16. https://doi.org/10.1044/persp1.SIG14.3

Cicak, M. (2011). Ethical rules in supervision. *Ljetopis Socijalnog Rada, 18*(2), 185–216.

Genesee, F. (2016). *At-risk learners and bilingualism: Is it a good idea?* Retrieved from https://www.colorincolorado.org/article/risk-learners-and-bilingualism-it-good-idea

Gutieérrez-Clellen, V. F., & Penña, E. (2001). Dynamic assessment of diverse children. *Language, Speech, and Hearing Services in Schools, 32,* 212–224.

King, D. (2003, May 27). Supervision of student clinicians: Modeling ethical practice for future professionals. *The ASHA Leader, 8,* 26.

Kohnert, K., Yim, D., Nett, K., Kan, P. F., & Duran, L. (2005). Intervention with linguistically diverse preschool children. *Language, Speech, and Hearing Services in Schools, 36,* 251-263.

Sherratt, S. (2018, June). *Person-centred care and whistleblowing: Can you have one without the other?* https://doi.org/10.13140/RG.2.2.20930.48325

Thordardottir, E. (2010). Towards evidence-based practice in language intervention for bilingual children. *Journal of Communication Disorders, 43,* 523-537.

Westby, C., Burda, A., & Mehta, Z. (2003). Asking the right questions in the right ways: Strategies for ethnographic interviewing. *The ASHA Leader, 8*(8), 4.

Articulation and African American English (AAE) — Dialect or Discrimination?

Alicia Fleming Hamilton and Jean Franco Rivera Pérez

PREBRIEF

African American English (AAE) is a language variation or dialect of Mainstream American English (MAE) that researchers have characterized as being spoken by some, but not all, African Americans as well as by other individuals within the United States. Not all African Americans speak AAE; some may speak AAE using only some of its features or vary its use among different social contexts, using a practice called code switching (Brice, 1997; Latimer-Hearn, 2019). AAE has its own set of rules for grammar, morphology, syntax, phonology, semantics, pragmatics, and paralinguistics (Hamilton, 2020). Speech-language pathologists (SLPs) should be able to identify features of this language variation when evaluating clients and be prepared to share information with others regarding the distinction between a linguistic variation and a disorder with regard to the use of AAE. Clinicians are encouraged to create positive, noncomparative descriptions when distinguishing between AAE and MAE, being aware of possible stigma related to AAE or not using MAE. This case highlights a situation in which the clinician's therapy recommendations may conflict with the parents' educational expectations for their child and provides possible suggestions on how to approach similar situations.

notes:

OBJECTIVES

- List AAE morphosyntactic and articulatory features.
- Select culturally appropriate evaluation strategies for the assessment of children who use AAE.
- Understand social beliefs and practices surrounding the use of AAE, MAE, and code switching.

CASE SCENARIO

Hannah is a White SLP who has just started working at a charter school, where she has a high population of African American students on her caseload. One student, Sam, is due for a reevaluation. Sam is 8 years old and currently has an individualized educational program (IEP) for an articulation disorder. As Hannah reviews his IEP, she notices that many of the sounds Sam is working on in therapy follow a pattern consistent with features of AAE. Hannah knows that AAE can be spoken by people who are in non-African American communities, and because Sam is African American, she is hesitant to make an assumption that Sam also speaks this dialect. Before analyzing Sam's language samples, Hannah researches the key grammatical and articulation features of AAE and calls Sam's parents to complete a parent interview. Hannah notices that Sam's speech is very much like the speech of his parents, and while speaking to them on the phone, she observes that they use the following phonologic characteristics of AAE: /r/ dropping in middle and final word position, as in /star/ [stah]. Sam's parents used /d/ for /ð/, such as /dɪs/ for / ðɪs/ and /f/ for /θ/ like in /bof/ for /boθ/. Hannah noticed the following morphosyntactical patterns, including use of the preterite "had" (e.g., "She had held the baby for the whole movie"), use of the indefinite article "a" (e.g., "I ate a egg for breakfast"), and the "zero plural" (e.g., "Dad got four new tire"). After completing the parent interview and receiving signed permission to evaluate, Hannah completes standardized testing and a language sample. Hannah reviewed the data and noticed that each pattern of response that differed from MAE that Sam produced was consistent with the features of AAE, and additionally, many of Sam's productions were consistent with patterns she noted in his parents' speech.

Hannah held a meeting to discuss Sam's evaluation results with the school principal and Sam's parents. She presented the data along with printed references outlining the characteristics of AAE. Her conclusions were that Sam should be dismissed from special education services because his speech patterns were not indicative of a disorder. While reporting, she shared that it was "great news" that Sam no longer qualified for special education services. She noted that because Sam's evaluation results indicate speech consistent with the rules of AAE he did not exhibit "disordered speech." Sam's principal, an African American man, was facilitating the meeting and paused when Hannah stated that AAE is a common language variation in the United States. The principal stated that African Americans do not speak "different" English when compared with White Americans and to state otherwise was a racist comment. Sam's parents appeared uncomfortable with the conversation and requested that the SLP just work on the sounds that were identified as "errors" in what she called "Mainstream American English." Sam's parents shared that they wanted their son to be successful in school and held to the same standards as all of the other students, where MAE is taught and spoken. Before Hannah could explain the role of special education and the idea of "difference versus disorder," the principal expressed his support of the parents' request and directed Hannah to change the IEP to indicate that the AAE features were "errors" and to address them as such in his educational goals. The principal reassured Sam's parents that he would still receive needed speech-language services for the coming year.

CRITICAL THINKING AND DEBRIEFING QUESTIONS

1. **What are some ways to respond to a situation in which your supervisor is insisting you modify your assessment results and educational goals?**
2. **Select one or two standardized tests you regularly use and determine whether they include AAE speakers in their sampling. After reviewing this case scenario and the results, how might you modify your assessment protocol?**
3. **What other evaluation strategies and tests could have been used to analyze Sam's speech and language skills?**

4. How might race be affecting this case study? What cultural considerations should be taken into account?

COMMENTARY

A survey of school SLPs conducted from 2015 to 2016 indicated that 76% of SLPs received minimal training to differentiate between dialect and disorder in children who speak AAE (Latimer-Hearn, 2019). The observable features of AAE may be misdiagnosed when SLPs do not have adequate training in identifying language variants of English.

In this scenario, the SLP was aware of the rules within the linguistic system of AAE. She researched them before her evaluation and noted the linguistic patterns during the parent interview and evaluation to confirm that Sam and his family spoke AAE. She gathered this information to ensure that she was analyzing his speech appropriately. One technique she used was performing a contrastive analysis of Sam's language samples. In doing so, Hannah compared patterns that occurred exclusively in AAE (contrastives) with patterns that were common to both AAE and MAE. Hannah then noted where true articulation errors occurred (noncontrastives), or productions that were not consistent with AAE or MAE. The SLP also administered culturally appropriate standardized tests normed on a population that included African American children who spoke AAE. When working with children who speak AAE and MAE, it is important to use several alternative assessment procedures to provide a rich profile of their languages. This may include modifications to available tests, contrastive analyses, or using diagnostic materials specifically designed for this population (Bland-Stewart, 2005).

Definition

AAE–a linguistic system with its own set of rules for grammar, morphology, syntax, phonology, semantics, pragmatics, and paralinguistics

Bias exists surrounding the use of AAE not only among non-African American individuals but also among African Americans. Like Sam's parents and the school principal, some individuals may value code switching and consider MAE the preferred language to use in school. Other opinions may see an emphasis to use MAE in school as a push for students to "assimilate" and discard the linguistic identity that exists within AAE. Historically, AAE speakers have been judged to have lower levels of education because of the misunderstanding that AAE patterns are errored speech, when in fact AAE patterns are indicative of a separate, sophisticated language variation. Both the principal and the parents expressed that the consistent use of AAE could function as a potential barrier to success and that it should be addressed through speech-language therapy. Although the principal's and parents' view that the consistent use of AAE could be a barrier for Sam, his use of AAE did not indicate the presence of an articulation disorder. Furthermore, research demonstrates that misidentification of students who speak a language variation and who are placed into special education can result in lost class time and placement in lower educational tracks (Latimer-Hearn, 2019).

Hannah faced a dilemma: Should she follow the directive from the school's principal to provide SLP services to the student? Or should she follow her training and her state's educational system best practices that guide her to document that Sam is using a linguistic variation and not exhibiting a disorder. Some states have published clear guidelines on who qualifies for services, and these guidelines provide clear direction on how to proceed. The American Speech-Language-Hearing Association's (ASHA's) practice portal also provides valuable guidance on how to proceed and support decision making (ASHA, n.d.).

In Hannah's case, it would be beneficial to have a candid conversation with Sam's parents about AAE and MAE. Hannah may share the linguistic value in maintaining both AAE and MAE and share specific strategies regarding code switching and its cognitive and cultural value. She could provide parents with the option of identifying private practitioners in their community, using ASHA's Pro Find, who would target their goals for addressing Sam's use of AAE. She may also consider further conversations with the principal to discuss AAE as a linguistic variation.

CRITICAL THINKING AND DEBRIEFING RESPONSES

1. **What are some ways to respond to a situation in which your supervisor is insisting you modify your assessment results and educational goals?**

There are many aspects that may influence the clinical decision-making process. Collaborators (e.g., parents) and other support personnel (e.g., teachers, para professionals, supervisors) are important agents during the assessment and intervention process, and they provide valuable information regarding a child's language use and practice at home and in the classroom. SLPs have the clinical expertise and training that lead to appropriate identification of a student's disability in the school setting. SLPs promote the educational growth of students in the school setting and advocate for appropriate services required by law (e.g., Individuals With Disabilities Education Improvement Act of 2004). Determining eligibility or the recommendation of services should be based on the individual needs of the students, along with state and federal requirements. Although it is important to note and discuss the personal beliefs of collaborators and guardians, these beliefs are not an indication for eligibility.

ASHA's (2016) *Code of Ethics*, Principle of Ethics I, Rule C, states that "individuals shall not discriminate in the delivery of professional services . . . on the basis of race . . . language, or dialect." Principle of Ethics 4, Rule B, also notes that "Individuals shall exercise independent professional judgment in recommending and providing professional services when an administrative mandate . . . prevents keeping the welfare of persons served paramount."

SLPs are clinical leaders who provide culturally competent services. In this case, the SLP can provide education for the parents, principal, and teachers to promote increased knowledge about the linguistic variations present in English. This information and other supports may include information about the specific rules and characteristics of AAE and ways to teach or support code switching in the classroom. Provision of written information that substantiates the clinical decision may also contribute to better understanding in the school community.

2. **Select one or two standardized tests you regularly use and determine whether they include AAE speakers in their sampling. After reviewing this case scenario and the results, how might you modify your assessment protocol?**

Personal responses will vary. Not all articulation differences are related to a speech or language disorder. Some differences are the result of linguistic variation within a language. When norm-referenced or standardized tests are used without contextual information (e.g., understanding community language influences, home language practices, and observations in the community), it can lead to incorrect identification of students who are exhibiting linguistic variation. It is important to review assessment manuals to understand the linguistic variations included in the norming sample and its diversity. When linguistic variations are not considered, when the normative data are not current, or when there is a lack of diversity in the normative sample, data from an assessment may lead to a misdiagnosis. Instruments for assessment that do not include AAE, or modifications for students who speak AAE, should be considered carefully because these instruments may not be representative of a student's speech and language abilities (Battle, 2012, p. 20).

3. **What other evaluation strategies and tests could have been used to analyze Sam's speech and language skills?**

There are many alternative methods to provide an accurate diagnosis in students who speak AAE (McLeod, Verdon, & The International Expert Panel on Multilingual Children's Speech, 2017). Culturally competent clinicians should consider the characteristics and features of a dialectical group to determine the use of a dialect versus a disorder (see Pollock et al., 1998). Contrastive analysis of speech between AAE and MAE is a strategy that helps to identify between features of AAE and an articulation/phonological error. Other alternatives include the use of language samples, dynamic assessment, observations in different environments, conversation with a variety of people, ethnographic interviews, and local norms measures. It is important to collect language samples across a variety of settings because clients may use code switching within different groups and situations.

4. **How might race be affecting this case study? What cultural considerations should be taken into account?**

The development of self-awareness and cultural humility are both characteristics of culturally responsive clinicians. A culturally competent clinician develops the ability to simultaneously appreciate cultural patterns and individual variations; engages in self-scrutiny to assess bias and improve self-awareness; uses evidence-based practice to include client characteristics, clinician expertise, and empirical evidence in clinical decisions; and understands the communication contexts and needs of clients by considering the social contexts in which they communicate (Kohnert, 2008, p. 39–41).

In this scenario, Hannah identified that race may have been a significant factor for Sam and his family. She understood the importance of appropriately researching AAE and its characteristics when preparing for Sam's evaluation. Another step Hannah may have taken would involve the concept of cultural humility. In this scenario, cultural humility may have looked like Hannah asking the family or principal more about their desires for Sam's language use in school. Consideration of the African American perspective and historical context and acknowledgment of injustices experienced across generations (Frattali & Kayser, 1997) can help provide context to family decisions and provide valuable learning opportunities for clinicians.

A culturally competent clinician develops the ability to simultaneously appreciate cultural patterns and individual variations; engages in self-scrutiny to assess bias and improve self-awareness; uses evidence-based practice to include client characteristics, clinician expertise, and empirical evidence in clinical decisions; and understands the communication contexts and needs of clients by considering the social contexts in which they communicate (Kohnert, 2008, p. 39–41).

TAKE AWAYS

- When evaluating students for speech and language disorders it is important to consider the influence of language variation. Observations, parent interview, and regional data can help inform characteristics of language variation.
- Not all African Americans speak AAE, and some people who speak AAE are not African American.

- Features of AAE are not considered errors and are not consistent with a diagnosis of speech and language disorder. Clients or their families who seek to address these linguistic variations may be directed toward resources that demonstrate the cultural value of retaining AAE and introduce the practice of code switching to address the need to use different linguistic variations across different situations.

REFERENCES

American Speech-Language-Hearing Association. (n.d.). *Speech sound disorders–Articulation and phonology.* Retrieved from https://www.asha.org/Practice-Portal/Clinical-Topics/Articulation-and-Phonology/

American Speech-Language-Hearing Association. (2016). *Code of Ethics.* Retrieved from https://www.asha.org/Code-of-Ethics/

Battle, D. E. (2012). The cultures of African American and other Blacks around the world. In *Communication disorders in multicultural and international populations* (pp. 20–36). Maryland Heights, MO: Mosby.

Bland-Stewart, L. M. (2005). Difference or deficit in speakers of African American English? What every clinician should know . . . and do. *The ASHA Leader, 10*(6), 6–31.

Brice, A. (1997). Code switching: A primer for speech-language pathologists. *Perspectives on Communication Disorders and Sciences in Culturally and Linguistically Diverse (CLD) Populations, 3*(1), 8–10.

Frattali, C., & Kayser, H. (1997). Outcomes measurement and management: Culturally diverse views of impairment, disability, and handicap. *Perspectives on Administration and Supervision, 7*(2), 5–8.

Hamilton, M.-B. (2020). An informed lens on African American English. *The ASHA Leader, 25*(1), 46–53.

Individuals With Disabilities Education Improvement Act of 2004, Pub. L. 108-446, 20 U.S.C. §§ 1400–1482.

Kohnert, K. (2008). *Language disorders in bilingual children and adults.* San Diego, CA: Plural Press.

Latimer-Hearn, D. L. (2019). *Training and perspectives of speech-language pathologists serving African American English-speaking students* (Doctoral dissertation). Available from ProQuest Dissertations and Theses database.

McLeod, S., Verdon, S., & The International Expert Panel on Multilingual Children's Speech. (2017). Tutorial: Speech assessment for multilingual children who do not speak the same language(s) as the speech-language pathologist. *American Journal of Speech-Language Pathology, 26,* 691–708.

Pollock, K. E., Bailey, G., Berni, M. C., Fletcher, J. M., Hinton, L. N., Johnson, I., & Weaver, R. (1998). *Phonological features of African American Vernacular English (AAVE).* Retrieved from http://www.rehabmed.ualberta.ca/spa/phonology/features.htm

ADDITIONAL RESOURCES

American Speech-Language-Hearing Association. (n.d.). *Multicultural affairs and resources.* Retrieved from https://www.asha.org/practice/multicultural/

Charity, A. H. (2008). African American English: An overview. *Perspectives on Communication Disorders and Sciences in Culturally and Linguistically Diverse (CLD) Populations, 15*(2), 33-42.

Connor, C. M. (2008). Language and literacy connections for children who are African American. *Perspectives on Communication Disorders and Sciences in Culturally and Linguistically Diverse (CLD) Populations, 15*(2), 43-53.

Hamilton, M. B. (2020). An informed lens on African American English: By reconceptualizing our approach to African American English, we can avoid misidentification of speech-language disorders, steer students to services that truly benefit them, and sustain cultural-linguistic identity. *The ASHA Leader, 25*(1), 46-53

Language and Life Project. (2015). *Talking Black in America* [DVD]. Available at https://languageandlife.org/documentaries/talking-black-in-america/

Latimer-Hearn, D. (2020). Don't get it twisted—Hear my voice. *The ASHA Leader, 25*(1), 54-59.

Multicultural Constituency Groups (MCCGs) https://www.asha.org/practice/multicultural/opportunities/constituency/

National Black Association for Speech-Language and Hearing (NBASLH) website: http://www.nbaslh.org

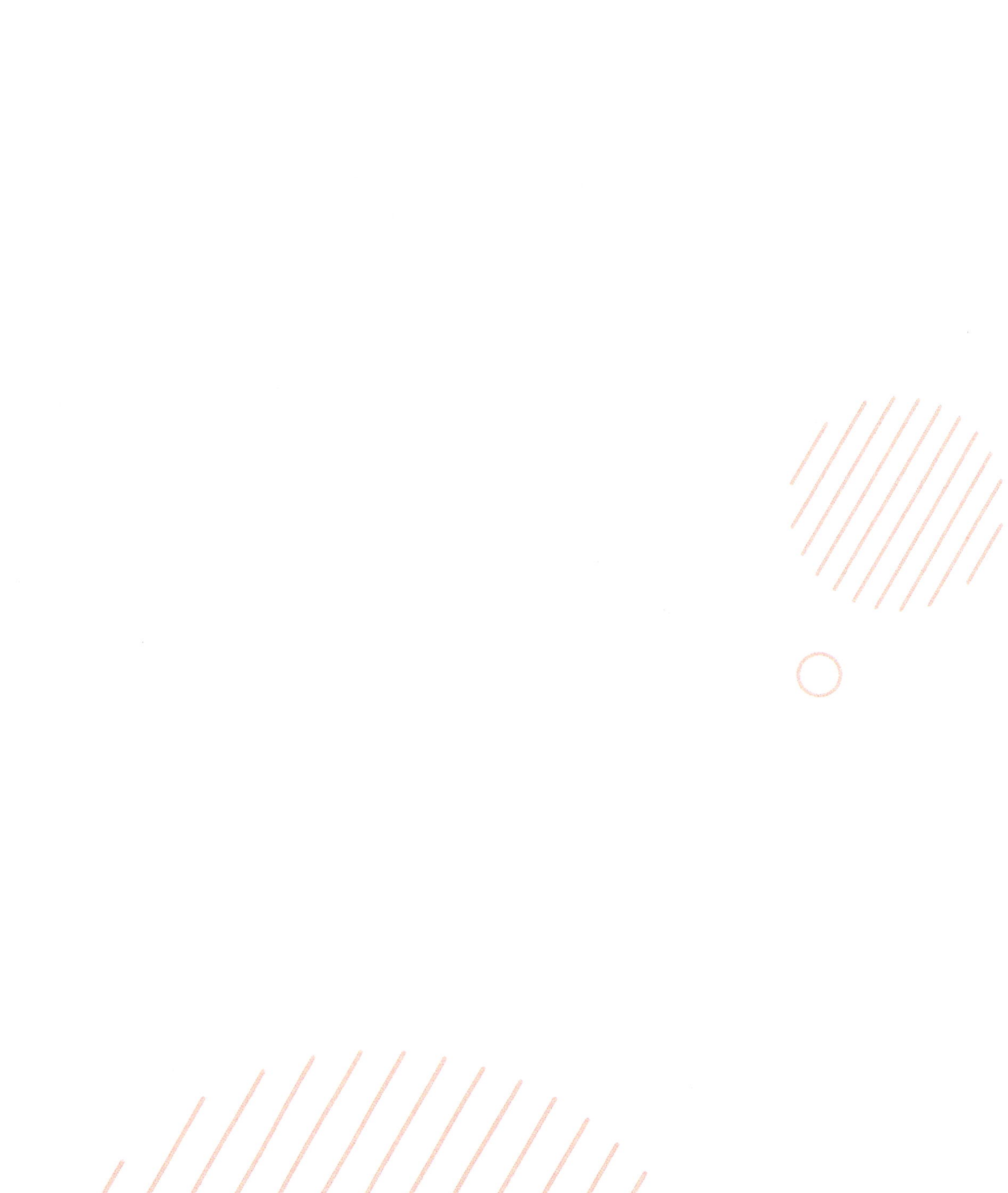

It Takes a Community

— Uniting Clinical and Cultural Practices to Capitalize on Intervention Outcomes

Alicia Fleming Hamilton

PREBRIEF

notes:

This scenario highlights cultural beliefs surrounding disability, with a focus on the Hmong culture. It discusses cultural traditions regarding healing and illustrates the difficulty that some families may encounter participating in the special education system. Finally, it provides alternative options for presenting information, especially when a family comes from a preliterate cultural tradition.

OBJECTIVES

- List alternatives to written communication that can be used with families who may prefer oral communication.
- Describe religious beliefs and rituals of the Hmong people and ways in which the professional can demonstrate sensitive and respectful acknowledgment of those practices.

CASE SCENARIO

Chao Yang is an 8-year-old Hmong girl who is currently in a second-grade classroom where English is the language of instruction. Chao's family speaks Hmong at home, and Chao is exposed to English in the community and at school. Chao is the youngest in her family and has four older brothers and sisters. Although Chao was born in the United States, her other siblings were born in refugee camps outside of the United States. Chao's parents completed some high school, and they have very basic literacy skills in English. They are preliterate in Hmong.

Chao first experienced school in kindergarten and was described as "very quiet." She appeared calm and liked to observe the busy classroom. Chao is a dual language learner (DLL) and started to receive DLL services in kindergarten. Her DLL teachers describe her as quiet, shy, and polite. Chao finished her kindergarten year knowing only the letters in her name and was able to count to 10 consistently, and to 30 with help. Although Chao was promoted to first grade, her kindergarten teacher shared concerns about her ability to access grade-level curriculum and recommended she receive additional supports. Chao completed first grade and remained behind her peers, even with extra DLL support.

When Chao started second grade, she was referred for a special education evaluation. Her teachers cited her continued difficulty reading sight words and identifying letters and numbers. Chao's DLL teacher also noted that she had difficulty answering questions, telling stories, and accurately producing the following sounds: /l, r, sh, th, ch, p, z, s, w/.

The special education assessment team–including Chao's current and previous grade teachers, DLL teacher, the special education teacher, and the speech-language pathologist (SLP)–scheduled a meeting with Chao's parents. A Hmong interpreter was present. The parents were provided with several documents in English detailing the evaluation process, including handouts and online resources they could access if they wanted additional information. The interpreter briefly provided an oral interpretation of these documents, and Chao's parents nodded in agreement. They stated they were in agreement with proceeding with an evaluation because of their concerns about Chao's development and their desire to give her as much help as possible.

The special education teacher noted that the process would take 30 school days to complete and that they could start as soon as the next day, if the family agreed and signed the documents. The interpreter explained this to Chao's family, and her parents paused. An energetic conversation between the interpreter and Chao's family ensued. The interpreter shared that Chao's parents were requesting that their Shaman perform a "soul-calling" ritual first, before any further evaluation was done. He explained that one of Chao's souls must be isolated or separated from her body, and they must perform the ritual so that her soul can be restored and she can heal (Fadiman, 2012). The family also requested that Chao's educational team be present for the communion meal after the soul-calling ritual and animal sacrifice and extended an invitation to each member.

CRITICAL THINKING AND DEBRIEFING QUESTIONS

1. **How could knowledge of the family's religious and cultural beliefs influence the SLP's and team's approach to communicating about the student's possible diagnosis and intervention?**
2. **What other alternatives to supplement written communications and documents would you suggest for this family?**
3. **Have you ever been invited to attend a client's celebration or ritual? Have you ever been offered food or been asked to participate in a cultural ritual? How might that experience have influenced/influence your knowledge of the client's culture and your subsequent approach to service delivery?**

COMMENTARY

When working with all families, it's important to identify their cultural values and preferences (Betancourt, Green, Carrillo, & Ananeh-Firempong, 2003). This information can help inform service delivery and provide context when making decisions as a group. It also helps to inform best practices when moving forward into treatment with families. In this particular scenario, knowledge of several aspects of the Hmong culture are required to fully understand the impact on processes and practices when providing care.

The Hmong espouse a strong oral tradition, which they use to tell stories and convey teachings. This family, given the parents' limited formal English education, may have preferred more time to discuss the concerns about their daughter and how to proceed. An anecdote or verbal example of the process may have been an appropriate approach to mirror their cultural practices. Although paperwork is a legal requirement, there are other possibilities for explaining the evaluation process (Barclay & Bowers, 2017). For example, a team might create visuals and brainstorm alternative means of communication with interpreters or liaisons to ensure that they are explaining the evaluation and special education process in a concise, informative, and less-intimidating way.

Expand Your Knowledge

The Hmong are people of Asian descent who form a distinct ethnic-cultural group originally from the mountainous regions of Laos. Many have migrated to the United States as refugees after the Vietnam War. Currently, Hmong families are settled primarily in California, Minnesota, Wisconsin, and North Carolina (Duffy, 2004).

Chao's classroom teacher identified several sounds that Chao had difficulty producing in English; however, a diagnosis of an articulation disorder would need to be made by a bilingual SLP, paired with an interpreter, reviewing Chao's production of English phonemes and a thorough review of the Hmong phonemic inventory. Difficulties with sound productions may be the result of language and phonemic differences between English and Hmong (Kan & Kohnert, 2005). There are many resources online and through the American Speech-Language-Hearing Association (ASHA) that can help clinicians distinguish between a speech sound difference and disorder (e.g., ASHA, n.d.).

Religious beliefs form an integral part of the cultural heritage that many families share (Cohen, Wu, & Miller, 2016). In this case, the parents felt that to heal their daughter, they needed to have healing ritual with their religious leader or shaman (Txiv Neeb). Their awareness of her difficulties, coupled with their cultural beliefs, led them to decide that a soul-calling ritual was the way to ensure positive outcomes from the school interventions. They felt that without this ritual, their child would not show progress or improvement. Acknowledging the central role of the team in their daughter's future service delivery, the family felt it was important for her educational team to be present for the ritual. However, the invitation placed the team members in a sensitive position. Some team members may have felt that if they accepted the invitation, they were sending a message that if the ritual is successful, Chao will show improvements, even if the staff does not believe this is the case. However, if the staff decline, they fear offending and alienating the family. Although the decision is ultimately a personal one, care must be taken to acknowledge the honor of the invitation. If a team member or members decide to attend, a prompt, timely arrival would be critical because otherwise the ritual would be considered interrupted by the shaman and participants.

Hmong families uphold strong values and traditions that enrich their culture and families. They also recognize the value of Western medicine and, in this case, educational interventions. The educational team and SLP must ensure that the roles and contributions of each team member are thoroughly explained regarding Chao's care and, when possible, attempt to collaborate with her family to incorporate cultural rituals into her care and educational plan.

CRITICAL THINKING AND DEBRIEFING RESPONSES

1. **How could knowledge of the family's religious and cultural beliefs influence the SLP's and team's approach to communicating about the student's possible diagnosis and intervention?**

Prior knowledge or research of the family's religious beliefs could provide the SLP and educational team with a broader context and understanding for the family's wishes. For example, understanding what a soul-calling ritual involves, why it is done, and how it is performed could give the team enough background to ask the family questions—if they felt that was appropriate—and to inquire how that ceremony or other practices may fit into the highly regulated special education process. By asking the family about their beliefs and traditions, the team invites the family into the process so that it becomes more collaborative.

2. **What other alternatives to supplement written communications and documents would you suggest for this family?**

The team could consider making visual flow charts, simplifying written material, or consulting with Hmong cultural liaisons or other families in special education to see whether they can suggest ways to adjust documents to make them more family and culturally friendly. The team could seek out multimedia online to provide the family with other opportunities to review the information.

3. **Have you ever been invited to attend a client's celebration or ritual? Have you ever been offered food or been asked to participate in a cultural ritual? How might that experience have influenced/influence your knowledge of the client's culture and your subsequent approach to service delivery?**

Personal response. If you have attended a cultural ritual or ceremony with a client or family, reflect on your feelings during the ritual and any preparation you may have completed before going. If you have never been to a client's cultural ritual or ceremony, reflect on how you would react to the invitation—Are there things you would do to prepare? How would you handle a situation in which you may not understand what is happening or may feel uncomfortable?

TAKE AWAYS

- It is important to consider each family's cultural practices when working with all clients. Attempts should be made to support and collaborate with families as well as with interpreters and cultural liaisons, whenever possible.
- When working with any family, team members should consider the literacy skills of the family as well as other cultural traditions regarding communication—including register and tone as well as developing or identifying tools that can better clarify the evaluation process for the families using visuals, text, and other easily accessible materials.
- When met with a cultural practice or tradition that is unfamiliar to you, use reputable resources to obtain more information. When possible, consult cultural liaisons and, if appropriate, the family.

REFERENCES

American Speech-Language-Hearing Association. (n.d.). *Phonemic inventories and cultural and linguistic information across languages.* Retrieved from https://www.asha.org/practice/multicultural/Phono/

Barclay, P. A., & Bowers, C. A. (2017, September). Design for the illiterate: A scoping review of tools for improving the health literacy of electronic health resources. *Proceed-*

ings of the Human Factors and Ergonomics Society Annual Meeting, 61(1), 545-549.

Betancourt, J. R., Green, A. R., Carrillo, J. E., & Ananeh-Firempong, O., II. (2003). Defining cultural competence: A practical framework for addressing racial/ethnic disparities in health and health care. *Public Health Reports, 118,* 293-302.

Cohen, A. B., Wu, M. S., & Miller, J. (2016). Religion and culture: Individualism and collectivism in the East and West. *Journal of Cross-Cultural Psychology, 47,* 1236-1249.

Duffy, J. (2004). *The Hmong: An introduction to their history and culture.* Washington, DC: Center for Applied Linguistics, Cultural Orientation Resource Center.

Fadiman, A. (2012). *The spirit catches you and you fall down: A Hmong child, her American doctors, and the collision of two cultures.* New York, NY: Farrar, Straus, and Giroux.

Kan, P. F., & Kohnert, K. (2005). Preschoolers learning Hmong and English. *Journal of Speech, Language, and Hearing Research, 48,* 372-383.

ADDITIONAL RESOURCES

American Speech-Language-Hearing Association. (n.d.). *Phonemic inventories and cultural and linguistic information across languages.* Retrieved from https://www.asha.org/practice/multicultural/Phono/

Bilinguistics. (n.d.). *Hmong speech and language development–Difference or disorder?* Retrieved from https://bilinguistics.com/hmong-speech-language-development/

Giger, J. N. (2017). *Transcultural nursing–E-book: Assessment and intervention.* Amsterdam, the Netherlands: Elsevier Health Sciences.

Hmongs and Native Americans. (2013, October 3). *Hmong traditions–Rituals & ceremonies: Soul calling* [Blog post]. Retrieved from http://www.hmongsandnativeamericans.com/hmong-traditions-rituals-ceremonies-soul-calling/

Kohnert, K. (2008). Second language acquisition: Success factors in sequential bilingualism. *The ASHA Leader, 13*(2), 10-13.

Vang, C. T. (2016). *Hmong refugees in the new world: Culture, community and opportunity.* Jefferson, NC: McFarland.

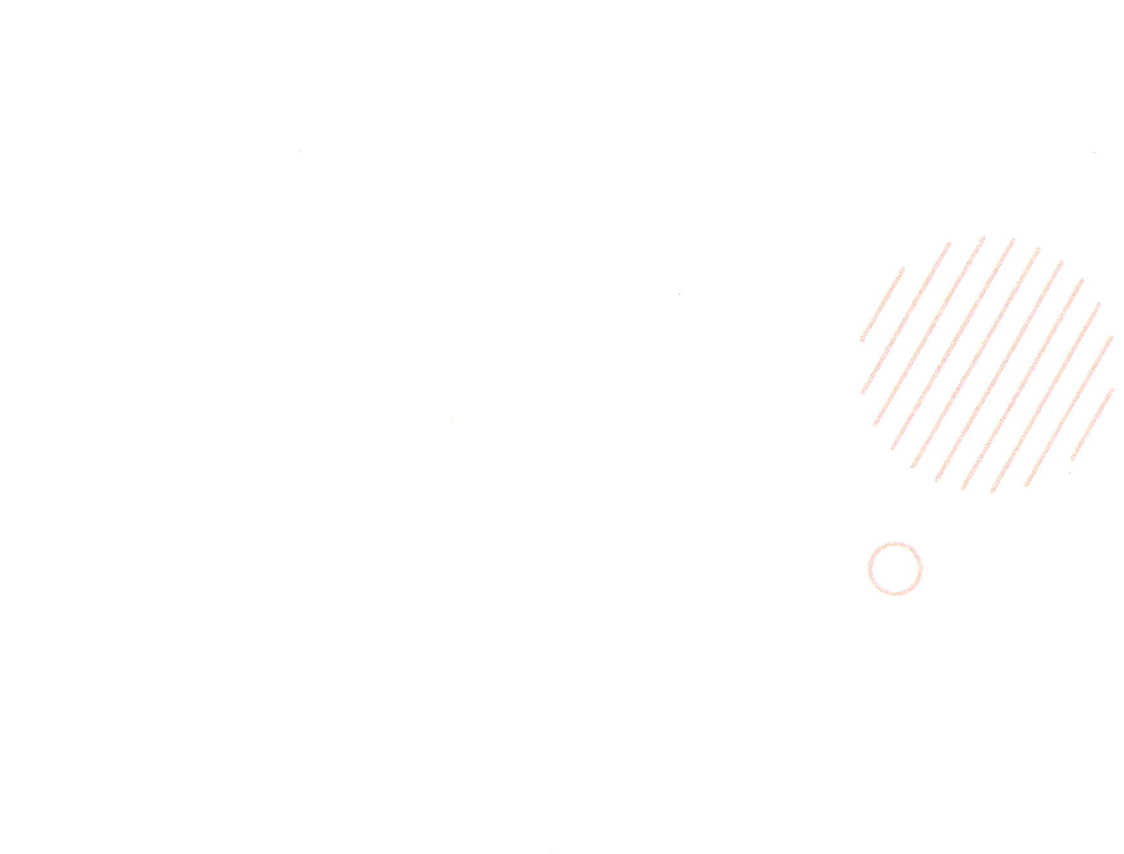

Lost in Translation

— Interpreting Special Education for Culturally Diverse Families

Wendyliza González and Alicia Fleming Hamilton

PREBRIEF

The language profile of students in schools is quickly changing to reflect the growing diversity of languages in our communities. More and more students speak a language other than English at home. Research suggests that speaking multiple languages has numerous benefits. Bilingualism has been linked to more flexible thinking, increased perspective-taking skills, and marketable business skills (Barac & Bialystok, 2011). Unfortunately, knowledge about the benefits of bilingualism is not universal, and often, school personnel and families have little understanding of how to support bilingual students. This is further complicated when working with bilingual children who present with communication and learning disorders. For those students with possible hearing, speech, and cognitive needs, it can be difficult to find skilled speech-language pathologists (SLPs), audiologists, or translators who are fluent in a student's native language or familiar with best practices when working with bilingual children. Moreover, families who speak a language other than English may perceive their child's needs differently from the educators who work in schools, resulting in miscommunications and differences in educational priorities. As you read this case, consider your own knowledge of bilingual language development and review federal requirements regarding the use of interpreters and appropriate assessment practices. Consider ways to explain the complex laws regarding special education to families in an accurate, accessible, and professional way that reflects health literacy.

OBJECTIVES

- Pinpoint key cultural elements needed to conduct a thorough and thoughtful parent interview while using an interpreter.
- Identify resources that can prepare a clinician to understand and address the family's specific cultural perception and concerns regarding special education services.
- Examine appropriate ways to advocate for students and families.

notes:

CASE SCENARIO

Adin is a 7-year-old male Muslim student, who is bilingual in English and Soninke, and is enrolled in a kindergarten integrated coteaching classroom, where students with and without individualized education plans are taught together. There are two teachers, one who has a focus in general education and one who has a focus in special education.

Adin was born in the United States and lives at home with his biological parents and three siblings, who all attend the same school. His parents are practicing Muslims from Senegal, and the family speaks Soninke at home. Adin has not been heard speaking Soninke at school in the classroom or with his siblings. His mother, who speaks conversational English, is the primary caregiver and the main contact with the school. His father works 12- to 16-hour days. On several occasions, the school has offered a translator via phone to communicate with Adin's mother, but she has refused saying that "English is fine."

Definition

Soninke—a language spoken mainly in the northeastern part of Africa by about 2.1 million people

Adin currently receives dual language learner (DLL) support in his classroom and has no special education supports. Adin received response to intervention (RTI; American Speech-Language-Hearing Association [ASHA], n.d.-b) speech services for 6 weeks after his classroom teacher raised concerns about his speaking fluency. These services included research-based interventions to teach Adin the specific concepts he lacked. Although the SLP who provided services was bilingually certified, she did not speak Soninke, and she provided services in English.

Before starting RTI speech services, Adin presented with a moderate-severe stutter in connected English speech, coupled with secondary characteristics that included eye rolling, facial grimacing, oral groping, and whole-body tension. Language screening showed that Adin was unable to label or identify any letters of the English alphabet. He struggled with categorizing items, answering questions, and sequencing tasks, and he had a limited vocabulary in English. He used fragmented sentence structures when describing pictures. On the basis of the SLP's recommendation, his parents agreed to RTI services to focus on fluency enhancing strategies and expressive language tasks.

After the 6 weeks of RTI services, which included strategies such as easy onset and "stretchy speech" and instruction in basic concepts, Adin started to use fluency strategies with maximal verbal and visual scaffolding. He showed improvements with basic concepts, such as big and little, and he labeled and categorized food. Despite these gains, his DLL and classroom teachers reported minimal progress related to his academic goals.

The bilingual SLP would like to recommend Adin for a speech-language evaluation for fluency and language, and Adin's teachers would like him considered for a comprehensive special education evaluation, but several issues have delayed this process. First, Adin's school administration does not "believe" in placing DLL students in special education, citing "overrepresentation of minority groups" in special education. The administration is afraid of overidentifying DLL students for special education but does not mention the underrepresentation of certain minority groups in the area of gifted education (Medina, 2017; Shifrer, Muller, & Callahan, 2011). Second, Adin's family continues to refuse translation services for meetings and evaluations. Because of a possible language barrier, the SLP is unsure that the family fully understands what will happen during the evaluation and the special education enrollment process if it is needed. This is because they continue to say "yes" to all suggestions and don't ask any questions.

CRITICAL THINKING AND DEBRIEFING QUESTIONS

1. What are some benefits to researching cultural aspects of the Soninke-speaking community?
2. What are possible approaches to overcoming the language barrier with Adin's family? How could you ensure access and consistency with an appropriate and culturally sensitive translator for Adin's family?
3. What are some possible difficulties when communicating with one parent, rather than both parents?
4. How might you work in alignment with the assessment team's approach to DLL students? How can the SLP best advocate for this student and his family?
5. What resources may be available to conduct a bilingual (English-Soninke) speech-language evaluation?

COMMENTARY

Across the United States, students whose primary home language is a language other than English are sometimes not introduced to English until they start school. In some cases, classroom teachers are aware of the benefits of bilingualism, including the common phases children go through as they are immersed in a totally new language and strategies that are useful in helping students achieve success in becoming bilingual. Other times, education professionals report feeling overwhelmed or ill-equipped to work with DLL students (Kritikos, 2003).

When working with families and students whose primary language is a language other than English, it is a clinician's professional and ethical duty to function as an advocate, educator, and ally (ASHA, 2016).

When working with families and students whose primary language is a language other than English, it is a clinician's professional and ethical duty to function as an advocate, educator, and ally (ASHA, 2016). One way to culturally advocate is by using strategies to facilitate open dialogue from the family's perspectives (Andrews & Andrews, 2000). Other ideas include providing information about typical bilingual development and disordered bilingual development.

There are several unknowns with this particular scenario. Without an appropriate translator, the SLP is unable to learn this family's perspective as they navigate educating their child. It is important to have some insight into how this Soninke-speaking, Muslim family views education and disability. Does the family consider their child in need of special education? Are disabilities acknowledged and discussed in their community? Do their religious beliefs influence the long-term goals they have for their child? Families may not be aware of the perceptions of disability in the United States or of the resources available through the school system. This family may also feel "pressured" to use the dominant language (English) when communicating with the school because they want to appear fully assimilated, or they do not want to feel indebted to the school by accepting extra assistance. Although an interpreter may be needed, the family may not feel comfortable accepting the help.

Creating a safe and welcoming space to present and discuss these issues helps to provide reassurance for the family as well as mutual understanding of cultural and educational expectations for all involved. Cultural information specific to the family provides context for the educational team as they move forward in developing a relationship with the family.

As language communities in the United States become more diverse, the clinical spectrum of care becomes more complex and dynamic. Young students and their families, with little exposure to English, are sometimes met with an educational system that, because of certain processes and procedures, may appear to not fully embrace bilingual or multicultural families. Ideally, families should trust that a school community understands the benefits of bilingualism and has the resources to provide adequate and evidenced-based instruction. When these families feel heard and included, the family and school community can work together to do what is best for the child.

CRITICAL THINKING AND DEBRIEFING RESPONSES

1. **What are some benefits to researching cultural aspects of the Soninke-speaking community?**

Researching cultural facts related to the regions where a language is spoken, the shared customs for greetings, and possible information on the incidence of literacy of those who speak the language may help to facilitate a rapport with the family and student, inform your questions for a parent interview, and create an atmosphere of comfort for all parties involved. It may also safeguard a clinician from making a cultural blunder and provide them with more confidence when working with a culture other than their own. Although customs and traditions may not be applicable to every person within a certain culture, because each individual is unique, information about cultural values can serve as a guide for planning assessment and intervention.

Gender roles in this community may stem from religious beliefs—for example, in Muslim families, women are often considered caretakers, whereas men are seen as the providers and decision makers (Battle, 2012). Women are respected but are expected to maintain their gender roles and responsibilities, even when they take on jobs outside of the home. This information may have been useful when trying to engage Adin's father in his educational decisions.

Disabilities in the Muslim culture are commonly accepted as fate (Hasnain, Shaikh, & Shanawani, 2008). Disabilities can bring to mind primarily physical ailments, for which there may be few accommodations, especially in the form of government support. Having a less visible disability—for example, language disorder—may be even less familiar to the general population; as a result, those with speech and language disorders may be seen as less intelligent. Because social supports are not as commonly available in their native countries, individuals and their families may believe there is no help available, even when a disorder is present, making the process of special education unfamiliar and bewildering.

2. **What are possible approaches to overcoming the language barrier with Adin's family? How can you ensure access and consistency with an appropriate and culturally sensitive translator for Adin's family?**

Federal law requires that part of an initial evaluation for special education be completed in a client's native language (Individuals With Disabilities Education Improvement Act [IDEA], 2004). Parents have a right, by law, to this information. The SLP and school staff should plan ahead and seek out a trained interpreter that can be committed to working with the team and family. The SLP and educational team should plan to brief the interpreter on their goals for the meeting and may want to ask for feedback on what is and is not culturally appropriate, given the interpreters background. In addition, general etiquette on how an interpreter is used should be reviewed with the family so that all parties have mutual expectations. For example, the interpreter will be used solely for language interpretation and not as a cultural mediator.

The team may also consider working with a cultural liaison or respected member of the community. This could include consultation with a religious leader regarding cultural views of disability and ways to appropriately inform the family of their rights. When working with a member of the community, the SLP should take measures to ensure that the family's anonymity and privacy are protected. Adin's mother declined an interpreter multiple times. In a situation like this, the SLP or team could invite an interpreter for their (the team's) own benefit and explain to the family that the interpreter is present as a team support or because of the requirements of the law, so as not to embarrass the family. This may be a nonthreatening alternative for all involved. This case requires significant preplanning and conferencing with the team and interpreter so that all parties (the interpreter, team, cultural liaison) are aware of the goals of the meetings and the different factors at play. When all are on the same page, it may be easier to understand the ways in which culture may affect the family's perspective on the meeting.

Federal law requires that part of an initial evaluation for special education be completed in a client's native language (Individuals With Disabilities Education Improvement Act [IDEA], 2004).

3. **What are some possible difficulties of communicating with only one parent, rather than both parents?**

The cultural implications of gender and family roles can have unforeseen consequences when communicating with only one parent. Whereas the mother may be more available and seen as the caretaker, the father may be viewed at the decision maker. The mother may be amenable to accepting the recommendations but unable to make a final decision because of the family structure and traditions. In this situation, it would be important to explain the special education evaluation timelines and how long the process can take in an attempt to convey a sense of urgency in communicating with the father to avoid unnecessary delays in evaluation and provide assistance quickly, if needed. Additionally, in all special education evaluations, both parents should be informed and included in the decision-making process, unless they are in agreement that one parent is making the decisions.

4. **How might you work in alignment with the assessment team's approach to DLL students? How can the SLP best advocate for this student and his family?**

Clinicians should safeguard against inaccurate identification of DLL students in special education; research indicates that DLL students are frequently underidentified (e.g., Artiles, Harry, Reschly, & Chinn, 2002). Striking a balance takes an increased commitment to preparation and research. The first step of identifying whether a student has a language difference or disorder is first learning about who the student is (Crowley, Washington, & El-Sawaf, 2015). Understanding how a student learns can be achieved through multitiered systems of support, which include RTI. This approach, coupled with appropriate use of a trained translator of the student's native language, will help safeguard against unwarranted categorization and referral of special education services. See below for more resources on conducting a dynamic bilingual assessment.

5. **What resources may be available to conduct a bilingual (English-Soninke) speech-language evaluation?**

Dynamic assessment is a tool that can be used in identifying the skills that a child has and their potential to learn new skills. The procedure focuses on the learning process and is interactive and process oriented (ASHA, n.d.-a). This, along with information from RTI services or other multi-tiered systems of support, will be critical in determining whether this student is exhibiting a delay (Hasson, Camilleri, Jones, Smith, & Dodd, 2013).

Other information from the cultural liaison, an in-depth parent report, and developmental expectations for bilingual children can all be used in making a clinical decision. Clinicians should consider the "tool for evidence-based practice," which includes research evidence; clinical expertise; and patient values, preferences, and characteristics (Sackett, Rosenberg, Gray, Haynes, & Richardson, 1996).

Definition

The response to intervention (RTI) process is a type of multitiered system of support (MTSS) for providing services and interventions to struggling learners at increasing levels of intensity. It includes

- Universal screening,
- High-quality instruction,
- Interventions matched to student need,
- Frequent progress monitoring, and
- The use of child response data to make educational decisions.

RTI should be used for making decisions about general, compensatory, and special education, creating a well-integrated and seamless system of instruction and intervention guided by child outcome data. An RTI process cannot be used to delay or deny an evaluation for eligibility under IDEA (ASHA, n.d.-b).

TAKE AWAYS

- Bilingualism benefits students (Bialystok & Viswanathan, 2009) and their families. As language experts, SLPs should continue to inform and encourage schools and families to speak their native languages at home and in their communities. They can encourage this by hosting trainings, creating and supplying handouts on bilingualism, and demonstrating an enthusiasm for the benefits of bilingualism with families and staff.
- Bilingualism does not cause language or learning disabilities and should not be seen as a deficit. In fact, bilingualism enhances a child's ability to use flexible thinking and to hold multiple perspectives. Later in life bilingualism can be a great asset in the workforce.
- There is no evidence that bilingual exposure causes additional language delays in children with existing speech and language disorders (Hambly & Fombonne, 2012).
- Federal law requires interpreters to be part of the initial evaluation process to protect families and practitioners (IDEA, 2004).

REFERENCES

American Speech-Language-Hearing Association. (n.d.-a). *Dynamic assessment: Basic framework*. Retrieved from https://www.asha.org/practice/multicultural/issues/framework/

American Speech-Language-Hearing Association. (n.d.-b). *Response to intervention (RTI)*. Retrieved from https://www.asha.org/SLP/schools/prof-consult/RtoI/

American Speech-Language-Hearing Association. (2016). *Code of Ethics*. Retrieved from https://www.asha.org/Code-of-Ethics/

Andrews, J., & Andrews, M. (2000). *Family-based treatment in communicative disorders: A systemic approach* (2nd ed.). DeKalb, IL: Janelle Publications.

Artiles, A. J., Harry, B., Reschly, D. J., & Chinn, P. C. (2002). Over-identification of students of color in special education: A critical overview. *Multicultural Perspectives, 4*(1), 3-10.

Barac, R., & Bialystok, E. (2011). Cognitive development of bilingual children. *Language Teaching, 44*(1), 36-54.

Battle, D. E. (2012). *Communication disorders in multicultural and international populations.* Maryland Heights, MO: Mosby.

Bialystok, E., & Viswanathan, M. (2009). Components of executive control with advantages for bilingual children in two cultures. *Cognition, 112,* 494-500.

Crowley, C. J., Washington, T., & El-Sawaf, D. (2015). *Innovative approaches to address disproportionate referrals to SPED in the nation's largest school district* [American Speech-Language-Hearing Association presentation]. Retrieved from https://www.leadersproject.org/2015/11/16/asha-2015-presentation-addressing-disproportionate-referral-of-diverse-students/

Hambly, C., & Fombonne, E. (2012). The impact of bilingual environments on language development in children with autism spectrum disorders. *Journal of Autism and Developmental Disorders, 42,* 1342-1352.

Hasnain, R., Shaikh, L. C., & Shanawani, H. (2008, January). *Disability and the Muslim perspective: An introduction for rehabilitation and health care providers.* Retrieved from https://digitalcommons.ilr.cornell.edu/gladnetcollect/460/

Hasson, N., Camilleri, B., Jones, C., Smith, J., & Dodd, B. (2013). Discriminating disorder from difference using dynamic assessment in bilingual children. *Child Language and Therapy, 29,* 57-75.

Individuals With Disabilities Education Improvement Act of 2004, Pub. L. 108-446, 20 U.S.C. §§ 1400-1482.

Kritikos, E. P. (2003). Speech-language pathologists' beliefs about language assessment of bilingual/bicultural individuals. *American Journal of Speech-Language Pathology, 12,* 73-91.

Medina, R. (2017). *The disproportionate representation of minorities in special education* (Master's thesis). Available from Theses and Dissertations database: https://rdw.rowan.edu/etd/2475

Sackett, D. L., Rosenberg, W. M. C., Gray, J. A. M., Haynes, R. B., & Richardson, W. S. (1996). Evidence-based medicine: What it is and what it isn't [Editorial]. *British Medical Journal, 312,* 71. https://doi.org/10.1136/bmj.312.7023.71

Shifrer, D., Muller, C., & Callahan, R. (2011). Disproportionality and learning disabilities: Parsing apart race, socioeconomic status, and language. *Journal of Learning Disabilities, 44*(3), 246-257.

ADDITIONAL RESOURCES

African Communities Together website: http://www.africans.us/

American Speech-Language-Hearing Association. (2020). *Dynamic assessment.* Retrieved from https://www.asha.org/practice/multicultural/issues/Dynamic-Assessment/

Hasnain, R., Shaikh, L. C., & Shanawani, H. (2008, January). *Disability and the Muslim perspective: An introduction for rehabilitation and health care providers.* Retrieved from https://digitalcommons.ilr.cornell.edu/gladnetcollect/460/

Javan, S. S., & Ghonsooly, B. (2018). Learning a foreign language: A new path to enhancement of cognitive functions. *Journal of Psycholinguistic Research, 47*(1), 125–138.

Lee-James, R., & Washington, J. A. (2018). Language skills of bidialectal and bilingual children. *Topics in Language Disorders, 38*(1), 5–26.

Mcleod, S., Verdon, S., & The International Expert Panel on Multilingual Children's Speech. (2017). Tutorial: Speech assessment for multilingual children who do not speak the same language(s) as the speech-language pathologist. *American Journal of Speech-Language Pathology, 26,* 691–708.

Mohr, K. A., Juth, S. M., Kohlmeier, T. L., & Schreiber, K. E. (2018). The developing bilingual brain: What parents and teachers should know and do. *Journal of Early Childhood Education, 46,* 11–20.

Sylvan, L. (2018). Tiers to communication success: How can SLPs join in the MTSS framework many schools are adopting to catch students' special education needs earlier and provide levels of intervention? *The ASHA Leader, 23*(8), 44–53.

We've Always Done It This Way — Implications of Audiological At-Home Remedies and Culturally Responsive Intervention

Karen L. Beverly-Ducker

PREBRIEF

notes:

In general, the discipline of communication sciences and disorders reflects a Western approach to health, wellness, and prevention that may not acknowledge and incorporate the influence of an individual's cultural background. At times, cultural beliefs and practices that differ from the majority view have been described in Western medical treatment as questionable, unorthodox, quackery, fringe medicine, primitive, and folk (e.g., Evans, 2001; Kronenfeld & Wasner, 1982). Although some practitioners may acknowledge complementary and alternative medicine (CAM) and homeopathic medicine, there may continue to be questions about their scientific evidence base and the quality of supporting research. Cultural factors may influence how individuals understand health concepts, how they make decisions about treatment options, and their compliance with professional recommendations. Many individuals accept and use multiple approaches to health care. It is important to provide the opportunity, across treatment, for clients to share their beliefs and practices so that their care can be coordinated, conflicts can be avoided, and treatment plans can be developed that are consistent with a patient's values.

Definition

CAM—healing and/or health practices not prescribed by health care professionals that patients feel will positively treat health conditions. Examples of CAM include acupuncture, herbal remedies, and healing rituals. Currently, families are combining CAM and evidence-based treatment practices to treat autism spectrum disorder. CAM can be used by any family regardless of culture, religious background, or socioeconomic status (Richmond, 2011).

OBJECTIVES

- Identify the role and influences of cultural beliefs and practice in health care.
- Learn ways to facilitate the open exchange of information when discussing cultural practices or beliefs.
- Review culturally appropriate ways to address and respond to health-related concerns, including CAM and homeopathic medicine.

CASE SCENARIO

Deja is an 8-year-old third grader who attended a community-based health fair with her grandmother. Both Deja and her grandmother expressed interest in the hearing screening booth at the fair. Deja's grandmother, who provides care for several of her grandchildren, was interviewed and shared that Deja recently failed her hearing screening at school. Deja's grandmother was surprised by the results of Deja's hearing screening and had not noticed any behaviors that indicated a hearing problem. She told the interviewer, "The children are all just loud!" Deja's grandmother did not recall any history of ear problems when Deja was younger or recall any family members with hearing loss. As far as she could remember, Deja "talked at about the right time," and there were no other language or learning difficulties.

As part of the hearing screening, the audiologist completed a visual examination that revealed an opaque, slightly thick substance on the right external ear canal as well as unidentified debris with redness noted, which prevented full visualization of the tympanic membrane. Deja did not respond to the screening threshold levels at any of the test frequencies when the pure tones were delivered to her right ear. Responses to tones delivered to her left ear were within normal limits. Air-conduction thresholds for the right ear were identified in support of the value of obtaining preliminary threshold levels as well as further orienting Deja to the behavioral responses needed for a complete audiologic evaluation. A pure tone average of 45 dB was obtained for the right ear, which meant that she failed the hearing screening because her response was outside the expected 20-dB-HL threshold.

The results of the visual and otoscopic examinations and the hearing screening results were discussed with the grandmother. The audiologist shared that throughout her career she has examined the ear canals of many children and adults. On some occasions she has found a variety of foreign items in her patients' ear canals. Some of the items were placed there accidentally, such as marbles and children's toys, and some were intentional. Some of the intentionally placed items were used for adornment purposes, whereas others were placed motivated by the belief of their medicinal and healing effects. The audiologist concluded her postscreening counseling by stating that although the different items may have been intended to serve a positive purpose, they also had the potential to impact hearing in a negative way. The audiologist noted that she could not be sure what caused the lack of response in Deja's right ear, but it could have been whatever debris was present. After some hesitation, Deja's grandmother revealed that she had recently placed warm sweet oil in Deja's ear, a common practice in their family for many years. After placing the sweet oil in Deja's ear, her grandmother had Deja lay her head on grandmother's lap. Her grandmother placed a small towel over Deja's ear, and then placed a plugged-in, "slightly warm" clothes iron over the towel. The thought was that the sweet oil would soothe the pain and the warmth of the iron would help to keep the oil warm and to "loosen things up." She has known sweet oil to be used as the remedy for several ear-related problems—including pain, infection, itching, ringing, hearing loss, and impacted cerumen—and has always found that it can "cure just about any problem with the ear."

CRITICAL THINKING AND DEBRIEFING QUESTIONS

1. **How might the clinician approach additional conversations regarding CAM and homeopathic practices and how they may be having an impact on Deja's hearing?**
2. **What is an appropriate decision-making process to use when identifying whether a practice or belief is questionable, potentially harmful, and in need of further investigation?**

3. What were some observable indicators in this case that CAM or homeopathic practices were a factor in Deja's care?
4. Have you ever used homeopathic treatments or CAM? How did you decide whether to use these approaches?

COMMENTARY

This scenario discusses the use of homeopathic treatments. Homeopathic treatments, along with CAM, are held under the umbrella term of alternative treatment practices. Home treatments are often incongruent with mainstream culture and practices and can be unfamiliar to practitioners.

The audiologist makes a hypothesis, on the basis of observations, that Deja's ear problems may be a result of something in the ear canal. Without directly asking or shaming the client, the audiologist shared that other clients had presented with similar complaints and opened a space for conversation by sharing with the client that she was not the only person who may have had a practice like this. This may have led Deja's grandmother to feel more comfortable divulging her use of sweet oil for medicinal purposes. Nungesser and Bierman-Mulvey (2003) cited that more than one third of patients indicate using homeopathic treatments for their health, and they noted that patients used such practices because they were more closely aligned with their beliefs and values. Additionally, hearing professionals were surveyed regarding their knowledge of homeopathic treatments, and more than 50% noted familiarity with the following remedies: sweet oil, cotton balls, rubbing alcohol, vinegar, and olive oil. These remedies were reportedly used across geographic areas, demographics, and age groups (Nungesser & Bierman-Mulvey, 2003).

Definition

Alternative treatment practices are defined broadly as "interventions that are not typically taught in medical school or used in medical facilities in the United States" (Nungesser & Bierman-Mulvey, 2003, p. 6).

In other fields, CAM is successfully used to complement Western treatments. For example, a recent study indicated that adults with cancer commonly use CAM for wellness or a combination of treatment and wellness (Rhee, Pawloski, & Parsons, 2019). The study stated that these patients indicated improved health-related, quality-of-life outcomes, making CAM a promising approach for enhancing health promotion and well-being among adults with cancer.

Communication sciences and disorders professionals may choose to enlist the practice of ethnographic interviewing to provide more opportunities to discuss medical and home practices (Westby, Burda, & Mehta, 2003). Opening up the space for this conversation can also help practitioners gauge a family's willingness to collaborate with or integrate Western medical practices alongside their homeopathic approaches. Although it may be difficult to approach the use of homeopathic practices, it is important to share current research and evidence, especially when a practice may cause harm or put a patient at risk.

CRITICAL THINKING AND DEBRIEFING RESPONSES

1. **How might the clinician approach additional conversations regarding CAM and homeopathic practices and how they may be having an impact on Deja's hearing?**

Because homeopathic practices are often related to personal beliefs and values, having a conversation regarding their use can be difficult, especially when a practitioner is trying to form a relationship with a new client. However, when the practice puts the patient at risk, there should be no hesitation in sharing risks, even in light of cultural beliefs. This difficulty may be magnified when the people involved are unfamiliar with one another and may have divergent views based on cultural background. Hearing professionals can help to diminish anxiety and create a more welcoming environment by sharing an awareness of the potential influence of one's cultural background and by demonstrating knowledge about homeopathic practices. Sharing a basic understanding of common homeopathic practices and their frequency, as the audiologist in the case scenario did, can help to create an environment that is open to sharing about cultural differences. Professionals can choose to adopt a practice of ethnographic interviewing, including asking open-ended questions and restating and summarizing comments to indicate understanding (Brown, 2017). Using these practices from the initial meeting can help lay a foundation for a collaborative relationship in which both parties feel respected. When difficult topics arise—for instance, when talking about a homeopathic treatment that may be harmful—the client may be more open to listening to a practitioner's rationale, knowing that they understand the value a client places on that practice.

2. **What is an appropriate decision-making process to use when identifying whether a practice or belief is questionable, potentially harmful, and in need of further investigation?**

Identifying questionable practices and potentially harmful behaviors can be complicated. It requires careful discernment between those practices or beliefs and those that reflect unfamiliar approaches that are culturally based. There must be an appropriate balance between acknowledging cultural differences and recognizing the need to intervene. When identifying whether a particular cultural practice or belief is questionable, it is helpful to consider the following:

- The cultural behaviors, beliefs, and practices of the client
- The variability in the acceptable range of cultural behaviors, beliefs, and practices of the client (i.e., what is within the range of "normal" for a particular culture. For example, when asking some children a question, there is the expectation that they will answer, whereas in certain cultures, the question is a warning or guide.)
- Whether the practice is actually doing harm to a client.

Expand Your Knowledge

In 2019, a study was done to determine the perspectives of audiologists in South Africa in regard to their clients' use of traditional healing (Pillay & Serooe, 2019). The study also looked at whether the audiologists engaged in the traditional healing practices. Overall, the study found that more than half of the surveyed audiologists were willing to collaborate with the traditional healers in their patient's care. In reference to holistic health care, Pillay and Serooe (2019) recommended that audiologists "should reflect on personal beliefs, thoughts, and assumptions that impact one's practice" and that they should "reevaluate the history taking process and consider the inclusion of questions pertaining to religious practices and belief systems" (p. 8).

3. **What were some observable indicators in this case that CAM or homeopathic practices were a factor in Deja's care?**

The signs noted by the audiologist that revealed possible homeopathic practices in Deja's case included an opaque, slightly thick substance on the right external auditory meatus with significantly different pigmentation of the surrounding skin. An otoscopic examination revealed an inability to visualize the tympanic membrane. Elevated hearing thresholds as well observations of debris and reddened ear canals led to the audiologist's conclusion that Deja had not passed the hearing screening and should be referred for further audiological testing and medical evaluation by an otolaryngologist.

4. **Have you ever used homeopathic treatments or CAM? How did you decide whether to use these approaches?**

Personal response. As you think about this, consider treatments such as ear candling/coning or acupuncture. Is there research to support the treatment? Do the treatments have the possibility to cause harm? If they don't have the possibility to cause harm, but have no credible evidence, should a client be counseled away from their use?

TAKE AWAYS

- Structure the case history so that the respondent has the opportunity to share about the variety of health approaches and treatments used. Consider using ethnographic interviewing practices.
- Increase your awareness of the cultural factors that may influence approaches to health care.
- Develop an effective, nonjudgmental communication plan for sharing information, content, and perspective that may not completely align with that of your client or patient.

REFERENCES

Brown, J. A. (2017). Impact of performance feedback in family-centered and culturally responsive interview instruction. *American Journal of Speech-Language Pathology, 26,* 1244–1253.

Evans, W. (2001). Mapping mainstream and fringe medicine on the Internet. *Science Communication, 22,* 292–299.

Kronenfeld, J. J., & Wasner, C. (1982). The use of unorthodox therapies and marginal practitioners. *Social Science & Medicine, 16,* 1119–1125.

Nungesser, N., & Bierman-Mulvey, N. (2003). Alternative medicine and hearing: Cultural influences, clinical implications. *The ASHA Leader, 8*(20), 6–7.

Pillay, D., & Serooe, T. (2019). Shifting and transforming the practice of audiology: The inclusion of traditional healing. *South African Journal of Communication Disorders, 66*(1), a635. https://doi.org/10.4102/sajcd.v66i1.635

Rhee, T., Pawloski, P., & Parsons, H. (2019). Health-related quality of life among US adults with cancer: Potential roles of complementary and alternative medicine for health promotion and well-being. *Psycho-Oncology, 28,* 896–902. https://doi.org/10.1002/pon.5039

Richmond, A. S. (2011). Autism spectrum disorder: A global perspective. *Perspectives on Global Issues in Communication Sciences and Related Disorders, 1*(2), 39–46. https://doi.org/10.1044/gics1.2.39

Westby, C., Burda, A., & Mehta, Z. (2003). Asking the right questions in the right ways: Strategies for ethnographic interviewing. *The ASHA Leader, 8*(8), 4-17.

ADDITIONAL RESOURCES

Agency for Healthcare Research and Quality, U.S. Department of Health and Human Services: Health Literacy Universal Precautions Toolkit, Second Edition: https://www.ahrq.gov/professionals/quality-patient-safety/quality-resources/tools/literacy-toolkit/healthlittoolkit2-tool10.html

American Speech-Language-Hearing Association practice portal: Cultural competence: https://www.asha.org/Practice-Portal/Professional-Issues/Cultural-Competence/

Stuttering and Stigma in a Somali Family — How Understanding Etiology Can Affect Choices in Intervention

Alicia Fleming Hamilton

notes:

PREBRIEF

The Americans With Disabilities Act of 1990 (ADA) is a civil rights law that prohibits discrimination against individuals with disabilities. The ADA defines an individual with a disability as "a person with a physical or mental impairment that substantially limits one or more major life activities, a person who has a history or record of such an impairment, or a person who is perceived by others as having such an impairment." Some cultures around the world view illness and disability as a manifestation of the spirit or a consequence of a family's past actions or missteps. Illness may be viewed as part of a deity's plan for one's life, an act of karma, or the result of a curse or ill feeling. In Somalia and surrounding geographical areas, disability is often equated with physical impairment, which may have been present from birth or the result of war or conflict injuries. Other disabilities—which may include language disorders, stuttering, and learning difficulties—are not as commonly addressed because they are less physically visible.

As you read through this case study, keep various cultural beliefs surrounding disability in mind. Look for ways in which these views and beliefs may affect assessment, evaluation, and treatment outcomes for students. Remember that although a family may be from a particular regional area, not all families adopt the same cultural beliefs or practices.

OBJECTIVES

- Identify cultural attitudes surrounding the term "disability," specifically regarding common beliefs in the Somali community.
- Consider appropriate evaluation planning practices when working with families who speak multiple languages.
- Understand the etiology of stuttering and the ways it presents in bilingual individuals.

CASE SCENARIO

Hamsa is a 9-year-old, third-grade student attending an English-speaking school. Hamsa's family are refugees from Somalia and live in a community where there are few other refugee families. There are two other Somali families in his school, and he is the only Somali student in his grade, which consists of predominantly White children. Hamsa has one older brother and two younger sisters, with whom he interacts in English and Somali. Hamsa has been exposed to Somali since birth. He began learning English as a toddler, when he was relocated to the United States as a refugee.

Hamsa was referred to his school speech-language pathologist (SLP) by his mother, Farrah, because of concerns that Hamsa has limited knowledge of Somali and that he repeats words often. She reported that Hamsa communicates using single words in Somali, but he uses phrases to communicate in English. Although Farrah does not use the word "stutter," she explained that Hamsa has repeated words and sounds since he started talking around 2 years old. This was also the time they came to the United States and Hamsa was first exposed to English. When he started kindergarten, she shared that he started to squeeze his face and hold sounds for a long time. Currently, she reported that this behavior has decreased, but he continues to repeat sounds and words, "like 10 times in a row." Farrah shared that Hamsa does this both in Somali and English. She noted that he does not repeat words or sounds when he is reciting lines from the Qur'an. Farrah asked their pediatrician about Hamsa's speech, and the pediatrician suggested that Hamsa was getting "confused" and that it may be beneficial for them to focus on "one language only." Farrah did not feel comfortable with this recommendation, and she continued speaking to Hamsa in Somali and English.

John, the SLP, contacted Farrah for permission to complete an observation of Hamsa. Farrah gave John permission to observe Hamsa in his classroom. After the observation, the SLP noted that Hamsa stuttered between 7% and 9% of the time and demonstrated secondary behaviors of hand shaking. He categorized Hamsa's dysfluencies as repetitions of initial sounds, blocks, and prolongations.

Results of dual language learning (DLL) placement tests showed that Hamsa's English skills were at a proficient level for his age, and as a result, he did not qualify for DLL services in his school. In English, Hamsa communicated in phrases of appropriate length and complexity. He was able to follow complex directions, understood academic concepts, and was at grade level for reading and writing skills. Hamsa's teacher described him as shy and reluctant to participate orally in class. In conversations, she said that he frequently holds sounds for a long period of time, or he opens his mouth without sound coming out for 3–5 seconds. She also noted that he waves his hand on the side of his body when he's speaking to a group of students or in front of class. She thinks he stutters more when he's nervous, excited, or upset. His second-grade teacher noted that his speech became worse as the year progressed.

On the basis of Hamsa's teacher's observations, his mother's concerns, and results of DLL testing, the SLP moves forward with testing for a fluency disorder. He contacted Hamsa's mother, Farrah, and father, Bashiir, who declined the use of an interpreter. The SLP scheduled an evaluation planning meeting and invited Bashiir and Farrah. The SLP called in the district Somali interpreter/cultural liaison in case there were any ideas or concepts he has difficulty explaining in English. He shared this rationale with Hamsa's parents, who seemed appreciative but reiterated that they did not need the interpreter for themselves.

The SLP started the meeting by explaining all of the special education paperwork. He noticed that each time he mentioned the word "disability," Hamsa's father, Bashiir, cleared his throat and shook his head side to side. John stopped and asked whether Bashiir or Farrah had any questions. Bashiir stated that he does not want to talk about "disabilities," that doing so is taboo in their culture. He continued, saying he thought they were there to talk about fixing Hamsa's speech. Bashiir shared that he does not want his son to have a "label," and Farrah began to cry. John apologized and asked the family to share more so he can better understand their perspective. Bashiir explained to John that in Somalia his uncle "talked like Hamsa," and he was ostracized and unable to find a job. As a result, his uncle relied on others' charity to survive. The family left him behind when they came to the United States, and they think that because they left Hamsa's uncle behind, the family is being punished by God, which is why Hamsa now talks like his uncle.

CRITICAL THINKING AND DEBRIEFING QUESTIONS

1. **What are your thoughts or beliefs regarding the parents' reactions in this case study? How might your thoughts or beliefs affect or influence service delivery?**
2. **How would you approach an assessment and treatment for this student?**
3. **What are ways the SLP could explain due process paperwork and potentially novel terms such as "special education" and "disability" in a culturally friendly way? How might the family's background influence the explanation?**
4. **What steps could you take before your meeting to learn about the Somali culture and ideas about disability, disorders, and stuttering?**
5. **How would you address the information from Hamsa's pediatrician about using "one language"?**

COMMENTARY

On the basis of clinical observations, parent reports, test results, and teacher information, Hamsa is presenting with a moderate fluency disorder. It appears that Hamsa has been presenting with these behaviors since he was 2 years old. Hamsa may not have been diagnosed earlier for a variety of reasons. Sometimes fluency disorders are not as widely identified by teachers and educational professionals, and stuttering may be confused or cited as a typical behavior for a child who is learning multiple languages. This belief can keep bilingual students from receiving needed services in a timely fashion. Both monolingual and multilingual populations of children present with fluency disorders from a young age with the same frequency.

Information from classroom observations revealed that Hamsa is aware of his stuttering and may be trying to hide it by avoiding public speaking and speaking in groups of his peers. Given Hamsa's family's experience with his uncle's stuttering, Hamsa may have strong emotional associations tied to his speech and stuttering. More observations of Hamsa's speech and discussions with his parents and teachers would be needed to determine whether this was the case. If so, the SLP should address Hamsa's feelings and attitudes surrounding stuttering. The SLP could teach Hamsa about people who stutter and are successful in a variety of different fields—including athletes, actors, and even high-ranking public officials.

Another aspect of this case that is important to discuss are the parents' reactions to and perceptions of special education and treatments for fluency disorders. Often, Western culture identifies a problem or disease, searches for an etiology, and seeks a treatment. There tends to be less emphasis on personal responsibility for disability or placing blame, and more emphasis on accessibility and resources. Other cultures may believe that disabilities, including fluency disorders and speech impairments, are caused by the actions of the mother while she was pregnant, mistakes made by the family, traumatic events, or karma. The manifestation of these disorders can bring out feelings of shame and guilt in a family. People with disabilities can be pitied, seen as an embarrassment to the family, and sometimes viewed as unable to contribute to society as a result of their differences (Rohwerder, 2018). In the scenario, observe how the mention of Bashiir's uncle and his stuttering is likely a contributing factor to the family's beliefs about fluency. They may feel that because they left his uncle behind, they brought Hamsa's fluency disorder on themselves. Their move to the United States also coincided with Hamsa's disfluency. Discussing the differences in views of disability between European American and other cultures, and making sure not to present one belief system as more valid, will be critical in framing treatment options for Hamsa.

It is important to talk about beliefs regarding bilingualism as well as research regarding bilingualism and stuttering. In this case, Hamsa's pediatrician suggested that his stuttering may be a result of the "confusion" of speaking two languages and recommended that the family choose one primary language for communication. This idea may have been reinforced to the parents because Hamsa moved to the United States and was exposed to English around the time when his stuttering started. SLPs should address this misconception and encourage parents and families to continue using their native languages at home in an effort to maintain cultural connections and provide rich language input for their children. The SLP would need to share that being bilingual does not and will not cause fluency or any other communication disorders and, in fact, is a benefit for Hamsa. A recent review of stuttering and bilingualism provides some suggestion that stuttering may be more prevalent in bilinguals when compared with monolinguals, but studies to corroborate this suggestion are lacking (Van Borsel, Maes, & Foulon, 2001). In addition, a small body of research indicates that it is likely that bilingualism can be a contributing factor to the development of stuttering, but other factors including linguistic input and social pressure play a role. Stuttering can impact one or both languages of a bilingual and may impact either language to varying degrees (Van Borsel et al., 2001). The authors also noted the importance of distinguishing dysfluency as a result of limited language proficiency by assessing language skills in all languages used.

Stuttering can impact one or both languages of a bilingual and may impact either language to varying degrees (Van Borsel et al., 2001).

Discussing cultural differences in an effort to bridge understanding is another critical component of this case. By taking the time to understand the family's beliefs and impressions regarding their son's diagnosis and the special education process, the SLP is providing an opportunity for the family to feel that their opinions are valued and to be collaborating members of the team. For example, it was beneficial for the SLP to stop the meeting and ask for clarification when Hamsa's parents appeared upset by the discussion. Taking time to address cultural beliefs and to clarify understanding for all parties is critical in creating collaboration. In future cases, it may be appropriate for the SLP to consult reputable online resources and consult a cultural liaison before meeting with the family to better understand possible cultural views of disability, gender roles, appropriate treatment goals and strategies, and suitable vocabulary to use when discussing the case. If Hamsa's family agreed to services, it would be beneficial for the SLP to educate Hamsa's teachers and other staff regarding the cultural beliefs surrounding disability as well as to provide more information on Somali history and culture.

CRITICAL THINKING AND DEBRIEFING RESPONSES

1. **What are your thoughts or beliefs regarding the parents' reactions in this case study? How might your thoughts or beliefs affect or influence service delivery?**

Personal answers. Consider your own personal beliefs regarding disability and consider the way other cultures may perceive disability. Reflect on those beliefs and how they may unknowingly affect service delivery from you—the clinician—and participation from the client. For this family, speaking about disabilities was taboo. Middle Eastern parents have dealt with their child's stuttering by praying for change, asking them to speak properly, completing their sentences, asking them not to speak in public, or sending them away to live with other relatives (Waheed-Kahn, 1998). Understanding these cultural attitudes can better inform a clinician when working with a family for treatment.

2. **How would you approach an assessment and treatment for this student?**

In this scenario, a clinician can start by interviewing the family, including an interpreter. To diagnose stuttering, the dysfluencies must be present in both languages, although they may vary in degree. Language testing would be appropriate to rule out lack of linguistic proficiency as a contributing factor to word-finding difficulty. The clinician would consider both structured and spontaneous language samples. Creating a video recording of the language samples, while the interpreter is present, would help the interpreter and clinician to identify true stuttering behaviors and not typical dysfluencies while reviewing the recording. Additionally, the video would be useful in looking for other physical concomitant behaviors or secondary characteristics. Hamsa's clinician may ask him to complete rating scales that gauge his perception of his stuttering and speech. These tools can be used in the future for progress monitoring.

Evaluating in both languages is crucial. The American Speech-Language-Hearing Association's (ASHA's) practice portal provides guidance on the use of interpreters, transliterators, and translators as well as a section on cultural competence. These resources have excellent information and suggestions for appropriate bilingual and culturally competent evaluations (e.g., ASHA, n.d.). There are also various foundations that provide information for specific disorders, including tips for parents and other pertinent research data. In this case, because Hamsa's SLP does not speak Somali, treatment at school would occur predominantly in English. The SLP would need to monitor the carryover of strategies, using an interpreter to gather data and working with Hamsa's parents to complete rating scales and report on Hamsa's progress at home and in the community.

In this scenario, Hamsa would likely receive treatment in English. Research has shown that treatment in one language results in spontaneous improvement in fluency in the untreated language (Rousseau, Packman, & Onslow, 2005). This will be important information to share with Hamsa's family as they continue through treatment. The SLP can also use information from the initial rating scales as well as continued language sampling in both Somali and English. The clinician should also consider the impact of Hamsa's culture on his stuttering treatment. The SLP may need to adjust treatment to allow for cultural differences. These adjustments may include using culturally appropriate stimuli, modifying instructions to accommodate the Somali language and its structure, using au-

Research has shown that treatment in one language results in spontaneous improvement in fluency in the untreated language (Rousseau, Packman, & Onslow, 2005).

dio and video exemplars in the home language of the child to involve the parents and family, and providing opportunities for practicing fluency in culturally relevant contexts and activities (Shenker, 2013).

3. **What are ways the SLP could explain due process paperwork and potentially novel terms such as "special education" and "disability" in a culturally friendly way? How might the family's background influence the explanation?**

When meeting with any client or family, it would be helpful to complete research on a given culture to provide a background and broad context for the client's possible belief systems. While doing this, it is important to remember that not all cultures are homogenous and each client presents with their own unique set of beliefs and interpretation of culture. For instance, a general statement about the Somali culture is that disabilities are stigmatized. Because of the history of war and its impact across many communities, disabilities are often connected to physical impairments. People with disabilities are commonly viewed with pity or excluded from general society. For children, this may include excluding those with disabilities so that they are not around other children, and believing that children with disabilities are not able to contribute to a household. Some communities believe that an illness or misfortune is the result of a spirit possession or is a form of punishment from God. However, this may not be the view of all people who are Somali. Understanding that using the word "disability" can evoke strong emotions with Somali clients, a clinician may be more sensitive when sharing results. It may also be beneficial to consult with a Somali cultural liaison and review the process for reporting special education results to see what culturally appropriate changes can be made.

Given this general information, a clinician may wish to present the special education process by talking about the percentage of students who receive special education in the United States, how the special education program works, and how students who complete the program or who receive services are successful. Discussing a client's goals for therapy or their speech may be useful at this point and could be used to tie back to other successful community members or well-known figures who stutter. Doing so may help to de-stigmatize stuttering and demonstrate that disability can be seen differently in the United States. You could also share that nothing in particular "causes" a stutter and provide the latest research regarding etiology.

Finally, it would be important to ask the family about their perceptions and beliefs regarding disability. It could be important here to talk about misconceptions about being bilingual and address the misinformation from their pediatrician—that Hamsa was stuttering because he was "confused" by two languages. This particular comment is covered in more detail in Question 5.

4. **What steps could you take before your meeting to learn about the Somali culture and ideas about disability, disorders, and stuttering?**

The SLP could seek out a cultural liaison within their district or plan extra time with the interpreter to provide better background for the assessment and to help understand the perception of disability and the special education process in this community. The SLP could send questions about cultural practices and beliefs to the interpreter before the meeting to help the SLP prepare with information and the interpreter prepare the necessary vocabulary for the meeting. This could include questions about general beliefs surrounding disabilities, the best words to use when describing disability or difference, and specific vocabulary words to use or that you may use during the conversation. It's common that terms do not directly transfer across languages, and it can be useful for interpreters to have information in advance so that they can adequately prepare for a visit. The clinician can search through reputable sites, some of which are listed in the Additional Resources section, for a basic understanding of how disability may be viewed within a culture.

5. **How would you address the information from Hamsa's pediatrician about using "one language"?**

According to Shenker (n.d.), no evidence has been found to suggest that speaking two languages at home since birth causes stuttering. Although information regarding bilinguals and stuttering has varied conclusions and is lacking in volume, it is incorrect to state that speaking two languages "confuses" a child or causes stuttering. Current evidence shows that bilingualism can influence stuttering in unpredictable ways, impacting the way that stuttering presents in an individual. Stuttering may also present itself differently across the languages that a client speaks—for instance, a client may stutter on function words in one language and content words in another. After hearing this statement to use "one language" from the family, the SLP could present research-based information affirming that children do not stutter as a result of confusion between languages (Shenker, 2013). Current research indicates that the causes of stuttering could be multifactorial. They may include genetic and neuropsychological factors and, in some cases, acquired neurogenic or psychogenic stuttering. The emergence of stuttering may also depend on environmental factors and child temperament in maintaining cultural and family ties—and at its most basic explanation, it is how someone communicates in their environment. Taking away one language for a client can mean taking away their ability to communicate and connect to their culture and community.

TAKE AWAYS

- A fluency disorder will present in all spoken languages, to varying degrees.
- Before meeting clients from a culture different than your own, it may be helpful to complete a basic review of cultural beliefs and values, especially surrounding disability.
- Being bilingual does not cause fluency disorders, and speaking more than one language does not exacerbate fluency disorders; moreover, a recommendation to only speak one language may be damaging to the client's cultural ties and overall communication (Shenker, 2013).

REFERENCES

American Speech-Language-Hearing Association. (n.d.). *Childhood fluency disorders.* Retrieved from https://www.asha.org/Practice-Portal/Clinical-Topics/Childhood-Fluency-Disorders/

Americans With Disabilities Act of 1990, Pub. L. 101-336, 42 U.S.C. §§ 12101-12213 (2000).

Rohwerder, B. (2018, January). *Disability in Somalia* (K4D Helpdesk Report). Retrieved from https://assets.publishing.service.gov.uk/media/5a744dbded915d0e8bf188ec/Disability_in_Somalia.pdf

Rousseau, I., Packman, A., & Onslow, M. (2005, June). *A trial of the Lidcombe Program with school age stuttering children.* Paper presented at the Speech Pathology National Conference, Canberra, Australia.

Shenker, R. (n.d.). *Stuttering and the bilingual child.* Retrieved from the Stuttering Foundation website: https://www.stutteringhelp.org/stuttering-and-bilingual-child

Shenker, R. C. (2013). Bilingual myth-busters series. When young children who stutter are also bilingual: Some thoughts about assessment and treatment. *Perspectives on Communication Disorders and Sciences in Culturally and Linguistically Diverse (CLD) Populations, 20*(1), 15–23.

Van Borsel, J., Maes, E., & Foulon, S. (2001). Stuttering and bilingualism: A review. *Journal of Fluency Disorders, 26*(3), 179–205.

Waheed-Kahn, N. (1998). Fluency therapy with multilingual clients. In E. C. Healey & H. F. M. Peters (Eds.), *Proceedings of the Second World Congress on Fluency Disorders* (pp. 195-199). Nijmegen, the Netherlands: Nijmegen University Press.

ADDITIONAL RESOURCES

American Speech-Language-Hearing Association. (n.d.). *Cultural competence.* Retrieved from https://www.asha.org/Practice-Portal/Professional-Issues/Cultural-Competence/

Americans With Disabilities Act of 1990: https://www.ada.gov/ada_intro.htm

Center for Applied Linguistics, Cultural Orientation Research Center. (n.d.). *The Somalis cultural profile.* Available at http://www.culturalorientation.net/library/publications/the-somalis-cultural-profile

Cruz-Ferreira, M. (2011, August 2). Recommending monolingualism to multilinguals—Why, and why not. *Leader Live.* Retrieved from https://blog.asha.org/2011/08/02/recommending-monolingualism-to-multilinguals-why-and-why-not/

Global Affairs Canada website: https://www.international.gc.ca/cil-cai/country_insights-apercus_pays/ci-ic_so.aspx?lang=eng

Langdon, H. W. (2002). Language interpreters and translators: Bridging communication with clients and families. *The ASHA Leader, 7*(6), 14–15.

Rohwerder, B. (2018, January). Disability in Somalia (K4D Helpdesk Report). Retrieved from https://assets.publishing.service.gov.uk/media/5a744dbded915d0e8bf188ec/Disability_in_Somalia.pdf

Shenker, R. (n.d.). *Stuttering and the bilingual child.* Retrieved from the Stuttering Foundation website: https://www.stutteringhelp.org/stuttering-and-bilingual-child

Stratis Health. (n.d.). Somalis in Minnesota. *Culture, Care, Connection.* Retrieved from http://www.culturecareconnection.org/matters/diversity/somali.html

World Health Organization. (n.d.). *World report on disability.* Retrieved from https://www.who.int/disabilities/world_report/2011/en/

Language Immersion Programs

— Professional Accountability in a Dual Language Setting

Alicia Fleming Hamilton

PREBRIEF

notes:

Dual language immersion programs in elementary schools are gaining popularity across the United States (Williams, 2017). Research demonstrates that enrollment in immersion programs can be beneficial to students, leading to more flexible thinking and marketable skills as future bilingual professionals (Zelasko & Antunez, 2000). As the popularity of immersion programs continues to grow, communication sciences and disorders professionals face difficulties when designing treatment for students in these programs with documented learning or language difficulties.

Research demonstrates that enrollment in immersion programs can be beneficial to students, leading to more flexible thinking and marketable skills as future bilingual professionals (Zelasko & Antunez, 2000).

As you read this case, consider the cultural perception regarding multilingualism, disability, and academic expectations. Review the federal requirements outlining the least restrictive environment as well as free and appropriate education for all students. Finally, consider the similarities and differences between the cultural viewpoints represented in this case study: German culture and mainstream American culture.

OBJECTIVES

- Understand that immersion programs instruct students both in language acquisition and cultural values, which may contrast with a family's home culture.
- Review federal regulations for students with disabilities or diverse learning needs and their rights to immersion in all education.
- Identify research that supports immersion settings for students with language or learning disabilities.

CASE SCENARIO

Liam is a White, fourth-grade student who attends a German immersion school. He has attended the school since kindergarten, and the program continues through senior year in high school. Liam was born on a military base in Germany, but he moved back to the United States when he was a toddler. Because of this experience, Liam's parents decided that they would like their son to continue learning German, even though they do not speak the language themselves. Liam's parents admired the way German families raised their children and aspired to instill similar values of structure, hard work, and industriousness in their son. They also valued the benefits of being bilingual, including increased mental flexibility and marketability later in life. Liam's parents are active members of his school's parent-teacher association (PTA).

Liam communicates with his parents in English, and they casually use German to name foods or greet each other. Liam's parents recognize that they are unable to assist Liam with his homework and report that his current assignments surpass their language abilities in German.

Liam began having problems at school in first grade. His teachers noted that he did not enjoy learning songs in German, seemed to "ignore" their directions, had difficulty sharing stories, and could not provide descriptions of items. His first-grade teacher shared that when Liam was given a multiple-step direction, he appeared to focus on what she was saying, but he was unable to repeat the direction or complete the task. Liam appeared distracted during less structured times of the day. After a referral to a developmental pediatrician, he was diagnosed with attention-deficit/hyperactivity disorder and a generalized anxiety disorder. As part of his comprehensive assessment, Liam was evaluated by a speech-language pathologist (SLP), in English only, and was diagnosed with a moderate language disorder. Liam also completed a hearing screening, and he passed. Since then, he has been receiving speech-language pathology services in a pull-out setting at his school, in English, because of his increased anxiety levels and his difficulty concentrating in the classroom.

During meetings with the special education team, Liam's parents have been told that Liam does well in math and excels in robotics. He also enjoys individual sports, such as running and swimming. Academically, Liam struggles with low performance in the areas of reading and writing. The special education team has shared that Liam is below his age level in reading and oral expression in both English and German. In fourth grade, his classroom is using a formula of 50% English and 50% German language exposure. His teacher is a native English speaker but has near-native proficiency in German, and the children in his class are all native English speakers. At the meeting with his special education team, his teacher noted that Liam is often late for class and does not complete his homework assignments in the exact way that she has assigned them. She says that he often "ignores" details. Liam reported that he feels "stupid" and "hates school." He also reported that he doesn't enjoy music class because he has difficulty singing "the right way." His parents were most concerned when he told them that he doesn't want to talk in German, "ever."

Liam is due for a 3-year reevaluation for special education services in the schools. The special education team speaks English. His evaluation will involve a review of his previous testing, current data on Liam's performance, and his present levels of functioning. His parents are concerned that with his increasing difficulties at school, his principal might recommend that Liam be transferred out of the German immersion program into an English-only curriculum. Liam's parents value bilingualism and would like him to receive the appropriate supports for his learning difficulties so that he can be successful in the German immersion setting. They expressed that they want Liam to have a positive attitude about school and that they have spent a significant amount of time and resources in keeping him in the school.

According to the principal, students in special education "have difficulty learning two languages" and suggests that Liam would do better in an English-only setting. The SLP does not feel comfortable speaking out, using current research and her training, to respond to the principal's opinion. She knows that under federal law, all students have a right to a free and appropriate public education in the least restrictive environment. She also knows that children with language impairments are capable of learning two languages and that learning a second language can sometimes provide a linguistic or cognitive advantage. The SLP knows that given appropriate supports, Liam can be successful in this setting (Peña, 2016; Restrepo, Morgan, & Thompson, 2013). She consults the audiologist with her observations and concerns, and the two of them work on creating an assessment plan to address Liam's needs. They schedule a meeting with Liam's parents to present information on bilingualism and immersion for children with language disorders, and they invite the principal. Their goal is to present current research regarding language disorders and the benefits of being bilingual. The principal's goal is to convince Liam's parents that he would be more successful in an "alternative setting."

CRITICAL THINKING AND DEBRIEFING QUESTIONS

1. **How would you modify Liam's initial evaluation?**
2. **What strategies can the audiologist and SLP use to educate the parents and principal regarding bilingual language acquisition, federal laws, and best practices?**
3. **What evidence can you cite to support immersion programs for students with language or learning disabilities?**
4. **How does the shared language (English) between Liam's family and his teachers affect their ability to advocate for him?**
5. **How might this situation be different for a family in which the language of instruction is the majority cultural language (English) but not the language of their home?**
6. **Reflection: Contrast this situation with those students for whom immersion learning is not a choice but their reality. How can professionals advocate for students whose home language and culture are not reflected in their community or school?**

COMMENTARY

In the United States, many students are in *total immersion* settings. This means that the student is immersed in the non-native language during 100% of their instruction. Consider a student who speaks Amharic at home but attends a school where information is presented in English only. Often, the language of instruction is not the child's first language or the language spoken at home. Other types of immersion, including the one mentioned in this scenario, use varying formulas to achieve bilingual instruction. Some involve partial immersion, in which students share time in English and the immersion language, or two-way immersion, in which native speakers of the targeted language and native speakers of the majority language are placed in a classroom together where there is instruction in both languages. In Liam's case, he is in partial immersion setting where he receives most instruction in German, with some instruction (including special classes such as science, technology, arts, and physical education) in English. For Liam, exposure to a second language occurs at school only.

The decision of Liam's parents to enroll him in an immersion setting, when English-only instruction is also available, indicates that they value bilingualism. Hearing the inaccurate comments made by the principal and negative comments from Liam's teachers may make Liam's parents feel as though they have made the wrong decision in his education. However, research indicates that children with language disorders are, indeed, capable of learning more than one language without negatively impacting second language acquisition (e.g., Restrepo et al., 2013). Some research has found that bilingual intervention helps to speed up the second language acquisition (Lugo-Neris, Jackson, & Goldstein, 2010; Rivera Pérez et al., 2019). Additionally, children with language disorders who were placed in an immersive setting performed better in the immersion language than children with language disorders who were taught a second language as a "specialized class" (Kay-Raining Bird, 2010). Kay-Raining Bird (2010) also noted that "if a child with a language and/or cognitive disorder needs to know two languages . . . it is not appropriate to recommend that the input be reduced to a single language" (Conclusions section, numbered list, Item 2). Providing this information to the parents may help them feel more confident in making placement decisions for their son.

Research indicates that children with language disorders can learn more than one language without negative impact on second language acquisition.

Another perspective is to consider the cultural implications in this case study. Both German and European American culture play a role. Typically, German culture values rules, punctuality, privacy, structure, hard work, and industriousness (Zimmermann, 2018). These values may clash when working with a child with Liam's needs. His teachers, who may have cultural expectations in line with German customs, may have made assumptions, because of Liam's observed difficulties, that he isn't "working hard enough" or that he was making a choice not to follow the routine and rules of the classroom. German culture also values perfection and precision, which can add another layer of difficulty in a language immersion setting where a student is struggling. The desire for precision may mean there is no allowance for errors, as there may be in English-only classrooms where independence and critical thinking/questioning are expected and valued. Typically, European American values include high academic achievement, independence, the ability to follow intrinsic expectations, and individual success. Without strategies to help Liam navigate the cultural expectations in his school, it is possible he may continue to feel unsuccessful. His parents and teachers could benefit from information on how unspoken cultural values may be adding more pressure to this situation. This information may indicate opportunities for classroom adaptations for Liam that can be documented on his individualized education plan.

CRITICAL THINKING AND DEBRIEFING RESPONSES

1. **How would you modify Liam's initial evaluation?**

Best practice for Liam's initial evaluation would be a review of all of his language skills in both German and English. If Liam demonstrated characteristics of language impairment in his native language (English), then he would also exhibit signs in his second language (German; Kohnert, 2010). It would have been important to measure Liam's capabilities in both languages to assist in measuring progress across his academic career. Finally, a full hearing evaluation would have been appropriate to rule out any possible hearing loss as a contributing factor in his difficulties.

2. **What strategies can the audiologist and SLP use to educate the parents and principal regarding bilingual language acquisition, federal laws, and best practices?**

The audiologist and SLP can share information on the benefits of being bilingual, specifically for students with language disorders. They can share information about federal laws, including the Individuals With Disabilities Education Improvement Act of 2004 and how it protects rights for all students, regardless of programming or abilities. They may add research about students with language disorders and other special needs and how they have been successful and have benefited from dual immersion programs, like Liam's. The team could consider planning an in-service or presentation at their school to educate staff on the benefits of learning multiple languages for students with language disorders or other special needs. See the References and Additional Resources sections for more specific details.

3. **What evidence can you cite to support immersion programs for students with language or learning disabilities?**

There are multiple studies that demonstrate how students with language or learning disabilities can be successful and even benefit from immersion programs (Steele et al., 2017). Regardless of placement, students will need supports based on their individual needs. Also, the law states that all students have the right to a free and appropriate public education in the least restrictive environment. Students should have access to all programming available, regardless of ability, with appropriate supports from their individualized education plan team.

4. **How does the shared language (English) between Liam's family and his teachers affect their ability to advocate for him?**

Liam's parents speak English and, because of their cultural upbringing, are well-versed in the cultural expectations in North American schooling practices. Liam's parents understand how to advocate for their son by requesting special education evaluations, services, and other academic supports. Liam's parents are also involved in the PTA and other school events. All of this information is a byproduct of knowing the cultural practices and expectations of North American schools and the rights one is afforded when attending such schools. The involvement of the family and their knowledge of these processes give them an advantage by making them just as aware of educational opportunities for Liam as his educational team is. Liam's family does not need these opportunities to be explicitly stated to understand and access them to support Liam's education. It is likely that Liam's parents are able to better advocate for him because of their shared language and cultural expectations with the team. They may also use socioeconomic and educational advantages, having grown up within this education system. As a result, they are able to ask questions for clarification, read resources in their home language, and know that they have protected rights in the public education system.

5. **How might this situation be different for a family in which the language of instruction is the majority cultural language (English) but not the language of their home?**

As referenced in the previous question, knowledge of implicit cultural expectations in a schooling environment is helpful in navigating that environment for your own child. In addition to the benefit of knowing the mainstream language, the cultural expectations, which are often not explicitly stated, can be difficult to navigate when a family did not grow up as part of the mainstream culture. Families who are unfamiliar with cultural practices in North American schooling may not be aware that they can challenge a teacher's or principal's recommendations for their child, do independent research on teaching approaches, and understand implicit expectations to volunteer on boards and in the classroom; therefore, these families may be at a disadvantage if these practices and expectations are not explained. An appropriate way to address this may be to pair mentors with all new families, produce brochures on how to be involved in their child's education, explicitly state expectations during parent-teacher conferences, and enlist the PTA to aim for the inclusion of a variety of cultural representatives in their association.

A family who is not part of the majority culture and does not speak the majority language may not know about these rights and responsibilities, and this can put them at a disadvantage when advocating for their child's education and navigating educational opportunities. Teams could work on explicitly stating cultural practices in the classroom, including having seat assignments, arriving promptly, greeting adults and peers, and participating in school events. Explicitly listing expectations for families can clear up confusion and provide all families with the knowledge and resources to advocate for their children.

6. **Reflection: Contrast this situation with those students for whom English immersion learning is not a choice but their reality. How can professionals advocate for students whose home language and culture are not reflected in their community or school?**

Personal responses may vary. Consider the additional difficulties that a family may encounter when communication and cultural barriers exist between the parents and staff.

TAKE AWAYS

- Although each situation is different, immersion settings are not detrimental to the language development of a child exhibiting a language disorder.
- Parents seeking immersion education for their child should consider the benefit of their child's development as a bilingual speaker and a bicultural person.

REFERENCES

Individuals With Disabilities Education Improvement Act of 2004, Pub. L. 108-446, 20 U.S.C. §§ 1400–1482.

Kay-Raining Bird, E. (2010, May 3). *Bilingualism and children with language and/or cognitive disabilities* [Blog post]. Retrieved from http://blog.bilingualtherapies.com/background-knowledge/bilingualism-and-children-with-language-andor-cognitive-disabilities/

Kohnert, K. (2010). Bilingual children with primary language impairment: Issues, evidence, and implications for clinical actions. *Journal of Communication Disorders, 43,* 456–473.

Lugo-Neris, M. J., Jackson, C. W., & Goldstein, H. (2010). Facilitating vocabulary acquisition of young English language learners. *Language, Speech, and Hearing Services in Schools, 41,* 314–327.

Peña, E. D. (2016). Supporting the home language of bilingual children with developmental disabilities: From knowing to doing. *Journal of Communication Disorders, 63,*

85-92.

Restrepo, M. A., Morgan, G. P., & Thompson, M. S. (2013). The efficacy of a vocabulary intervention for dual-language learners with language impairment. *Journal of Speech, Language, and Hearing Research, 56,* 748-765.

Rivera Pérez, J. F., Creaghead, N. A., Washington, K., Guo, Y., Raisor-Becker, L., & Combs, S. (2019). Using audio prompting to assist monolingual speech-language pathologists to teach English-Spanish vocabulary to English learners. *Communication Disorders Quarterly, 41*(1), 3-11.

Steele, J. L., Slater, R., Zamarro, G., Miller, T., Li, J. J., Burkhauser, S., & Bacon, M. (2017). *Dual-language immersion programs raise student achievement in English.* Retrieved from https://www.rand.org/pubs/research_briefs/RB9903.html

Williams, C. (2017, December 28). The intrusion of White families into bilingual schools. *The Atlantic.* Retrieved from https://www.theatlantic.com/education/archive/2017/12/the-middle-class-takeover-of-bilingual-schools/549278/

Zelasko, N., & Antunez, B. (2000). *If your child learns in two languages: A parent's guide for improving educational opportunities for children acquiring English as a second language.* Washington, DC: National Clearinghouse for Bilingual Education.

Zimmermann, K. A. (2018, March 9). German culture: Facts, customs and traditions. *Live Science.* Retrieved from https://www.livescience.com/44007-german-culture.html

ADDITIONAL RESOURCES

American Speech-Language-Hearing Association. (n.d.-a). *Central auditory processing disorder: Treatment.* Retrieved from https://www.asha.org/PRPSpecificTopic.aspx?folderid=8589943561§ion=Treatment

American Speech-Language-Hearing Association. (n.d.-b). *Learning two languages.* Retrieved from https://www.asha.org/public/speech/development/learning-two-languages/

Bilinguistics. (2019, October 7). *What the law and ASHA say concerning best practice for evaluating bilingual children.* Retrieved from https://bilinguistics.com/evaluating-bilingual-children/

Lowry, L. (n.d.). *Can children with language impairments learn two languages?* Retrieved from http://www.hanen.org/Helpful-Info/Articles/Can-children-with-language-impairments-learn-two-l.aspx

Paradis, J. (2007). Bilingual children with specific language impairment: Theoretical and applied issues. *Applied Psycholinguistics, 28,* 551-564. https://doi.org/10.1017/S0142716407070300

Paradis, J., Genesee, F., & Crago, M. B. (2011). *Dual language development and disorders: A handbook on bilingualism and second language learning.* Baltimore, MD: Brookes.

Thordardottir, E. (2006). Language intervention from a bilingual mindset. *The ASHA Leader, 11*(10), 6-21. https://doi.org/10.1044/leader.FTR1.11102006.6

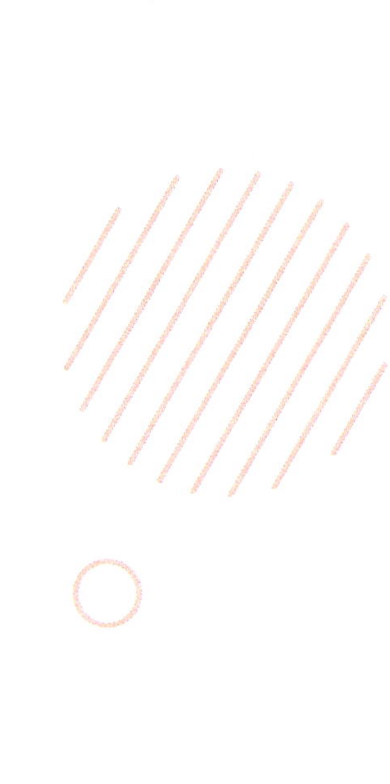

Where Do I Begin?

— Undertaking Language Disorder and Language Difference Interventions in the Classroom

Ivan Campos and Alicia Fleming Hamilton

PREBRIEF

notes:

Dual language learners (DLLs) present with many different levels of mastery in the languages they are exposed to and speak. These language skills can present differently depending on the situation. A student may be comfortable and appear fluent in a social situation but struggle with providing a response to an academic topic in the classroom. Although it is important to identify DLL children who require extra support, it is equally important to understand typical DLL development so as not to over refer this population for special education testing if they are showing patterns of language acquisition that is different from monolingual expectations. Speech-language pathologists (SLPs) play a critical role in identifying "typical" versus "disordered" language behavior and providing support to school teams. This case illustrates a common scenario and discusses several approaches as solutions.

OBJECTIVES

- Refer colleagues to helpful resources on working with DLL students.
- Differentiate, using resources, a language "difference" versus "disorder."

CASE SCENARIO

Miriam is a 13-year-old, seventh-grade student in a general education English classroom. At home, Miriam's parents speak to her and her siblings in Spanish, which is also the language Miriam prefers to use. Her parents reported that she uses well-formed sentences in Spanish, and they have no concerns about her ability to use or understand language. Miriam was born in the United States and attended day care, preschool, and kindergarten programs in English until her family moved back to Mexico during the middle of her first-grade year to take care of family members. Back in Mexico, Miriam received academic instruction in Spanish for 4 years. Her family returned to the United States during the beginning of fifth grade. Miriam has received academic instruction in English since her return to the United States.

In the sixth grade, Miriam was referred to the assessment planning team by her classroom teacher because of language and academic concerns. The team consisted of the special education teacher, the school psychologist, the SLP, the occupational therapist, the social worker, and the physical therapist. She received general education interventions for 8 weeks in English in the areas of reading, writing, and math. Miriam's parents were supportive of the extra help that she was receiving, but they did not express any concerns with Miriam's academic or language abilities when they were asked. Miriam's reading intervention teacher reported that she reads in English at a third-grade level and has difficulty writing a complex sentence in English. In math, she was able to solve age-appropriate math facts, but she has significant difficulty with word problems.

Before entering the seventh grade, her sixth-grade teacher shared concerns about Miriam joining the seventh-grade class. Her concerns included worries about her being able to communicate with peers in English, difficulty "keeping pace" with other students in her class, and the teacher's own lack of access to "Spanish" resources. Now that Miriam has started in seventh grade, her new teacher reports that Miriam does not appear to understand what is said to her and does not initiate conversation with peers or adults. She also reported that Miriam appeared to withdraw from recess and play by herself, and she was very quiet during group work time in the classroom.

After a year of interventions with minimal progress, her classroom teacher referred Miriam for full special education testing toward the end of her seventh-grade year. Special education academic testing was completed by a special education teacher, and psychoeducational testing was completed by a school psychologist in English, without an interpreter. Results from testing indicated that Miriam obtained scores 2 standard deviations below the mean, indicating significant difficulties. Before obtaining speech and language evaluation results, the individualized education plan team was considering the eligibility areas of intellectual disability and specific learning disability for Miriam. After an evaluation completed by the bilingual SLP in both English and Spanish, results indicated low average English language scores and Spanish language scores within the typical or solid average range for a bilingual student. This pattern prompted additional referrals for testing Miriam's academic and cognitive skills in Spanish initiated by the school psychologist and special education teacher. Additional academic and psychoeducational testing was completed, and—along with parent information—it revealed that Miriam was exhibiting average scores in Spanish in the areas of academics and language.

The evaluation team met and reported the conclusions of the evaluation, which stated that Miriam did not meet eligibility for special education services. Miriam's parents were relieved to find out that their child did not have a learning disability. However, the classroom teacher was furious that Miriam did not meet eligibility for special education services and asked, "What am I supposed to do with her? It took you 2 years to even evaluate her and now you're saying she's typical? You can't continue to expect me to teach all these students English, too! I'm not a DLL teacher! Why do we even have special education teams?"

CRITICAL THINKING AND DEBRIEFING QUESTIONS

1. How can you address the classroom teacher's concerns about "teaching students English"?
2. What are some steps to take before a referral to special education for a DLL student?
3. Is it appropriate to complete comprehensive testing in English only when a child is

exposed to multiple languages?

4. Do you believe that Miriam's referral to special education assessment was overdue, or was it timely?
5. As an SLP, how would you explain to the teacher the difference between language disorder and the normal process of mastering a second language?

COMMENTARY

DLLs are characterized by a wide variety of patterns of language acquisition and levels of language mastery. Miriam is an example of a child with early exposure to English who, after a family transition, returned to the United States and demonstrates limited language proficiency in social and academic language.

SLPs should approach assessment of referred DLL students in a systematic way by addressing two basic questions (Cummins, 2008): (1) Is there a clinically significant difference between a child's performance in their primary language versus English in any of the language modalities tested? (2) Is there a discrepancy between basic interpersonal communication skills and cognitive academic language proficiency?

This SLP's findings supported the classroom teacher's observations on Miriam's performance on academic subjects with high language dependency (Aguilar-Mediavilla, Buil-Legaz, Lopez-Penadés, Sánchez Azanza, & Adrover-Roig, 2019). Although the SLP's results were straightforward and conclusive, greater support and guidance may have been provided to the classroom teacher on the process of language acquisition of bilingual children and current services available to support language instruction in the classroom. An empathetic ear by the SLP to reassure the teacher that it is indeed a significant responsibility to work with these children would help ease the teacher's concerns.

Expand Your Knowledge

According to the U.S. Department of Health and Human Services (2017), DLLs are children "who are learning two or more languages at the same time" or children who are "learning a second language while continuing to develop their first language" (p. 1). Although many terms have been used to describe this group of children, DLL is preferred because it is meant to be broader to encompass the other, commonly used terms, including English language learning, multilingual learner, bilingual, minority language children, and children with limited English proficiency. DLL is preferred because it weighs the two languages that a child is learning equally, and it promotes the development of both. This study reported that in 2017, 22% of school-age and 27% of birth to age 5 children in the United States can be categorized as DLL (U.S. Department of Health and Human Services, 2017).

The SLP could also emphasize the teacher's unique role and influence on the student's progress by providing information on how to support DLL students as they master communication in the language of instruction. Including suggestions on how to adjust the length and complexity of the teacher's language when communicating with students to account for their level of language acquisition can help to keep children engaged and allow for their participation in the task. The SLP could also share ideas and strategies on scaffolding to ensure DLL students are supported across interactions. The SLP could encourage bilingualism and biliteracy by promoting the reading of bilingual books and encourage students to create their own bilingual books (Giambo & Szecsi, 2015). The SLP could team with the DLL teachers to work on social groups that may pair children with similar languages together in an effort to provide them with opportunities to use their native language during the school day.

Finally, SLPs, as members of the assessment team, can offer evidenced-based guidance to classroom teachers on the wide range of abilities and needs bilingual students have and the best placement and services to address them.

CRITICAL THINKING AND DEBRIEFING RESPONSES

1. **How can you address the classroom teacher's concerns about "teaching students English"?**

Part of educational state standards include the instruction of Mainstream American English. Given this information, it is the role and responsibility of the classroom teacher to instruct all students in the appropriate use and production of Mainstream American English. Although this teacher may be overwhelmed or frustrated by the additional support DLL students may need, the SLP has an opportunity to provide information and ideas for supporting typically developing DLL students. Additional explanation of the stages of language acquisition and the importance of giving a student time could also be useful in this case to provide the teacher with more context regarding the amount of time it took to complete the referral and evaluation.

2. **What are some steps to take before a referral to special education for a DLL student?**

Appropriate steps would include response to intervention services that target the skills that the student is "lacking." This provides a student with appropriate learning time and intensive instruction, along with multiple data points to determine whether the student can learn the given concepts with extra support. An SLP could also use the dynamic assessment approach to teach skills a student may not have been exposed to, given different schooling environments, and use data to demonstrate whether the student does not know a concept because it has not been taught or because there is something interfering with their ability to learn new language concepts (Roseberry-McKibbin, 2019).

3. **Is it appropriate to complete comprehensive testing in English only when a child is exposed to multiple languages?**

No. Testing should be completed in all languages a student is exposed to, and this is part of federal law for initial evaluations to determine whether a student is eligible for special education services (Individuals With Disabilities Education Improvement Act of 2004). A team may choose to add the following: using a language sample, conducting a dynamic assessment, using an interpreter, approaching the family with an interpreter to obtain case history information, and conducting a language inventory describing the history of a student's language acquisition. They may use standardized assessments in the students' native languages if the constructs or design of the assessments are appropriate and the students are represented in the norming or standardization sample. An introduction to information on best practices for DLL evaluation and intervention by Sheng (2019) cites promising new research regarding nonlinguistic processing tasks as well as robust intervention approaches.

4. **Do you believe that Miriam's referral to special education assessment was overdue, or was it timely?**

Although the teacher in the end of the scenario may have disagreed, the time that Miriam was given to acclimate was appropriate. When working with students who are learning multiple languages, it is essential for special education teams to consider the difference between a language learning need and a true disability. The timeline of this referral seemed appropriate given Miriam's time in the United States since moving back from Mexico. When students have transitions from different schools or even schooling systems, it is best to give them enough time to acclimate to their new environment. Given that there were no concerns when Miriam was previously in the United States, it was appropriate to wait until she completed prereferral interventions. The SLP may want to work with the team in creating and measuring interventions to ensure that they are effective and using best practices to teach targeted concepts. When the results are reviewed, the team can be sure they are reliable when considering the appropriate response to a special education referral.

5. **As an SLP, how would you explain to the teacher the difference between language disorder and the normal process of mastering a second language?**

SLPs have extensive training in the areas of communication, including typical and disordered language development. A benefit of working on a team is collaborating and sharing information. An SLP may choose to share information regarding basic interpersonal communication skills and cognitive academic language proficiency (Baker, 2006) to (a) explain the difference between social communication and academic language learning and (b) discuss the differences in those two skills. SLPs may also use references from websites and other resources to illustrate that bilingualism is fluid—that is, proficiency in either language may vary on the basis of the situation, emotions, topics, and other factors. Additionally, the input and output of language(s) may vary across a student's lifetime. This underscores the importance of looking at all languages a student is exposed to across a variety of tasks.

TAKE AWAYS

- When evaluating students who speak or are exposed to multiple languages, it is critical to evaluate skills in a variety of ways across all the languages they are exposed to. Evaluation tasks should include tasks that describe academic, language, and social skills.
- SLPs have extensive training in typical and disordered language development. This training provides opportunities to serve as resources and to collaborate with classroom teachers and paraprofessionals in learning strategies that can maximize and support the language skills of children who are bilingual.
- Parent input, language acquisition history, and language samples are critical pieces of information in an assessment and provide rich data when evaluating children who are bilingual.

REFERENCES

Aguilar Mediavilla, E., Buil-Legaz, L., Lopez-Penadés, R., Sánchez Azanza, V. A., & Adrover-Roig, D. (2019). Academic outcomes in bilingual children with developmental language disorder: A longitudinal study. *Frontiers in Psychology, 10,* 531.

Baker, C. (2006). *Foundations of bilingual education and bilingualism* (4th ed.). Clevedon, England: Multilingual Matters.

Cummins, J. (2008). BICS and CALP: Empirical and theoretical status of the distinction.

Encyclopedia of Language and Education, 2(2), 71–83.

Giambo, D. A., & Szecsi, T. (2015). Promoting and maintaining bilingualism and biliteracy: Cognitive and biliteracy benefits and strategies for monolingual teachers. *The Open Communication Journal, 9*(Suppl. 1), 56–60.

Individuals With Disabilities Education Improvement Act of 2004, Pub. L. 108-446, 20 U.S.C. §§ 1400–1482.

Roseberry-McKibbin, C. (2019, November 26). Utilizing comprehensive preassessment procedures for differentiating language difference from language impairment in English learners. *Communication Disorders Quarterly.* Advance online publication. https://doi.org/10.1177/1525740119890314

Sheng, L. (2019). Introduction to the forum: Innovations in clinical practice for dual language learners, Part 1. *American Journal of Speech-Language Pathology, 28,* 929–931.

U.S. Department of Health and Human Services. (2017, January 5). *Policy statement on supporting the development of children who are dual language learners in early childhood programs.* Retrieved from https://www.acf.hhs.gov/sites/default/files/ecd/dll_policy_statement_final.pdf

ADDITIONAL RESOURCES

Penn State College of Education. (n.d.). *How can I support ELLs in my classroom?* Retrieved from https://ed.psu.edu/pds/elementary/intern-resources/esl-handbook/supporting-ells

Roseberry-McKibbin, C., & Brice, A. (2000). Acquiring English as a second language. *The ASHA Leader, 5*(12), 4–5, 7.

U.S. Department of Education, Office for Civil Rights. (2003, July 28). *First Amendment: Dear colleague.* Retrieved from https://www2.ed.gov/about/offices/list/ocr/firstamend.html

I Stutter and Have an Accent—Can I Be Your Speech-Language Pathologist? — Clinical Education Approaches to Supervision of Student Clinicians With Speech and Fluency Disorders

Mark Guiberson, Rachel M. Williams, and Alicia Fleming Hamilton

PREBRIEF

notes:

Clinical education and supervision are key components of graduate programs for speech-language pathologists and audiologists. As we strive to make our discipline more diverse, supervisors must be prepared to work with a variety of students who represent many different cultures and abilities. Supervisors must have knowledge of the basic distinctions between dialect, accent, and speech sound disorders. They must also understand how power dynamics play a role across cultures and in the professional preparation of students. When a supervisee exhibits possible characteristics of communication disorders, it is critical to consider the multiple factors at play when providing guidance and training.

OBJECTIVES

- Reflect on your perception of working with professionals who exhibit disabilities.
- Review and understand appropriate American Speech-Language-Hearing Association (ASHA) resources on discrimination and clinical competency.
- Consider how cultural practices may affect a clinician's behavior within the clinician-clinical supervisor relationship.

CASE SCENARIO

Jan is a 24-year-old Asian American male student clinician in his first semester of clinical assignments. Jan traveled to the United States to complete his undergraduate degree in communication sciences and disorders. While studying full time, he maintained contact with his local Chinese community in the United States and relatives at home in China. He is being supervised by a White female supervisor, Professor Thompson. Jan's supervisor is aware that Jan has a fluency disorder because he disclosed this information to her as part of their initial supervisory meeting.

Jan grew up and attended high school in Hong Kong. Since birth, Jan has been exposed to Cantonese and English, both of which he speaks and understands. According to Jan, he began having problems with his speech in early primary school when it was first noticed by his teachers. His teachers shared with his parents that Jan was demonstrating stuttering moments in both English and Cantonese, noting he repeated sounds and words. Jan's parents believed that his stuttering brought shame and embarrassment to the family, and he spent most of his childhood trying to hide his stuttering to make them happy. Because of his family's beliefs and attitudes about his stuttering, Jan was never enrolled in speech services while living in Hong Kong.

At the recommendation of his undergraduate clinical supervisor, Jan was evaluated and received speech-language therapy to address his stuttering. Jan was also asked to consider accent modification to increase his intelligibility. Jan obliged and continued with speech fluency therapy and consultative services for his accent throughout his undergraduate degree program where he excelled as a student. Jan was admitted to a different graduate program to pursue his master's degree in speech and hearing sciences.

During Jan's first semester of clinical practicum, he was assigned a pediatric client, Stephen. Stephen was a second-grade student who was working on improving his literacy skills, including reading fluency and phonemic awareness—specifically, segmentation, blending, and rhyme. During Jan's and Stephen's first therapy session, Jan's clinical supervisor, Professor Thompson, entered the cubicle multiple times to correct Jan's production of English phonemes. After the session was over, Professor Thompson informed Jan that he needed to work on improving the accuracy of his articulation of English sounds before he could resume his clinical sessions with his assigned client. When Jan asked whether there were any online or audio resources to help him, the supervisor encouraged him to research these on his own and to demonstrate more clinical independence. Jan spent the following week practicing phonemes that were not present in his native language but were present in English only in an attempt to decrease his perceived accent.

Jan felt as though he was improving in his English production, but he became very anxious knowing that his supervisor may interrupt his session at any moment. As a result, although Jan's intelligibility increased, so did his dysfluencies. During his next session, Professor Thompson interrupted him after he stuttered, and she modeled a fluency strategy for him in front of his client. She asked Jan to attempt the fluency strategy during the session before he could continue working with his client on the next activity. After the session, Professor Thompson shared that it was important for Jan to maintain fluency during therapy sessions and during his interactions with others in the clinic by applying the specific fluency strategies she modeled to him. Jan, however, had difficulty with consistently implementing these specific modeled fluency strategies, and he felt more comfortable using other strategies he had learned during his previous therapy intervention while an undergraduate. Jan felt unsure of how to proceed. He felt as though he could not decline using the strategies proposed by Professor Thompson because he feared retaliation, either through impact on his clinical grade or progression through the program. At times he felt as though his anxiety and stuttering behaviors actually increased when he was around his supervisor.

His supervisor held a meeting with him and the clinical director. She stated that for Jan to successfully complete the program he must complete ASHA Certification Standard V-A, "Demonstrated Speech and Language Skills in English." She stated that she interprets this standard to mean that Jan must be fluent most of the time and must speak using clear and intelligible diction in Mainstream American English. Jan reported he was incorporating all of the strategies he has learned to his best ability, but he believed that his clinical supervisor's bias will affect his overall grade and put him in jeopardy of not completing his master's program. Jan is conflicted as to whether he can mention this to the director because he does not want to embarrass his supervisor by sharing this information.

CRITICAL THINKING AND DEBRIEFING QUESTIONS

1. How can Jan address the difficulties he is experiencing with his supervisor?
2. What resources are available to clinical supervisors when supporting student clinicians?
3. How might the essential functions developed by the Council of Academic Programs in Communication Sciences and Disorders (CAPCSD) be useful in this case?
4. What can the program do to support Jan if he cannot fluently or accurately produce cues and prompts to support his client?
5. How could Jan's cultural beliefs and traditions affect his supervisory relationship?
6. Reflect on a time when you may have had beliefs and attitudes that influenced your interactions with someone because of their race, ethnicity, sex, gender identity/gender expression, sexual orientation, age, religion, national origin, disability, culture, language, or dialect. What did you do to address those beliefs and attitudes? What are approaches you would take now?

COMMENTARY

Admission to graduate school for audiology and speech-language pathology programs is a highly competitive process, making it difficult to secure a spot. Programs are rigorous and have many highly qualified applicants. Once admitted, students are asked to form working relationships with their assigned supervisors. These relationships have an inherent power differential in which the students depend on their supervisors for instruction in their field and program, guidance, recommendations, and—ultimately—their final grade. The relationship also leaves a student feeling vulnerable because of their lack of knowledge in a field where they require training.

In this particular situation, the power differential creates an expectation for Jan to follow the supervisor's recommendations related to implementation of her suggested fluency and articulation strategies. Although it may be appropriate to expect Jan to model his best speech, including clear articulation and mostly fluent speech, it is unrealistic to expect him to have perfect diction and use of fluency strategies all of the time. Additionally, it may be more appropriate for Jan to use strategies that he is comfortable with implementing or have been more effective for him in the past. The department may want to have a policy and procedure for communication sciences and disorders students who require speech-language services.

Another factor to consider in this relationship dynamic is Jan's cultural values. Jan was raised in Hong Kong, where education holds high value. Part of Jan's Chinese culture involves the adherence to rules and working hard to remove perceived linguistic or cultural barriers so that they can be successful. Teachers are held in high regard, and if a child is successful in school, it brings honor to the entire family (Cheng, 2012). Additionally, Chinese culture has a history of using high-context communication, in which the communication style relies on information that is expressed through physical contexts and inference, with less emphasis placed on direct communication. This contrasts with low-context communication, common in European American culture, in which most of the message lies in the explicit message and values clarity and effectiveness in a communication exchange (Park & Kim, 2008). Religious traditions and values of Confucianism may also influence communication, with a focus on developing and maintaining harmony with others. Communicative exchanges may appear more obliging and avoiding than direct, which is typical of a European American communicative expectation. Perceived status can also play an important role in how people of Chinese heritage communicate. They may use more indirect communication with superiors and not subordinates, possibly to protect the superior from embarrassment or disagreement (Park & Kim, 2008). In reviewing Jan's indirect communication style and hesitancy to challenge his supervisor, he is demonstrating communication patterns more consistent with his cultural upbringing and low-context communication.

This case scenario asks us to consider our own views and beliefs about whether a clinician can be effective if they also exhibit a speech sound disorder, accent, or fluency disorder. As certified professionals, we are guided by ASHA's (2016) *Code of Ethics* to avoid "discriminat[ion] in the delivery of professional services or in the conduct of research and scholarly activities on the basis of race, ethnicity, sex, gender identity/gender expression, sexual orientation, age, religion, national origin, disability, culture, language, or dialect" (Principles of Ethics 1, para. C). We are also told that certified individuals should not engage in any form of harassment, power abuse, or sexual harassment. The *Code of Ethics* is an excellent guidepost for reflection on professional and clinical practices and expectations.

In any supervisory relationship, a supervisor will hold power over their supervisee. This can include the power to delay or deny the completion of a requirement for a program or even the ability to seek employment (ASHA, 2017). In the case of a conflict, there should be clear paths to allow students to express their views without retaliation by including anonymous evaluations or feedback, providing clear evaluation rubrics to reduce subjective judgments, using team supervision, and offering forums or opportunities for students to share any concerns or conflicts without fear of retribution. When you initially read this case study, if you did not observe a power difference, please read it again and reflect on moments when the power imbalance was present, and how it may have affected Jan's actions. Consider Jan's cultural heritage and practices while reviewing.

CRITICAL THINKING AND DEBRIEFING RESPONSES

1. **How can Jan address the difficulties he is experiencing with his supervisor?**

Given Jan's cultural background, it may be difficult for him to directly approach his supervisor regarding her comments and guidance related to his stuttering. Jan may feel more comfortable demonstrating her fluency strategies, even though they didn't work for him, instead of challenging her suggestions. He may also prefer to ask for help outside of the clinic to address his stuttering. It would be helpful if his program outlined a process for addressing disagreements with supervisors. Depending on his level of comfort, he may choose to schedule a private meeting with his supervisor or clinical director to discuss alternative approaches to addressing his fluency needs, such as referrals to other clinical supervisors who would be able to provide intervention while maintaining confidentiality. Jan may also want to address her comments regarding his "accent" and speak to the clinical director about any specific requirements or even supports they may have for Jan so that he can successfully complete his program.

2. **What resources are available to clinical supervisors when supporting student clinicians?**

The program director may consult ASHA's (2011) Professional Issues Statement titled *The Clinical Education of Students With Accents.* This statement contains an overview of literature followed by strategies for supporting students when there are concerns about their accents. Strategies include providing early support, providing an accent modification/intelligibility enhancement plan, avoiding communicating inferiority, being respectful of what the student brings to the profession, focusing on the client's perception of accent, addressing any client concerns regarding a student's accent, choosing external placements with care, promoting the acquisition of self-awareness by students, and encouraging students to seek some outside support and guidance (ASHA, 2011).

This guidance also includes actions for the supervisor. Specifically, the supervisor must avoid communicating to the student that their accented speech is viewed as inferior. The supervisor in this scenario may benefit from evaluating her own beliefs about accented speech and cultural differences and how those beliefs may impact the student's clinical experience. Supervisors should take care when providing feedback to ensure that it is appropriate and culturally sensitive (Bonner, 2014). The supervisor may choose to highlight student's strengths, including their benefit as a bilingual provider and the benefit of time in developing improved skills. The supervisor should be open to learning from the student and may ask them to present information on their native language, accent modification, or another related topic.

University programs would benefit from making grievance procedures highly visible and accessible for students when they need to access them. Jan's history of stuttering and his attempts to decrease his accent should be self-disclosed after acceptance to a program, if he would like reasonable accommodations, but cannot be required. Appropriate and timely disclosure of his fluency disorder is important so that the program may benefit from time to prepare any necessary accommodations. Considerations regarding his accent should be separate from those used to address his fluency disorder. The program director may choose to observe Jan's session to help provide another perspective, especially if Jan feels that his supervisor has a bias toward him.

Supervisors should take care when providing feedback to ensure that it is appropriate and culturally sensitive (Bonner, 2014).

There are differing opinions as to whether to disclose and when to disclose. Disclosure is required to obtain reasonable accommodations. Considerations and responses to concerns related to his accent should be separate from those related to his fluency.

If a student elects not to disclose or to disclose and not seek accommodations, then it should be documented in case there are future concerns.

3. **How might the essential functions developed by the Council of Academic Programs in Communication Sciences and Disorders (CAPCSD) be useful in this case?**

CAPCSD's (n.d.) essential functions were developed to identify the needed foundational knowledge and skills in the discipline. The essential functions serve as guiding principles and are a resource for programs, but they are not a requirement. The essential functions identify core skills and attributes in five areas: communication, motor, intellectual/cognitive, sensory/observational, and behavioral/social. This resource may provide Jan, the clinical director, and his supervisor with opportunities to brainstorm accommodations and modifications to his program by reviewing the core skills and attributes in the five areas

(Horner et al., 2009). Not all programs use the essential functions; some have developed their own, modified those from CAPCSD, or do not have any in place. It is important to note that the list of essential functions does not indicate how or to what degree a student needs to demonstrate the function.

If they are used in this program, the essential functions may provide an opportunity to discuss Jan's speech and fluency disorders in the context of his performance as a practitioner in his program and field (Martin, Johnstone, & Hedrick, 2015).

The rights of students with disabilities are protected by the Americans With Disabilities Act of 1990 (ADA) and Section 504 of the Rehabilitation Act of 1973. The team needs to consult the ADA and work with the University's Office of Disability Services to ensure that Jan is receiving any needed accommodations.

4. **What can the program do to support Jan if he cannot fluently or accurately produce cues and prompts to support his client?**

Suggestions from ASHA's (2011) *The Clinical Education of Students With Accents* include providing support early. This involves notifying clinical supervisors or directors about specific characteristics of a student's accent after they are observed. Supervisors can note difficulties with intelligibility, vocabulary, or grammar and encourage students to keep a notebook of changes that need to be made. Discussion of previous accent modification or therapies should also occur to review whether the student continues to use the strategies, if they were effective, and if a new plan needs to be made. Jan may also benefit from videotaping or audiotaping sessions to review the interaction afterward, minimizing pressure and possible feelings of shame or embarrassment by using an "online" correction. Goals should be clearly outlined, and all parties should note that it may be inappropriate to expect native proficiency (Bonner, 2014).

Definition

CAPCSD's essential functions rubric identifies core skills and attributes in five areas: communication, motor, intellectual/cognitive, sensory/observational, and behavioral/social (Martin et al., 2015).

5. **How could Jan's cultural beliefs and traditions affect his supervisory relationship?**

Jan's cultural background is different from his supervisor's. A review of cultural dimensions demonstrates many instances of dissonance between Jan and his supervisor (ASHA, n.d.). Specific topics include individualism versus collectivism. Jan was raised in a collectivist society where conflict is avoided and harmony is valued. He may not feel comfortable challenging or confronting his supervisor when her actions are affecting his clinical practice. Jan and his supervisor also have a power distance where, in his culture, he was taught to value obedience and to refrain from expressing disagreement or challenging his supervisor. As a result, his supervisor may view his deference as a lack of interest of involvement in his clinical training and have no reason to suspect that he is unhappy with her actions or suggestions. Finally, because of possible internal feelings of embarrassment, guilt, or shame as it relates to his history of stuttering, Jan may feel more pressure to perform and be successful to please his supervisor and family.

6. **Reflect on a time when you may have had beliefs and attitudes that influenced your interactions with someone because of their race, ethnicity, sex, gender identity/gender expression, sexual orientation, age, religion, national origin, disability, culture, language, or dialect. What did you do to address those beliefs and attitudes? What are approaches you would take now?**

Personal response. We suggest reviewing cultural resources and information on developing cultural competence.

TAKE AWAYS

- An individual should not be discriminated against on the basis of race, ethnicity, sex, gender identity/gender expression, sexual orientation, age, religion, national origin, disability, culture, language, or dialect.
- Accented speech is not a speech disorder. Individuals may seek modification of their accent when their intelligibility is reduced.
- Clinical programs should notify students of available accommodations in their training program when there is an applicable disability.
- Clinical educators may refer to ASHA's (2011) *The Clinical Education of Students With Accents* for information on how to support student clinicians exhibiting accented speech.

REFERENCES

American Speech-Language-Hearing Association. (n.d.). *Examples of cultural dimensions.* Retrieved from https://www.asha.org/Practice-Portal/Professional-Issues/Cultural-Competence/Examples-of-Cultural-Dimensions/

American Speech-Language-Hearing Association. (2011). *The clinical education of students with accents.* Retrieved from https://www.asha.org/policy/PI2011-00324/

American Speech-Language-Hearing Association. (2016). *Code of Ethics.* Retrieved from https://www.asha.org/Code-of-Ethics/

American Speech-Language-Hearing Association. (2017). *Issues in ethics: Responsibilities of individuals who mentor clinical fellows in speech-language pathology.* Retrieved from https://www.asha.org/Practice/ethics/Responsibilities-of-Individuals-Who-Mentor-Clinical-Fellows-in-Speech-Language-Pathology/

Americans With Disabilities Act of 1990, Pub. L. 101-336, 42 U.S.C. §§ 12101-12213 (2000).

Bonner, J. (2014). Facilitating clinical success for students with accents. *e-Hearsay, 4*(1), 68–80.

Cheng, L. (2012). Asian and Pacific American languages and cultures. In D. E. Battle (Ed.), *Communication disorders in multicultural and international populations* (4th ed., pp. 37–60). St. Louis, MO: Elsevier.

Council of Academic Programs in Communication Sciences and Disorders. (n.d.). *Essential functions in communication sciences and disorders.* Available from http://www.capcsd.org

Horner, J., Schwarz, I., Jackson, R., Johnstone, P., Mulligan, M., Roberts, K., & Sohlberg, M. M. (2009). Developing an "essential functions" rubric: Purposes and applications for speech-language-hearing academic programs. *Journal of Allied Health, 38*(4), 242–247. https://www.ncbi.nlm.nih.gov/pubmed/20011824

Martin, K., Johnstone, P., & Hedrick, M. (2015). Auditory and visual localization accuracy in young children and adults. *International Journal of Pediatric Otorhinolaryngology, 79*(6), 844–851.

Park, Y. S., & Kim, B. S. (2008). Asian and European American cultural values and communication styles among Asian American and European American college students. *Cultural Diversity and Ethnic Minority Psychology, 14*(1), 47–56.

Rehabilitation Act of 1973, Pub. L. 93-112, 29 U.S.C. §§ 701-7961.

ADDITIONAL RESOURCES

American Speech-Language-Hearing Association. (n.d.). *Clinical education and supervision.* Retrieved from https://www.asha.org/Practice-Portal/Professional-Issues/Clinical-Education-and-Supervision/

American Speech-Language-Hearing Association. (2008). *Clinical supervision in speech-language pathology.* Retrieved from https://www.asha.org/content.aspx?id=10737450495

American Speech-Language-Hearing Association. (2019, February). *Final report: Ad Hoc Committee on Language Proficiency.* Retrieved from https://www.asha.org/uploadedFiles/AHC-Language-Proficiency.pdf

Cheng, L. R. (2007). Codes and contexts: Exploring linguistic, cultural, and social intelligence. *The ASHA Leader, 12*(7), 8–33.

Ip, M. L., St. Louis, K. O., Myers, F. L., & Xue, S. A. (2012). Stuttering attitudes in Hong Kong and adjacent Mainland China. *International Journal of Speech-Language Pathology, 14,* 543–556. https://doi.org/10.3109/17549507.2012.712158

Jackson, R., Johnstone, P., & Mulligan, M. (2008, April). *Essential functions in speech-language pathology.* Paper presented at the annual meeting of the Council of Academic Programs in Communication Sciences and Disorders, Palm Harbor, FL. Retrieved from https://wordpressstorageaccount.blob.core.windows.net/wp-media/wp-content/uploads/sites/1023/2019/06/Essential-Functions-Presentation-2008.pdf

Rose, M. L., & Best, D. L. (Eds.). (2005). *Transforming practice through clinical education, professional supervision, and mentoring.* St. Louis, MO: Elsevier Health Sciences.

Schwarz, I., Horner, J., Jackson, R., Johnstone, P., Mulligan, M., Roberts, K., & Sohlberg, M. (2007). Defining essential functions for a diverse student population: Summary. *Perspectives on Issues in Higher Education, 10*(2), 6.

Speech Pathology Graduate Programs. (n.d.). *Do you speak with an accent? . . . You can still be an outstanding SLP.* Retrieved from https://www.speechpathologygraduateprograms.org/do-you-speak-with-an-accent-you-can-still-be-an-outstanding-slp/

Sudler, K. (2012). *Accent, attitudes, and the speech-language pathologist.* Retrieved from https://scholarworks.wm.edu/honorstheses/491/

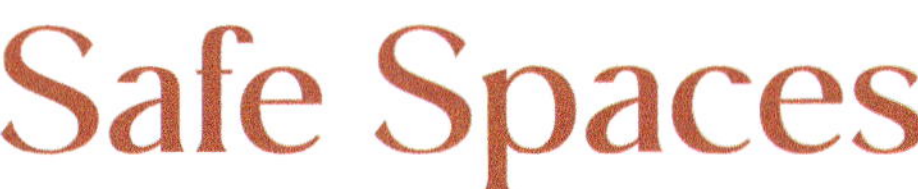

Safe Spaces

— Creating an Inclusive Environment for Gender Diverse Individuals

CARMEN ANA RAMOS-PIZARRO

PREBRIEF

notes:

Gender diverse populations may seek gender-affirming speech-language services to achieve a more authentic voice that better aligns with their gender identity or internal knowledge of their self (American Speech-Language-Hearing Association [ASHA], n.d..). Speech-language pathologists (SLPs) who work with this population will benefit from training to help them communicate with their clients using sensitive and culturally appropriate language within a lesbian, gay, bisexual, transgender, and other gender diverse identities (LGBT+) friendly environment (Hancock & Haskin, 2015). Gender diverse individuals feel that their gender identity is not in congruence with traditional, binary ideas of masculinity and femininity. Consequently, they feel using binary pronouns (i.e., he/him and she/her) when referring to themselves does not adequately align with their personal sense of gender. Instead, these individuals may feel that gender-neutral pronouns (them/their or others such as zi, hir, and xe) better reflect their gender identity (Lesbian, Gay, Bisexual, Transgender, Queer Plus Resource Center at University of Wisconsin-Milwaukee, n.d.). The following case explores how personnel in a voice clinic worked to fully support a client who identified as gender nonbinary. The use of the pronouns them/theirs throughout the writing is intentional in response to the client's request.

OBJECTIVES

- Explain the concept of gender as a continuum and how it may influence gender identity.
- Enumerate at least three ways a culturally responsive SLP may modify clinic procedures to make them more compliant with Safe Space recommendations.
- Explain the various ways a gender diverse individual may incorporate voice changes as part of their evolving gender expression.

CASE SCENARIO

Gender diverse individuals may use gender-neutral pronouns that better align with their gender identity. This is the case of Samantha, a 26-year-old gender-nonconforming individual who contacted a private voice clinic to inquire about their advertised gender-af-

Definitions

The following definitions are drawn from multiple advocacy resources and are intended as guide for the reader:

Gender fluid, gender nonconforming, gender nonbinary, or gender diverse–Terms used sometimes interchangeably to describe individuals who define their gender outside of the culturally established binaries of male versus female.

Cisfemale/cismale–Individuals who identify with the sex they were assigned at birth.

Transgender–An umbrella term to include individuals whose gender identity does not correspond to the gender assigned at birth. For example, transfeminine people identify as female but were assigned male at birth. Trans individuals may or may not seek additional interventions to reach better congruence between their gender identity and their primary and secondary sex characteristics.

Gender identity–A person's sense of being male, female, neither, or somewhere along a continuum. A person's gender identity does not always align with the sex that was assigned at birth.

Gender expression–External expressions of gender that include behavior, clothing, speech patterns, nonverbal communication, and gender roles. An individual's gender expression may or may not conform to society's expectations of male versus female genders.

Gendered pronouns–On the basis of binary male/female point of view–for example, he/him/his versus she/her/hers.

Authentic self–A phrase that captures each gender-diverse individual's true sense of themselves as opposed to what others' perceptions might be.

Gender-neutral pronouns or gender-inclusive pronouns–Pronouns that align with each individual's authentic self and not necessarily with the sex assigned at birth. Examples of gender-neutral pronouns include them/their and others used less frequently, such as zi, hir, and xe.

Misgendering–When an incorrect pronoun is used to refer to a gender diverse individual on the basis of gender expression or physical characteristics, such as facial hair or voice.

LGBT+–Lesbian, gay, bisexual, transgender, and other gender diverse identities that are abbreviated by some groups using the plus (+) and include queer or questioning, intersex, asexual, among others.

firming communication services. Samantha let the clinic staff know that they would like to be addressed by their chosen name, not their legal name, which was masculine, and requested the use of the pronouns "they, them, and theirs." Initially, this created some confusion for the clinic staff who consistently referred to the client using "she," a gendered pronoun that was consistent with her feminine name, when discussing clinical issues during supervisory meetings and in written communications. Although not intentional, these instances of misgendering were not in alignment with the client's wishes and could have been offensive to Samantha. On one occasion, Robert, the clinic's administrative assistant, misgendered Samantha while they were present, and he did not immediately realize his mistake. Although Samantha did not correct Robert, they crossed their arms and seemed to visibly distance themselves from the interaction.

During Samantha's initial intake interview, they shared that seeking gender affirming voice or communication services was one of the first steps in their journey of gender affirmation, and they wanted to rely on the guidance of a trained SLP to help them through it. Samantha shared that they were assigned male at birth. They elected to use gender nonspecific or androgynous clothing, jewelry, and hairstyles with the clear intent to avoid denoting binary genders (i.e., cisfemale or cismale). Samantha wanted to have options to express their voice with more typically feminine voice characteristics in select situations, including when they socialized with transgender women. Samantha was specifically interested in exploring voice therapy techniques to produce a higher pitch and wider pitch range.

Samantha's clinician targeted the exploration of higher pitches through pitch glides and the selection of a target pitch that would best convey the desire of the client to develop (a) the flexibility to sound more or less feminine given their communication partners and communicative situations and (b) a more frontal resonance consistent with patterns observed in cisfemales. Samantha attended only three sessions and appreciated the opportunity to explore their voice's capabilities.

After Samantha's intervention concluded, the clinic staff held a meeting to discuss instances in which they had not effectively served their client and set goals to make their office more welcoming and inclusive for the LGBT+ community in general. A Safe Space training for the clinic was organized (e.g., Campus Pride, n.d.). This workshop provided an opportunity for all clinicians and staff to learn basic concepts related to the gender identities of LGBT+ individuals and their needs. The Safe Space training also explored the concepts of prejudice, bias, and privilege related to working with the LGBT+ population as well as how to provide a welcoming space in the clinic for LGBT+ individuals.

During the training, the clinicians and office staff completed a thorough evaluation of clinical procedures and practices and, in conjunction with the Safe Space trainers, generated a list of recommendations to make the clinic more inclusive and welcoming. The clinic adopted policies that stated verbal and written communications were expected to consistently agree with expressed client wishes, including pronoun identification. Additionally, other administrative changes were instituted, such as updated questionnaires and intake forms, scripts for the receptionist, guidelines for all clinic documentation including submissions and billing to insurance companies, and a process to verify the name to use for official paperwork.

CRITICAL THINKING AND DEBRIEFING QUESTIONS

1. **Did reading about this scenario make you feel confused or uncomfortable? Have you worked with this population before?**
2. **What ideas about gender does this scenario challenge?**
3. **How might personal beliefs related to gender impact or influence service delivery?**
4. **What are potential challenges when adopting the use of the pronoun "they" and "theirs" or other nongendered pronouns?**
5. **What were positive changes that occurred as a result of seeing this client in the voice clinic?**
6. **Which, if any, of the changes listed above would you consider implementing in your own practice?**

COMMENTARY

Gender-affirming communication therapy offers a unique opportunity to create a partnership between an SLP and a transgender or gender diverse client and to provide support in their journey to achieve congruence (World Professional Association for Transgender Health, 2011).

Although general awareness of the needs of LGBT+, gender diverse, and transgender individuals has increased over the last decade, studies show that more work is needed by SLPs to improve their knowledge and skills to serve the needs of these populations (Hancock & Haskin, 2015; Ramos-Pizarro, Alcaraz, Piñeiro-Valentín, & Cortés-Vélez, 2018). This scenario reveals a critical aspect of service delivery related to best practices when working with the gender diverse population: pronoun use. Samantha had expressed their wish to be addressed with the pronouns "they/them," which better reflected their current identity. When Samantha was misgendered, whether it was intentional or unintentional, they may have perceived it as a microaggression. Samantha was placed in an uncomfortable position by staff. Ideally, Robert should have addressed his mistake with a brief apology and the use of more intentional language going forward. Further reflection on his actions and

Definition

Microaggressions are brief, subtle, intentional or unintentional, verbal, or environmental indignities that indicate the presence of bias. These microaggressions may elicit emotional reactions of anger, betrayal, distress, hopelessness, and exhaustion as well as feelings of being invalidated and misunderstood (Nadal, Davidoff, Davis, & Wong, 2014).

the identification of any conscious or unconscious bias could help Robert to improve his future practices and prevent further microaggressions (Marcelin, Siraj, Victor, Kotadia, & Maldonado, 2019). By following up with Robert and providing staff education, the clinic personnel took effective action with steps to address the concern of misgendering and to identify the need for additional training.

Safe Space training has been described as a structured, well-defined endeavor to provide background information on gender terminology, LGBT+ culture, and the specific health care or educational needs of the transgender and gender diverse community (Campus Pride, n.d.). In-person workshops may also provide opportunities for participants to practice their communication strategies with transgender or gender diverse individuals. Ideally, communication sciences and disorders specialists should seek Safe Space training from individuals familiar with their specialty area who individualize the content to their clinical setting. All aspects involving client interactions—from intake phone calls, surveys, and questionnaires to written and verbal professional communication and reports—may be evaluated for best practices. Clinical staff in this scenario correctly targeted the many instances in which sex information was requested on their clinical paperwork and replaced it with data on gender.

The clinician who worked with Samantha was trained in voice techniques to work not only an elevation of the pitch and range but also in recognizing that targeting a frontal resonance would add additional gender cues to the voice. Other communication areas—such as vocabulary, written communication style and word choice, nonverbal mannerism, and nonvocal productions that could provide cues for gender—were not addressed in therapy on the basis of the client's choice (Davies, Papp, & Antoni, 2015). There are many resources available online to help a clinician learn more about the service delivery needs and options available for this population. Clinicians desiring to work with gender diverse individuals who feel their mastery of basic skills is at novice level are encouraged to seek mentoring from experienced clinicians in their community, local universities, or ASHA's Special Interest Groups (Special Interest Group 3: Voice and Upper Airway Disorders).

Evolving characterizations of gender are prompting a reevaluation of those aspects that define a person's gender identity. It is within our scope of practice as SLPs to provide gender-affirming communication therapy that will assist gender diverse and transgender people in finding alignment between their voice and their own gender identity.

Clinicians can structure their clinical environment and interview processes to allow for these conversations to happen in a welcoming setting. According to ASHA's (2016) *Code of Ethics,* SLPs are required to provide culturally and linguistically competent service. If unsure of correct terminology or what is culturally appropriate with this population, clinicians may consider seeking out training to prepare them to address the needs of an often discriminated against and vulnerable population. With the help of appropriate resources, and cultural humility, it is possible for clinicians to provide sensitive, high-quality care.

CRITICAL THINKING AND DEBRIEFING RESPONSES

1. **Did reading about this scenario make you feel confused or uncomfortable? Have you worked with this population before?**

If this is the first time you have read about gender diverse individuals and their communication needs, it might prompt a variety of feelings. The purpose of this case scenario is to encourage personal reflection on the subject.

2. **What ideas about gender does this scenario challenge?**

This scenario challenges culturally reinforced binary gender constructs and accepts that gender reflects a more inclusive continuum extending beyond just male or female.

It also challenges assumptions that are made regarding gender on the basis of voice, communication, hairstyle, clothing, and other forms of gender expression. Finally, it brings to light how binary gender representation is prevalent across all aspects of organizational systems, including office administrative protocol and even traditional grammatical patterns (i.e., pronoun use).

3. **How might personal beliefs related to gender impact or influence service delivery?**

Personal beliefs guide personal ethics. Practitioners should evaluate whether their beliefs are compatible with the decision to provide gender-affirming voice therapy. Part of the decision-making process perhaps could include seeking additional training on LGBT+ cultural background knowledge, health needs, and disparities as well as seeking mentorship from more experienced clinicians on professional aspects. If, after deliberate thought, clinicians find that the degree of dissonance is too great to personally engage in clinical practice with this population, they should refer clients to other professionals who would be able to provide competent services (Hancock & Haskin, 2015).

More importantly, ASHA's (2016) *Code of Ethics* provides explicit guidance on the need to avoid discrimination in the practice and provision of clinical services to all individuals seeking our help. Intentional misgendering and use of incorrect names or pronouns hinder the clinical partnership by affecting the productive therapeutic environment.

4. **What are potential challenges when adopting the use of the pronoun "they" and "theirs" or other nongendered pronouns?**

The use of nongendered pronouns may be unfamiliar for both clinicians and administrative staff. However, it is important to respect a client's wishes regarding their pronouns. If you do misgender a client in their presence or when speaking with a colleague, correct yourself as soon as possible, offer a brief apology, and continue your conversation. Be mindful not to over apologize or put the individual in a position to reassure you. The best apology is to learn from your mistake. Cultural responsiveness is a process, and recognizing your mistake is a sign that you are committed to the process. If you find that misgendering and other microaggressions are occurring in your presence, ensure that you signal the error, promoting best nondiscriminatory language in your workplace. Consider whether further discussion is merited with the individual(s) at a later time.

5. **What were positive changes that occurred as a result of seeing this client in the voice clinic?**

Several positive changes were instituted in this scenario, including the scheduling of a Safe Space training with administrative staff and revising telephone scripts and intake questionnaires in accordance with systematic recommendations to guide everyday decision making. Other environmental modifications that could be considered may include making gender neutral bathrooms available, having the clinic's nondiscrimination policy prominently displayed in the waiting room along with a Safe Space sign, and evaluating artwork or reading material that is displayed for explicitly or implicitly represented gendered messages.

Clinicians can seek out further information through continuing education, ASHA's Special Interest Groups, and working with more experienced professionals. In university training facilities, it rests on supervisors and faculty to provide clinical training for student clinicians that includes concepts related to cultural responsiveness and cultural competence related to LGBT+ populations, modeling the use of inclusive language, and opportunities for implicit bias identification.

6. **Which, if any, of the changes listed above would you consider implementing in your own practice?**

It is recommended that clinicians become informed on the antidiscrimination policies at their workplace before implementing Safe Space recommendations. Nonetheless, the practice of inquiring for pronouns is easily incorporated into exchanges with clients and their families. Being open to changes in clinical practice—in an effort to maximize patient relationships and comfort, along with personal reflection regarding our own beliefs—are key pieces to culturally responsive practices.

TAKE AWAYS

- As you evaluate the quality of the services you provide to gender diverse populations, expand your view to include administrative and clinical processes. Corroborate that all documentation as well as scripts comply with preferred practices.
- Share that you are an ally of the LGBT+ community by displaying a Safe Space banner that will let everyone know your practices support them.
- Discuss with your client their expectations regarding treatment; do not assume all LGBT+ clients will seek the same goals.
- Be respectful of boundaries and only ask questions that are pertinent to the treatment you are providing.
- Seek additional training opportunities to improve on your knowledge and skills to partner with your gender diverse clients to achieve a more authentic voice and communication.

REFERENCES

American Speech-Language-Hearing Association. (n.d.). *Voice and communication services for transgender and gender diverse populations.* Retrieved from https://www.asha.org/Practice-Portal/Professional-Issues/Transgender-Gender-Diverse-Voice-and-Communication/

American Speech-Language-Hearing Association. (2016). *Code of Ethics.* Retrieved from https://www.asha.org/Code-of-Ethics/

Campus Pride. (n.d.). *Online Safe Space training.* Retrieved from https://www.campuspride.org/safespace/onlinesafespace/

Davies, S., Papp, V. G., & Antoni, C. (2015). Voice and communication change for gender nonconforming individuals: Giving voice to the person inside. *International Journal of Transgenderism, 16*(3), 117–159. https://doi.org/10.1080/15532739.2015.1075931

Hancock, A., & Haskin, G. (2015). Speech-language pathologists' knowledge and attitudes regarding lesbian, gay, bisexual, transgender, and queer (LGBTQ) populations. *American Journal of Speech-Language Pathology, 24,* 206–221. https://doi.org/10.1044/2015_ajslp-14-0095

Lesbian, Gay, Bisexual, Transgender, Queer Plus Resource Center at University of Wisconsin-Milwaukee. (n.d.). *Gender pronouns.* Retrieved from https://uwm.edu/lgbtrc/support/gender-pronouns/

Marcelin, J. R., Siraj, D. S., Victor, R., Kotadia, S., & Maldonado, Y. A. (2019). The impact of unconscious bias in healthcare: How to recognize and mitigate it. *The Journal of Infectious Diseases, 220*(Suppl. 2), S62–S73. https://doi.org/10.1093/infdis/jiz214

Nadal, K. L., Davidoff, K. C., Davis, L. S., & Wong, Y. (2014). Emotional, behavioral, and cognitive reactions to microaggressions: Transgender perspectives. *Psychology of Sexual Orientation and Gender Diversity, 1*(1), 72–81. https://doi.org/10.1037/sgd0000011

Ramos-Pizarro, C. A., Alcaraz, L., Piñeiro-Valentín, L., & Cortés-Vélez, A. (2018, November). *Barriers to access voice transition services faced by transgender individuals in Puerto Rico: SLPs' perspective.* Poster presented at the American Speech-Language-Hearing Association Convention, Boston, MA.

World Professional Association for Transgender Health. (2011). *Standards of care for the health of transsexual, transgender, and gender nonconforming people* (7th version). Retrieved from https://www.wpath.org/media/cms/Documents/Web%20Transfer/SOC/Standards%20of%20Care%20V7%20-%202011%20WPATH.pdf

ADDITIONAL RESOURCES

Adler, R. K., Hirsch, S., & Pickering, J. (2018). *Voice and communication therapy for the transgender/gender diverse client: A comprehensive clinical guide* (3rd ed.). San Diego, CA: Plural Publishing.

American Speech-Language-Hearing Association. (n.d.-a). *Providing transgender voice services.* Retrieved from https://www.asha.org/Practice/multicultural/Providing-Transgender-Transsexual-Voice-Services/

American Speech-Language-Hearing Association. (n.d.-b). *Special Interest Group 3, Voice and Upper Airway Disorders.* Retrieved from https://www.asha.org/SIG/03/

Bennett, J. (2016, January 30). She? Ze? They? What's in a gender pronoun. *The New York Times.* Retrieved from https://www.nytimes.com/2016/01/31/fashion/pronoun-confusion-sexual-fluidity.html

Gender Spectrum. (n.d.). *Understanding gender.* Retrieved from https://www.genderspectrum.org/quick-links/understanding-gender/

GLAAD. (2016, October). *GLAAD media reference guide* (10th ed.). Retrieved from http://www.glaad.org/sites/default/files/GLAAD-Media-Reference-Guide-Tenth-Edition.pdf

Hancock, A. B. (2015). The role of cultural competence in serving transgender populations. *Perspectives on Voice and Voice Disorders, 25*(1), 37–42. https://doi.org/10.1044/vvd25.1.37

Human Rights Campaign. (n.d.). *Sexual orientation and gender identity definitions.* Retrieved from https://www.hrc.org/resources/sexual-orientation-and-gender-identity-terminology-and-definitions

McLemore, K. A. (2014). Experiences with misgendering: Identity misclassification of transgender spectrum individuals. *Self and Identity, 14*(1), 51–74. https://doi.org/10.1080/15298868.2014.950691

Multicultural Constituency Groups (MCCGs) https://www.asha.org/practice/multicultural/opportunities/constituency/

PFLAG. (2019, July). *PFLAG national glossary of terms.* Retrieved from https://pflag.org/glossary

Self-Treatment in Adult Fluency Disorders — The Tip of the Iceberg

Jean Franco Rivera Pérez

PREBRIEF

notes:

This scenario discusses different ways dysfluency may be perceived across cultures. It also highlights the emotional aspects of stuttering and how speech-language pathologists (SLPs) can address those feelings of embarrassment and shame during treatment and counseling. The scenario presents sociocultural and religious views that may impact treatment. As you read, consider your thoughts about how this client attempted to "manage" his stuttering and reflect on whether you would address those alternative management techniques in your practice.

OBJECTIVES

- Understand the emotional aspects of stuttering and how they may be different across languages and cultures.
- Identify the importance of assessing a client in all languages they use.
- Review treatment tools that target the multifaceted needs of a person who stutters and, if necessary, identify the need for outside referral sources.

CASE SCENARIO

Mobuto is a 28-year-old male who was seen in a private clinic for a fluency evaluation. Mobuto is multilingual, speaking French, Lingala, and English. He grew up in the Democratic Republic of the Congo (DRC). On the basis of Mobuto's intake interview, his native or primary languages are Lingala and French, and he uses a combination of both to communicate with his family, and uses English in his community and work setting. Mobuto's parents still live in the DRC, and he currently resides with his brother and niece in the United States. There is no family history of stuttering reported. Mobuto mentioned that his family does not know he attends therapy for stuttering because he does not want them to know that stuttering affects his life so drastically.

Mobuto learned how to read and write English when he was 16 years old and living in the DRC. He used English in school but primarily spoke French and Lingala in his community. Mobuto increased his use of English when he moved to the United States to attend a graduate program. He is currently attending a university where he is completing his third year in a doctoral program in physics. Mobuto reported he was not as concerned about his stuttering while residing in his home country because it seemed more common there, so he felt more confident in speaking situations in which he might have stuttered (e.g., Gillespie & Cooper, 1973). In fact, people rarely noticed or commented on his stuttering in the DRC. Mobuto reported experiencing disfluencies in all three of the languages he speaks, but he noted that they seem to occur more frequently in French and English.

Mobuto has been in the United States for 4 years, and he continues to feel self-conscious about his speech. He reports feeling anxious in speaking situations and, as a result, avoids speaking to others and in groups. He shared that his stuttering increases during public speaking situations, and he is worried that his stuttering may affect his grade on an upcoming presentation for his doctoral program. Mobuto described his stutters as "holding sounds and repeating words."

After a detailed background history, Mobuto is assessed using perceptual rating scales and an analysis of conversational speech in each language with the help of both French and Lingala interpreters. His speech in all languages exhibited disfluencies, including part-word repetitions, prolongations, and tense pauses consistent with diagnostic criteria for fluency disorder (American Psychiatric Association, 2013). A bilingual clinician conversed with Mobuto in French and confirmed that he used interjections and prolongations and spoke with a rapid rate. Analysis of Mobuto's conversational speech revealed a fluency disorder with moderate severity rating across languages. Mobuto and the SLP discussed his results. The SLP asked whether he had any feelings he associated with stuttering. Mobuto shared that he typically feels nervous, embarrassed, and ashamed and that his quality of life is significantly affected by his stuttering. These feelings of anxiety and shame have increased since he has lived in the United States.

After his evaluation, Mobuto agreed to attend therapy once a week for an hour. English conversational speech was targeted in intervention because this was the language Mobuto had the most difficulty with and needed for his work, and there were no bilingual SLPs available for therapy. Treatment focused on decreasing Mobuto's overall self-perception of stuttering and associated feelings of stress and anxiety through the use of cognitive-behavioral therapy (Menzies, Onslow, Packman, & O'Brian, 2009). Fluency shaping techniques (easy onset) and voluntary stuttering were also used in therapy. Mobuto was coached to create and use a self-disclosure statement regarding his stuttering. Because he was taking a course in which he often had to give presentations, the clinician targeted communication skills—including rate of speech, body language, pitch, and volume—that would be helpful during his presentations.

During therapy, the clinician noted that Mobuto disclosed the following avoidance behaviors: avoiding peers, not going to restaurants, and not talking when running errands. Mobuto said that he chose his current career because it did not require much speaking, although he's not passionate about his field of study. Mobuto reported that he drinks alcohol "every day" to "relax himself" because he feels great amounts of anxiety. Mobuto says that he thinks the alcohol helps him relax and makes his speech more fluent. Additionally, Mobuto talked about attending different healing services in an effort to "cure" his stuttering.

At the end of his semester in treatment, Mobuto met and surpassed his goal of utilizing a self-disclosure statement with unfamiliar listeners in the clinical environment. He noted he wanted to use his self-disclosure at the beginning of his academic presentations and in restaurants and grocery stores. Mobuto reported increased confidence across multiple rating scales. Observations of his social interactions demonstrated improvements in his communication skills and advancement in his self-perception of people who stutter. Mobuto did not feel comfortable using easy onsets or voluntary stuttering, stating that they made him uncomfortable because they did not "feel natural" and that it was likely he would not use these strategies outside the therapy setting. An analysis of Mobuto's speech samples at the end of the semester yielded a mild severity rating, whereas Mobuto continued to rate the impact of stuttering on his life as moderate. The clinician addressed Mobuto's self-reported alcohol use and, with his permission, referred him to other professionals, including substance abuse counselors, to create an integrated plan to help meet his needs.

CRITICAL THINKING AND DEBRIEFING QUESTIONS

1. **How would you assess the fluency skills of a client who speaks a language that is less prevalent in the United States, such as Lingala?**
2. **What factors may have been initially overlooked during assessment? What important details became more apparent during treatment? Was there a way to learn about these details during the intake process, or was it better to have them revealed after the clinician and client developed rapport?**
3. **Would it be necessary to address Mobuto's attendance at healing services as a means to "cure" his fluency disorder? If so, how would you approach this with cultural sensitivity?**

COMMENTARY

This case illustrates the many factors involved when working with a client who presents with a fluency disorder. Fluency disorders impact both a client's daily communications and their overall quality of life.

Mobuto did not grow up in the United States and had different perspectives on the causes and treatments of fluency disorders. He reported that his fluency disorder wasn't as big of a problem for him in the DRC because many people there presented with speech disorders, and it seemed as though it was something that the community just accepted. This statement seemed to be in contrast to his desire to keep his fluency disorder and treatment from his family because he did not want them to know how much his stuttering affected his life. Per his disclosure, his feelings of anxiety and shame affected his relationship with his family and his ability to openly seek help. The complex emotions surrounding his stuttering were an important aspect to address during therapeutic sessions to better understand the true impact that stuttering had on all areas of his life.

Mobuto reported feeling less anxious about his stuttering while in the DRC. This could have been for a variety of reasons. Perhaps it was more acceptable or commonplace there, perhaps he was more comfortable speaking in French and Lingala and felt more fluent as a result, or perhaps he felt less pressure living in a culture he was familiar with. Additionally, Mobuto was enrolled in a competitive graduate program that required frequent presentations, something he was not aware of, adding more pressure to his speech and elevating his levels of anxiety. These feelings further increased the demands on his communication skills. With little family or community support, Mobuto turned to self-medication (alcohol) to relieve his anxiety.

All of these factors are important when helping a client to learn strategies that will help their overall communication.

Although it is important to focus on strategies that are specific to disfluencies, it is also important to focus on behaviors and strategies outside of the clinic that the client can use to decrease feelings of anxiety and shame. Particularly in this case, some behaviors were helpful, such as going to healing ceremonies, and some were not, such as Mobuto's substance misuse. Creating a positive, open client-clinician relationship may provide a space for clients to share the strong feelings that may accompany a communication disorder. Luterman (2017) identified several characteristics of effective counseling. The competent SLP—in the role of counselor—is genuine, and the client experiences a mutually respectful, nonjudgmental attitude and unconditional positive regard in the therapeutic relationship. The counselor yields power to the client, who establishes their own goals for work and thus retains the responsibility to effect change in their own life. In the safety of this supportive atmosphere, the client can risk the expression of difficult feelings, being free to express emotions, including loss, anxiety, anger, and shame. Acknowledging these feelings allows the client to use cognition to guide their behavior to make more adaptive choices. In this case, the client's beliefs and goals were the focus through the assessment and therapy, and although the client continued to rate his stuttering as moderate, by focusing on adaptive behavior and strategies, he was able to participate more fully in his career and social life.

CRITICAL THINKING AND DEBRIEFING RESPONSES

1. **How would you assess the fluency skills of a client who speaks a language that is less prevalent in the United States, such as Lingala?**

Lingala is a tonal language and is spoken primarily in the DRC. During his language history, Muboto noted he grew up speaking both French and Lingala and then learned English as an adolescent. He reported more difficulty with English, and because of the demands of his graduate program and occupation, it would be appropriate to target his therapy in English. During the initial evaluation, it was apparent that Mobuto's disfluencies were present in all of the languages he used per observation and his interview. In a fluency assessment, if the client speaks more than one language, disfluencies will persist across all languages a client speaks, although they may present differently (Lim, Lincoln, Chan, & Onslow, 2008).

During the assessment process, it may have been valuable to look into the perception of stuttering in the DRC before the initial intake appointment. Having information regarding Muboto's cultural experiences before his first clinic visit may have helped to open up the conversation to discussing cultural beliefs about stuttering. The clinician may have shared information about successful professionals in the United States who stutter, attempting to help with any feelings of shame or stigma and to demonstrate positive instances of stuttering in the United States.

2. **What factors may have been initially overlooked during assessment? What important details became more apparent during treatment? Was there a way to learn about these details during the intake process, or was it better to have them revealed**

after the clinician and client developed rapport?

A factor that became apparent during treatment was Mobuto's self-report of drinking alcohol to "improve his fluency and decrease his anxiety." Although it would have been useful to know about Mobuto's substance use at the beginning of his treatment session, he may have felt uncomfortable providing this information initially because of the cultural difference between Mobuto and his clinician (Bradshaw & Randolph, 2016). Once known, this information provided the clinician with further insight regarding the high anxiety that Mobuto felt while stuttering, his perceptions of strategies that helped to increase his fluency, and the need for possible referrals to outside professionals.

If a client speaks more than one language, disfluencies will persist across all languages a client speaks, although they may present differently (Lim, Lincoln, Chan, & Onslow, 2008).

Given the information he shared regarding feelings of shame and embarrassment surrounding his stuttering, the clinician may consider adding an anxiety rating scale to the intake forms. These scales could be used as data points on the efficacy of treatment and provide opportunities to talk with a client about their anxiety and what tools or strategies they may use to manage it. The clinician may also consider adding a question about beliefs or practices that the client feels may "help" their stuttering. The addition of these tools to the intake interview may have provided opportunities for further disclosure of Mobuto's substance use, visits to healing ceremonies, and other cultural beliefs regarding stuttering and its treatment.

Another successful component of creating a client-clinician relationship is the cultivation of interpersonal soft skills. Soft skills are associated with increased professional success (Shollenbarger, 2019). Working on these soft skills can help the clinician in the future to enhance clinical interactions and job performance, creating stronger client relationships and, hopefully, improved treatment outcomes.

3. **Would it be necessary to address Mobuto's attendance at healing services as a means to "cure" his fluency disorder? If so, how would you approach this with cultural sensitivity?**

Addressing all practices meant to "cure" or decrease stuttering should be addressed in therapy. If a specific technique provides a way for the client to decrease their anxiety, shame, or other negative emotions surrounding stuttering, and does not cause harm, it may be appropriate to explore these as supplemental activities for the client. In this case, it was important to maintain sensitivity toward Mobuto's beliefs. This included his choice to attend healing services. During their therapy sessions, the clinician offered Mobuto literature and resources that discussed the causes of stuttering and also described other cultures' beliefs regarding stuttering and speech impediments. For example, in some Latino cultures, the "mal de ojo" may be the cause of a person's stutter. This occurs when someone gives a person (generally a child) the "evil eye," which can later affect their overall health (Bayles & Katerndahl, 2009). Although the clinician did not encourage attendance at the healings, the clinician found no professional reason to discourage his attendance. Other behaviors—including drinking alcohol to make his speech more "fluent"—were viewed as detrimental to Mobuto's health and addressed accordingly.

Definition

Soft skills—a "combination of interpersonal skills, emotional intelligence, and personal attributes [that] include work ethic, professionalism, courtesy, initiative, and communication" (Shollenbarger, 2019, para. 3).

TAKE AWAYS

- Clients may exhibit differing patterns and levels of severity of stuttering across languages. This underscores the importance of assessing each language that a client speaks to obtain an accurate picture of the severity and types of disfluencies presented.
- Cultural beliefs surrounding disability and its etiologies are important in framing the impact of a disability for a client. It is important to discuss these beliefs and provide culturally appropriate education regarding the etiology of communication disorders. It can also be beneficial to illustrate members of the community who have communication disorders and who are achieving their goals or are viewed as "successful."
- Understanding the socioemotional impact of stuttering on a client can help a clinician determine the best course of treatment, including projected impact of treatment, level of support from family and community, and the cultural attitudes surrounding disclosure of a fluency disorder.

REFERENCES

American Psychiatric Association. (2013). *Diagnostic and statistical manual of mental disorders* (5th ed.). Arlington, VA: American Psychiatric Publishing.

Bayles, B. P., & Katerndahl, D. A. (2009). Culture-bound syndromes in Hispanic primary care patients. *The International Journal of Psychiatry in Medicine, 39*(1), 15–31.

Bradshaw, J. L., & Randolph, C. C. (2016). Multiple perspectives in counseling for culturally and linguistically diverse populations. *eHearsay, 6*(2), 4–15.

Gillespie, S. K., & Cooper, E. B. (1973). Prevalence of speech problems in junior and senior high schools. *Journal of Speech and Hearing Research, 16,* 739–743.

Lim, V. P., Lincoln, M., Chan, Y. H., & Onslow, M. (2008). Stuttering in English-Mandarin bilingual speakers: The influence of language dominance on stuttering severity. *Journal of Speech, Language, and Hearing Research, 51,* 1522–1537.

Luterman, D. M. (2017). *Counseling persons with communication disorders and their families.* Austin, TX: Pro-Ed.

Menzies, R. G., Onslow, M., Packman, A., & O'Brian, S. (2009). Cognitive behavior therapy for adults who stutter: A tutorial for speech-language pathologists. *Journal of Fluency Disorders, 34*(3), 187–200.

Shollenbarger, A. (2019, May 28). The importance of soft skills for professional success. *Leader Live.* Retrieved from https://blog.asha.org/2019/05/28/the-importance-of-soft-skills-for-professional-success/

ADDITIONAL RESOURCES

International Fluency Association (IFA) website: http://theifa.org

Lukong, J. (2007). Speech therapy services to be provided to emerging self-help groups for people who stutter in Africa under the framework of the International Speech Project-Stuttering. *The ASHA Leader, 17*(1), 16–18. https://doi.org/10.1044/ffd17.1.16

Nsabimana, D. (n.d.). *Lesson from Rwanda: Using technology to provide access to therapy.* Retrieved from the International Stuttering Association website: http://isad.isastutter.org/isad-2017/papers-presented-by/research-therapy-and-support/lesson-from-rwanda-using-technology-to-provide-access-to-therapy/

Robinson, T. L. (2012). Cultural diversity and fluency disorders. In D. E. Battle (Ed.), *Communication disorders in multicultural and international populations* (4th ed., pp. 164-173). St. Louis, MO: Elsevier.

Shenker, R. (n.d.). *Stuttering and the bilingual child.* Retrieved from the Stuttering Foundation website: https://www.stutteringhelp.org/stuttering-and-bilingual-child

Stuttering Foundation. (n.d.). *Translations*. Retrieved from https://www.stutteringhelp.org/translations

Yaruss, J. S. (1997). Clinical measurement of stuttering behaviors. *Contemporary Issues in Communication Science and Disorders, 24,* 27-38.

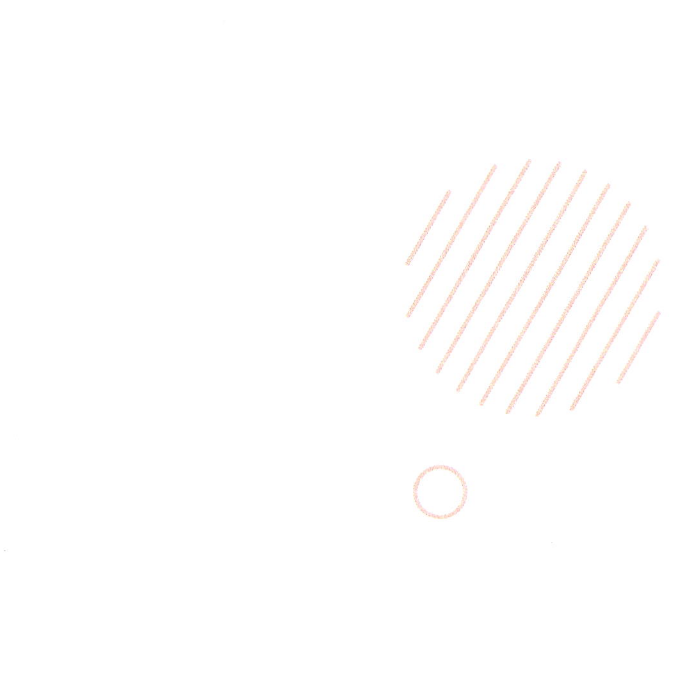

Marrying Cultural and Clinical Practices — Adapting Clinical Practices to be Inclusive of Cultural Beliefs

Carmen Ana Ramos-Pizarro

PREBRIEF

Some highly visible cultural and religious practices, such as wearing religious attire (e.g., the Muslim hijab, the Catholic mantilla veil, the Jewish yarmulke/kippah, or the Sikh turban), may physically affect service delivery because of a need to remove or adjust while also having an influence as the result of a conscious or implicit bias (e.g., having negative thoughts or misperceptions about a racial/ethnic group identifiable from their apparel). It is important for clients to feel respected and that their cultural practices and values are accommodated when receiving therapy services. Clinicians can benefit from continued education regarding other cultures and self-reflection practices to help identify conscious bias and implicit bias. This case provides suggestions for strategies that may be implemented in a speech-language pathology or audiology clinic that help to acknowledge and support unique expressions of culture.

notes:

OBJECTIVES

- Describe cultural patterns of some traditional Muslim individuals and how they may impact family dynamics.
- Develop recommendations for clinical practices to accommodate cultural/religious preferences of Muslim families.

CASE SCENARIO

Mrs. Ibrahim, a 33-year-old Muslim woman, came to clinic accompanied by her husband and two children, ages 14 and 8, seeking voice therapy services. The family arrived 45 minutes past the appointment time and were surprised when the receptionist explained they would have to reschedule the evaluation because of a strict policy about arriving on time. Mr. Ibrahim explained they were not used to such strict rules about punctuality and would wait in the lobby until there was an opening. The administrative staff told them this was not possible. As the family was ready to leave, the staff received a phone call, and because of a last-minute cancellation, Mrs. Ibrahim was able to be seen that afternoon. Mrs. Ibrahim's husband completed all administrative forms and was the primary interviewee during the intake. He explained that her primary complaint was a complete loss of her voice. When offered an interpreter, Mr. Ibrahim stated that he spoke English fluently and said that his wife knew "enough English to get by." They shared that the family speaks Punjabi at home.

Mr. Ibrahim explained that their family had relocated to the United States in the last year from Pakistan when he was accepted as a graduate student at a local university. Mr. Ibrahim was concerned because his wife was very healthy until 3 months ago when she developed severe hoarseness and general fatigue. A visit to a physician a few weeks after the onset of her symptoms documented Mrs. Ibrahim's use of whispered speech, prompting a referral to a speech-language pathologist for a full voice evaluation.

Mr. Ibrahim expressed concerns about his wife's loss of voice affecting her ability to work as an Arabic tutor for university students and her ability to socialize with other Pakistani women in their community. Throughout the interview, when questions were addressed to Mrs. Ibrahim, she gazed toward her husband who would respond for her, and she would nod while looking down. After the initial interview with all family members present, Ms. Carter, the speech-language pathologist, and her male student clinician, Mark, invited Mrs. Ibrahim to accompany them on her own to an examination room.

While in the exam room, a full voice evaluation was completed: Noninstrumental observations of breathing, posture, and muscle tension were gathered while Mrs. Ibrahim attempted production of sustained vowels at comfortable pitch and loudness, at soft and loud levels, and at low and high pitches. To assess more functional speech, the clinician asked Mrs. Ibrahim to read standard sentences and the Rainbow Passage as well as speak about her voice problem. Mrs. Ibrahim fully cooperated with all requests using a whispered voice. For the final task of the evaluation, under the supervision of Ms. Carter, Mark politely requested that Mrs. Ibrahim remove her hijab for a manual examination of her neck area. She declined the exam. At that point, Mark explained that the procedure would help the clinicians clarify whether displacement, pressure, and massage of the muscles in the neck area could release any muscle tension that may be contributing to her voice loss. After Mark explained the rationale, Mrs. Ibrahim accepted the explanation and completely removed her hijab. During the manual examination and trial therapy, Mrs. Ibrahim was able to produce brief, but clear, speech elicited after sustained laryngeal massage. The massage appeared to be effective in reducing some of the extrinsic laryngeal muscle tension that was previously identified and contributed to her aphonia.

After the trial, Mr. Ibrahim was asked to join his wife along with Ms. Carter and Mark in the exam room. The results of the evaluation were explained. The clinicians reported that Mrs. Ibrahim presented with muscle tension dysphonia as originally diagnosed and that manual circumlaryngeal techniques, including laryngeal massage used in trial therapy, were successful in helping Mrs. Ibrahim produce some voicing. Mrs. Ibrahim was invited to demonstrate her progress in phonating to her husband. Mrs. Ibrahim removed her hijab and demonstrated speech production during the laryngeal massage. Mr. Ibrahim asked the clinicians several questions regarding the treatment. Mr. and Mrs. Ibrahim thanked the team, and they scheduled their next appointment before leaving the clinic.

The following week, Mrs. Ibrahim missed her clinic appointment. The clinic conducted a follow-up phone call and were notified by Mr. Ibrahim that his wife would not be returning for treatment. Mr. Ibrahim did not share any reasons for this decision.

CRITICAL THINKING AND DEBRIEFING QUESTIONS

1. How comfortable would you feel working with female patients who wear hijab or other covering that may require physical touch or removal of their covering?
2. What positive cultural practices were implemented by the clinicians in this case study?
3. Considering your gender, what might you do differently if you were in the same situation as the clinicians in this case study?
4. What are some possible reasons that the patient has decided not to return for treatment?

COMMENTARY

The cultural and religious traditions and practices of our clients are woven into their daily lives and influence the way that they approach therapy (Reeves & Azam, 2012). Addressing patient values early in the clinical process provides critical information for service delivery and can be a starting point for clinician-patient conversations. However, it is important to note that each patient may express their own cultural and religious traditions in different ways. Relying on generalizations and failing to recognize individual differences in cultural practices may be interpreted as cultural stereotyping and may lead to clinical interactions that do not feel welcoming or respectful to the client.

Cultural practices that are highly visible may affect aspects of clinical practice, whether through implicit or explicit bias. *Explicit bias* includes prejudicial thoughts and behaviors that manifest a bias verbally or through one's actions. *Implicit bias* is a form of bias or prejudice that is beyond the awareness of the individual. It can be in direct contradiction to a clinician's beliefs and values and may affect their behavior or clinical conduct during service delivery. Each clinician should critically evaluate their own beliefs and understand how those beliefs may impact service delivery or interactions with clients. Aspects of this scenario appear to reflect generalizations associated with people from Muslim cultural backgrounds. For example, it is typical to see several members of a family attend a medical appointment and remain involved during the interview and evaluation process.

Clinicians are advised to observe and gain valuable information from these interactions and map family dynamics that could contribute to the initial assessment and diagnosis. A possible approach could include conducting a cultural ecogram with the client (Yasui, 2015). Although this may require additional visits or time spent with a client, making an effort to understand a client's cultural influences may help with adherence to future appointments. In Mrs. Ibrahim's case, aspects of her interactions with her husband during the initial interview might have motivated the clinicians to explore possible causative factors of Mrs. Ibrahim's aphonia by creating opportunities to observe the couple together as well as apart. These details may have come out during the cultural ecogram.

The clinic staff in this scenario did not demonstrate an awareness of cultural time orientation when they initially did not accommodate the late arrival of the patient and her family (Giger, 2017). They did not understand that this family may not have been acculturated to the expectation of punctuality in the European American culture. The last-minute cancellation presented an opportunity for clinicians or

Definition

Cultural ecogram can be described as "a clinical engagement tool designed to facilitate the development of a culturally anchored shared understanding ... (it) applies the use of visual tools to gather information about the ethnic minority family's culture and context ... with a central goal of establishing a shared understanding through the use of pictorial cues that guide an open discussion of areas of the clients' lives that influence parenting practices and experiences of families (Yasui, 2015).

the receptionist to emphasize clinic expectations related to attendance and punctuality as well as an explanation of the appointment system. However, the clinicians appeared knowledgeable regarding gender roles for this family by following their lead and addressing the male in the family during the initial interview. The team identified and followed Mrs. Ibrahim's nonverbal communication cues of turning toward her husband and directing her gaze to the floor. While still maintaining cultural sensitivity, clinicians could have acknowledged Mrs. Ibrahim during the initial interview by inquiring of both adults in the family as to how to make the visit more comfortable for them.

This scenario highlights the practice of wearing hijab. Hijab is known most commonly as a headscarf or covering worn over the head and neck of Muslim females. More specifically, hijab also represents a set of religious guidelines that are in place to ensure that both men and women maintain modesty. It is typically recommended that clinicians of the same gender provide services to Muslim patients to avoid potential cultural missteps and to accommodate a patient's need for modesty (Attum, Waheed, & Shamoon, 2020).

The clinicians could have accommodated the patient's cultural background and religious belief in other ways. As the visit progressed, the team could have engaged the family in a conversation about cultural background and practices, which may have demonstrated the team's cultural humility and desire to accommodate the family's requests (Tervalon & Murray-Garcia, 1998). Ms. Carter, the clinical educator, could have offered a description of the tests and procedures that would be part of the voice evaluation, providing the rationale for each step to both the patient and her husband. Inserting pauses would have allowed them to ask questions and, most importantly, for Mrs. Ibrahim to provide consent free from undue influence. This strategy would demonstrate respect for the autonomy of the patient and their unique cultural and religious practices. Equipped with the information, Mrs. Ibrahim may have been offered alternatives to complete removal of her hijab: to partially remove the hijab, accommodating the examination under the cover of the hijab, or to have her husband present during the examination (Harris, Mukati, & Ghandchi, 2012). Cultural knowledge of patriarchal family dynamics and a strict observance of hijab may have helped the clinicians prevent the loss of Mrs. Ibrahim to follow-up. Although well-intentioned, efforts by the clinicians to acknowledge the religious practices of their patient were not completely effective and did not allow the patient full participation.

After the Ibrahim family declined further service, it would be prudent for the team to reflect on the experience. Some options could be accessing resources through the American Speech-Language-Hearing Association's (n.d.) cultural competence practice portal page and researching ways to promote additional culturally responsive practices pertaining to Muslims in the clinic, which could include the following:

- cultural ecograms,
- specific questions in intake questionnaires to capture a patient's cultural or religious practices and ways to accommodate them,
- providing a handout with a description of the procedures that would take place during the assessment to identify potential issues with appropriate time to discuss alternatives,
- verbally confirming with both the patient and spouse that they understand the procedures to take place, and

- having alternative plans for patients who decline working with clinicians of a specific gender.

Finally, in clinical situations that end in miscommunication or confusion, it is important for clinicians and clinics to attempt to understand what aspects of practice can be improved. This practice is consistent with the idea of cultural humility. Tervalon and Murray-Garcia originally defined cultural humility as "a lifelong commitment to self-evaluation and critique, to redressing power imbalances . . . and to developing mutually beneficial and non-paternalistic partnerships with communities on behalf of individuals and defined populations" (Greene-Moton & Minkler, 2019, p. 142). Cultural humility allows a patient to be the expert of their own experiences and fosters a respectful curiosity in a clinician to learn about a client's culture and to adapt practices and techniques to best suit the unique needs of the client. All of these steps can help clinicians and clinics be more culturally responsive to the needs of all clients who seek their service.

CRITICAL THINKING AND DEBRIEFING RESPONSES

1. **How comfortable would you feel working with female patients who wear hijab or other covering that may require physical touch or removal of their covering?**

This question requires an individual answer, but clinicians are encouraged to research cultural and religious traditions related to hijab. Greater familiarity with these specific cultural practices may lead to improved sensitivity and understanding when providing services to this population.

2. **What positive cultural practices were implemented by the clinicians in this case study?**

When working with this conservative Muslim family, the clinicians correctly addressed the husband while still attempting to engage the female patient. During the laryngeal examination, the male student clinician requested verbal consent before proceeding to palpate the female patient's neck, which required removing her hijab. By offering the option of declining the examination, they demonstrated some degree of sensitivity to her cultural views. The team could have considered the impact of power differentials (i.e., expert vs. client) and how that may have affected Mrs. Ibrahim's willingness to remove her hijab. They may have also considered that Mrs. Ibrahim might have preferred a female speech-language pathologist, especially if the requirement for treatment was removal of her hijab.

3. **Considering your gender, what might you do differently if you were in the same situation as the clinicians in this case study?**

Different responses are possible depending on your gender. For females, one possibility is to take the lead in the consent process. Before initiating the laryngeal palpation, a full explanation of the procedure could have been provided to the patient asking whether there was a way to make her more comfortable. Options offered may have included examination by the female supervisor, inviting the husband back into the exam room while the procedure was conducted, or attempting to complete the palpation under the hijab covering.

As a male clinician, the voice examination of the patient would require increased responsiveness. At no point should the male clinician remain alone with his unaccompanied Muslim female patient (Harris et al., 2012). Carefully pursuing exploratory questions during the intake would have given the patient an opportunity to share her desire to have her family in the exam room with her and to remain covered in the presence of male health care providers. The male clinician could also defer to a female clinician for that specific procedure if the patient declined being seen by a male speech-language pathologist.

4. **What are some possible reasons that the patient has decided not to return for treatment?**

Multiple factors could have influenced the patient's decision not to return to clinic for follow-up. Because the report was provided by the husband, one possibility is that he did not agree with his wife's interaction with the male student clinician because he was not mahram or family (Bennett, 2013). Another possibility is that during the initial visit, the patient did not feel she could decline the examination and save face and ultimately preferred not to return. It may be beneficial for the clinic to complete a follow-up call acknowledging the errors they made and to ask whether there may be another approach that is more appropriate, should the family be open to coming back.

TAKE AWAYS

- Acknowledge that in some cultures, patriarchal family dynamics mean that male family members are the decision makers. This can influence the interactions, clinical partnerships, and intervention outcomes of the female family members they represent.
- Provide options for patients who wear hijab or head covering if your exam requires them to remove their covering by offering to have a female clinician conduct the examination or other possible alternatives, including half removal or offering another sort of covering.
- Develop clinical procedures that explicitly acknowledge accommodations for a variety of cultural, religious, or personal practices and provide appropriate training to staff regarding implementation.

REFERENCES

American Speech-Language-Hearing Association. (n.d.). *Cultural competence*. Retrieved from https://www.asha.org/Practice-Portal/Professional-Issues/Cultural-Competence/

Attum, B., Waheed, A., & Shamoon, Z. (2020, February 17). *Cultural competence in the care of Muslim patients and their families.* Retrieved from https://www.ncbi.nlm.nih.gov/books/NBK499933/

Bennett, M. J. (2013). Stereotypes/generalizations. Entry in C. Cortes (Ed.), *Multicultural America: A multimedia encyclopedia.* New York, NY: Sage. Retrieved from https://www.idrinstitute.org/resources/stereotypes-generalizations/

Giger, J. N. (2017). *Transcultural nursing: Assessment and intervention.* St. Louis, MO: Elsevier.

Greene-Moton, E., & Minkler, M. (2019). Cultural competence or cultural humility? Moving beyond the debate. *Health Promotion Practice, 21*(1), 142–145. https://doi.org/10.1177/1524839919884912

Harris, O., Mukati, A. S., & Ghandchi, N. (2012, October 1). What SLPs need to know when working with Muslim patients. *The ASHA Leader, 17*(13). https://doi.org/10.1044/leader.FTR2.17132012.np

Reeves, T. C., & Azam, L. (2012). To wear hijab or not: Muslim women's perceptions of their healthcare workplaces. *Journal of Business Diversity, 12*(2), 41–58.

Tervalon, M., & Murray-Garcia, J. (1998). Cultural humility versus cultural competence: A critical distinction in defining physician training outcomes in multicultural education. *Journal of Health Care for the Poor and Underserved, 9,* 117–125.

Yasui, M. (2015). The cultural ecogram: A tool for enhancing culturally anchored shared understanding in the treatment of ethnic minority families. *Journal of Ethnic and Cultural Diversity in Social Work, 24*(2), 89–108.

ADDITIONAL RESOURCES

Ahmad, N. B., & Quraishi-Landes, A. (2019, March 15). Five myths about hijab. *Washington Post.* Retrieved from https://www.washingtonpost.com/outlook/five-myths/five-myths-about-hijab/2019/03/15/d1f1ea52-45f6-11e9-8aab-95b8d80a1e4f_story.html

American Speech-Language-Hearing Association. (2016). *Code of Ethics.* Retrieved from https://www.asha.org/Code-of-Ethics/

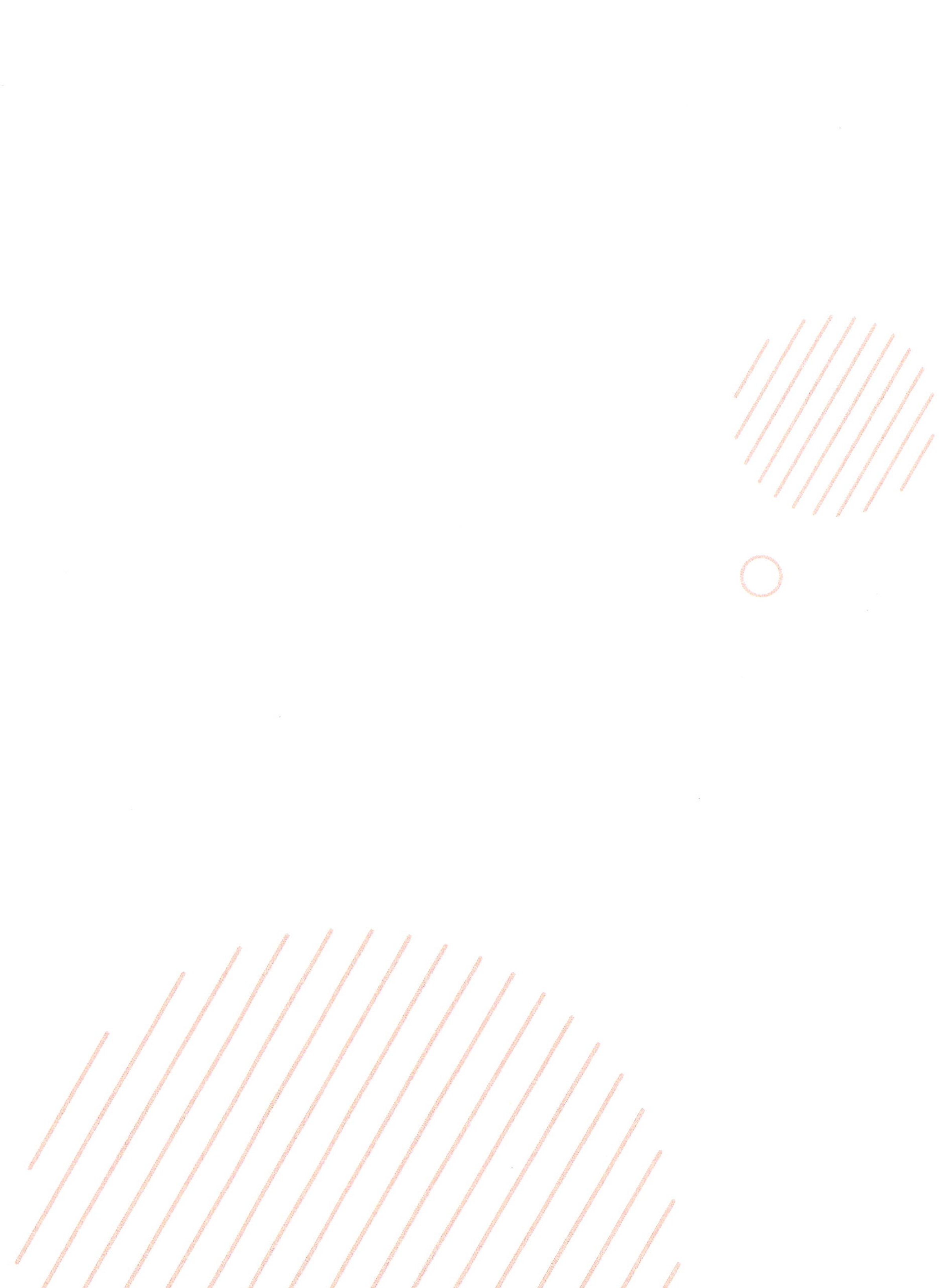

A Token of Gratitude

— Can Culturally Responsive Practices Become a Conflict of Interest?

Carmen Ana Ramos-Pizarro, Alicia Fleming Hamilton, Puja Goel, and Ivan Campos

PREBRIEF

There may be times during every clinician's career when they will encounter situations that pose ethical questions. Although ethical decisions vary on the basis of a variety of factors, the American Speech-Language-Hearing Association's (ASHA, 2016) *Code of Ethics* can be used along with a clinician's own ethical compass and values for guidance in making these decisions. In this scenario, a wife offers gifts to her spouse's clinician. While reading, consider the actions of the client, clinician, and other colleagues and reflect on how professionals may sensitively approach similar situations while maintaining ethical and professional standards.

OBJECTIVES

- Identify possible ethical dilemmas involved in accepting gifts from clients.
- Establish guidelines that determine which gifts may be accepted without incurring a potential ethical violation.
- Draft a possible response to clients who offer gifts that do not meet ethical guidelines.
- Recognize cultural factors and how they may influence gift exchanges.

CASE SCENARIO

Mr. Spencer is a clinician who has accepted his first clinical fellow (CF), who will work under his supervision for the next 9 months. Tyler, the CF, is an engaging young clinician who grew up in Singapore until he moved to the United States to complete his undergraduate and graduate degrees. Tyler expressed great interest in working with adult populations in outpatient clinics. During his first week, Mr. Spencer provided an initial orientation to Tyler regarding the clinical and administrative aspects of his new position and was impressed with the level of mastery he showed.

Tyler was assigned his first client, Mr. Susanto. Mr. Susanto was from Indonesia and was referred for a full speech and language evaluation following a stroke. Tyler's clinical educator asked him to take the lead on the case and was impressed with how he engaged the family both in English and some short phrases in the patient's native Bahasa Indone-

notes:

sian. Tyler was familiar with the family's cultural background because he came from a neighboring country, and Mr. Susanto's family was happy to make small talk with Tyler. The family was greatly appreciative of Tyler's efforts to reference their culture, and during the next visit to discuss the assessment results, they brought Tyler traditional sweets from their country. Tyler gladly accepted and shared the treats with his CF clinical educator and all of his colleagues on the therapy unit.

As Tyler continued providing language therapy for Mr. Susanto, he made sure to address the family with a short greeting in their language and involve the client's wife in the session to ensure that she would learn how to provide support for her husband as he recovered. At the end of each session, Mr. Susanto's wife would gift Tyler a bagful of sweets or other traditional confections. As in previous occasions, Tyler continued to share the treats with his CF clinical educator and other colleagues in the unit.

On the final day of the patient's clinic intervention, the client's wife listened attentively to all further recommendations and profusely thanked Tyler for his services, promising to stay in touch. As they left the clinic, with Mr. Spencer present, the family handed Tyler a meticulously hand-carved wooden ornament as a token of appreciation. Tyler was honored, but he was also caught off-guard and hesitated to accept the gift. Tyler knew that, culturally, it may be viewed as disrespectful to decline, but he also knew that the clinic guidelines forbade him from accepting gifts of significant monetary value. The client's wife insisted several times that Tyler accept until Mr. Spencer explained that although lovely and thoughtful, because of clinic rules, Tyler was not allowed to accept the gift. The family left the otherwise positive encounter looking confused and embarrassed.

CRITICAL THINKING AND DEBRIEFING QUESTIONS

1. **What is the clinical educator's role in this situation? Could the clinical educator have taken a different approach in addressing the family giving gifts to Tyler?**
2. **When a family or client bring candy and treats to a clinician, what are some acceptable responses that are consistent with ASHA's *Code of Ethics?***
3. **Are there situations in which accepting a more expensive gift is acceptable?**
4. **What alternatives were there to declining the final gift? Might there have been certain procedures in place to mitigate the situation?**

COMMENTARY

Gift-giving practices vary across cultures. In a clinical setting where clients and clinicians are forming a relationship to work on communication outcomes, gifts can represent a physical expression of appreciation or gratitude. It is possible that in some cultures or situations, given the timing or value of the gift, a gift may carry other motivations. These motivations may be related to seeking some sort of an advantage or preferential treatment, or they may be another way of expressing appreciation and gratitude for the services received. As culturally responsive clinicians, it is important to seek to understand as much as possible about our clients' and coworkers' cultural backgrounds, including practices related to gift giving, to better understand a situation in which a gift may be given. This information may also help to create policies and guidance for clients and clinicians.

In 2018, ASHA revised an "Issues in Ethics" statement originally published in 2004 to address issues regarding matters concerning conflicts of professional interest. Principle of Ethics III, Rule of Ethics B, specifically prohibits conflicts of professional interest (ASHA, 2016). A conflict of interest can be defined as an

> *opposition between the private interests and the official or professional responsibilities of a person in a position of trust, power, and/or authority. Such conflicts may result in a situation in which personal, financial, and/or nonfinancial considerations have the potential to influence or compromise professional judgment in clinical service, research, consultation, instruction, administration, or any other professional activity. (ASHA, 2018, Introduction section, para. 3)*

Any perceived conflict of interest has the possibility of diminishing the public's trust and confidence in the profession of communication sciences and disorders at large.

ASHA's (2018) statement goes on to note that although an individual may personally believe that their judgment is not affected by a gift, that belief is not enough to protect against a perceived conflict of interest. The influence of a gift may be subtle, and the receiver may be unaware of the way in which their judgment has been impacted by the kind gesture. Research in social sciences has shown that when a gift is received, it can create a sense of obligation to reciprocate that is unrelated to the value of the gift (DeRuiter & Rao, 2012). For these reasons, it is recommended that workplaces establish policies for employees that minimize professional conflicts of interest and have clear guidelines regarding the giving and receptions of gifts. These policies should be shared with clients and employees before services start to help alleviate potentially uncomfortable situations before they arise.

Any perceived conflict of interest has the possibility of diminishing the public's trust and confidence in the profession of communication sciences and disorders at large.

ASHA (2018) provides some guidance in this area and suggests three appropriate actions when faced with potential professional conflicts of interest: avoid, disclose, and recuse.

Avoidance does not indicate a policy in which nonwage benefits may be accepted; it suggests that all gift offers should be scrutinized. Accepted gifts should clearly demonstrate one or more of the following:

- Primarily contribute to the welfare of people served professionally,
- Do not reasonably appear to bias professional judgment,
- Enhance one's professional knowledge and skills, and/or
- Do not diminish the dignity or autonomy of the professions.

Using these criteria to understand the motive behind a gift can be useful in assessing a situation appropriately.

Disclosure involves the clinician demonstrating full transparency with the client, or the one giving the gift, by explaining gift giving/receiving policies. It also includes disclosing gifts received with employers. Any disclosure should be honest and complete to remain consistent with the code.

Recusal involves withdrawal from a situation in which one's participation creates a bias.

Additional guidelines from ASHA (2018) and the American Medical Association (2016) have noted that gifts or economic benefits of significant value may be accepted by the individual if they primarily benefit the people served professionally. Gifts or economic benefits of token or trivial value may be accepted if they are appropriate to the individual's professional practice. Cash gifts should not be accepted.

In this scenario, there were two instances of gift giving. The first was the offer of candies and confections that were low in value and considered a basic token of appreciation for the clinician and staff to enjoy. This gift appeared to express gratitude from the family, but clinicians should also consider whether such gifts create a potential bias or expectation to reciprocate. A recipient should evaluate whether the gift is a consumable that can be shared among the staff. For future situations, the clinic may seek to define the nature of acceptable gifts—possibly classifying them as "nondurable" or "consumable" versus "consumable" or "durable." This would indicate whether something can be used up or adds benefit to the staff/clinician. This decision-making process would benefit from value thresholds to signal a potentially problematic gift.

When the estimated value of the final gift turned out to be exponentially higher, the clinical educator felt as though it was his responsibility to decline the gift on Tyler's behalf.

In some cultures, declining a gift for any reason is considered offensive, and every effort should be made to help the giver save face by profusely and repeatedly thanking them for the thoughtful offering. It is important to note that in some cultures, accepting an offered gift or even food or drink when first offered is considered distasteful, so declining once or twice initially before accepting is the norm. As we saw in this case, Tyler initially declined the beautiful carving, and Mrs. Susanto continued to offer it several more times. During home visits, declining an offered gift (such as food or drink) can be offensive and may negatively affect the therapeutic relationship (Roseberry-McKibbin, 1997). Additionally, gift giving can be an important practice in collectivistic societies to indicate gratitude for an action, service, or assistance you have provided (Battle, 2012).

Gift giving can be an important practice in collectivistic societies to indicate gratitude for an action, service, or assistance provided (Battle, 2012).

Tyler indicated at the onset of Mr. Susanto's therapy that he was familiar with the family's cultural practices. Given his understanding of the culture, Tyler could have attempted to communicate the cultural practices surrounding gift giving with this clinical educator after the first gift—the sweets—was given. This information may have helped his clinical educator to understand the intent behind the gift. It also may have given Tyler and the clinical educator an opportunity to confer privately and encourage Tyler to thank the family profusely but politely decline the gift while explaining the clinic's "no gift" policy. Another possible alternative could have been to have Tyler ask whether the gift could be displayed in the clinic, for all of his coworkers and their future clients to enjoy. Given that this was the end of the client's therapeutic sessions, perhaps Tyler could have used the guidance from ASHA and may have determined that accepting this gift (a) may have contributed to the welfare and good feelings of the couple as an expression of their gratitude, (b) would not have created a bias in judgment because the family was no longer coming for services, (c) would not have enhanced Tyler's knowledge or skills, and (d) would not have diminished the dignity of the professions. Although there is no "correct" answer in this situation, it could be possible to find a better outcome in which the clients do not leave the situation feeling embarrassed by their generous and seemingly innocent act.

Although it might be possible to accept small gifts deemed as tokens of gratitude for services provided, each clinician should evaluate the timing, nature, value, and motivation behind each gift before accepting it. It is crucial to remember that even the perception that a conflict of interest has occurred is damaging for the reputation of our professions. Outlining and disclosing policies for gift giving that cite conflict of interest policies are beneficial to both clients and clinicians.

CRITICAL THINKING AND DEBRIEFING RESPONSES

1. **What is the clinical educator's role in this situation? Could the clinical educator have taken a different approach in addressing the family giving gifts to Tyler?**

In this scenario, it was important for the clinical educator to guide and support Tyler in an unfamiliar situation in which a conflict of interest could have presented itself. Conflicts of interest, including even perceived conflicts of interest, have ethical implications and affect the way in which a profession is viewed. Even the acceptance of small gifts can be perceived as a "favor" or an action that could imply some sort of reciprocated response. Social science research has noted that those who receive such gifts feel (consciously or unconsciously) a need to reciprocate in some way that may not even be related to the value of the gift. Mr. Spencer, Tyler's clinical educator, would be remiss in not addressing this situation with Tyler to discuss the ways to reflect on the gift, with the ASHA's (2016) *Code of Ethics* as guidance, to come to a mutually agreed on decision. Culture is an additional layer in this situation, and Mr. Spencer may choose to have Tyler review some research in this area to better understand how gift giving varies across cultures, or to ask Tyler about his culture and how gift giving is viewed. Finally, this may be a good opportunity for Tyler, his clinical educator, and the department to review and develop, if needed, policies related to gift giving and receiving and to note how they are presented to clients.

2. **When a family or client bring candy and treats to a clinician, what are some acceptable responses that are consistent with ASHA's *Code of Ethics?***

If Tyler and his clinical educator have reviewed the ethical guidance from ASHA (2016, 2018) and determined that the candies and sweets (1) primarily contribute to the welfare of the client, (2) do not reasonably appear to bias professional judgment, (3) enhance one's professional knowledge and skills, and (4) do not diminish the dignity or autonomy of the professions, then it would be appropriate to accept the treats. Tyler and his clinical educator could implement a protocol in which they discuss conflicts of interest at the beginning of working with a client. This way the information is known to all parties before they do something that may make them feel embarrassed. They can relate the refusal of offered gifts as part of their desire to not demonstrate a conflict of interest, emphasizing that the true reward is the work itself.

3. **Are there situations in which accepting a more expensive gift is acceptable?**

This would be a question in which a clinician would benefit from reviewing the ethical guidance from ASHA (2016, 2018). There is no clear answer in this situation, but if a clinician can carefully scrutinize a gift, given the aforementioned set of questions, and determine that the gift has little to no impact on judgment, expectations, or reciprocation, it may be acceptable. The clinician may also want to consider the timing of the gift. In this case, it was at the end of treatment, which would show less of a desire from the client to curry "favors" with the practitioner (Caddell & Hazelton, 2013). Each decision must be made on a case-by-case basis. However, cash gifts should not be accepted.

4. **What alternatives were there to declining the final gift? Might there have been certain procedures in place to mitigate the situation?**

Ideally, this scenario would have started with a review of the ethical obligations by the clinician to the client before treatment began. This brief conversation would have been an excellent time to provide the client with information regarding acceptance of gifts and conflicts of interest. Addressing this subject at the beginning of the relationship may have alleviated future issues. However, a client may still want to show their gratitude with a gift. In that case, Tyler's suggestion of displaying the gift in the clinic was an appropriate alternative that would benefit other professionals and clients in the future.

TAKE AWAYS

- When considering whether or not to accept a gift, clinicians should consider the timing, nature, value, and motivation behind the gift.
- Gift-giving practices are often linked to cultural and social traditions, and a refusal may be seen as offensive to the giver.
- In any professional situation, it is important to understand and share gift giving and gift acceptance policies with all parties to avoid possible conflicts and misunderstandings.

REFERENCES

American Medical Association. (2016). *AMA principles of medical ethics: Chapter 1: 1.2.8: Gifts from patients.* Retrieved from http://bit.ly/2kZICRe

American Speech-Language-Hearing Association. (2016). *Code of Ethics.* Retrieved from https://www.asha.org/Code-of-Ethics/

American Speech-Language-Hearing Association. (2018). *Issues in ethics: Conflicts of professional interest.* Retrieved from https://www.asha.org/Practice/ethics/Conflicts-of-Professional-Interest/

Battle, D. E. (2012). *Communication disorders in multicultural populations—E-book.* St. Louis, MO: Elsevier.

Caddell, A., & Hazelton, L. (2013). Accepting gifts from patients. *Canadian Family Physician, 59*(12), 1259–1260.

DeRuiter, M., & Rao, A. (2012). More than overseeing. *The ASHA Leader, 17*(14), 22–25.

Roseberry-McKibbin, C. (1997). Understanding Filipino families: A foundation for effective service delivery. *American Journal of Speech-Language Pathology, 6*(3), 5–14.

ADDITIONAL RESOURCES

American Medical Association. (2016). *AMA principles of medical ethics: Chapter 1: 1.2.8: Gifts from patients.* Retrieved from https://www.ama-assn.org/sites/ama-assn.org/files/corp/media-browser/code-of-medical-ethics-chapter-1.pdf

Caddell, A., & Hazelton, L. (2013). Accepting gifts from patients. *Canadian Family Physician, 59*(12), 1259–1260.

DeRuiter, M., & Rao, A. (2012). More than overseeing. *The ASHA Leader, 17*(14), 22–25.

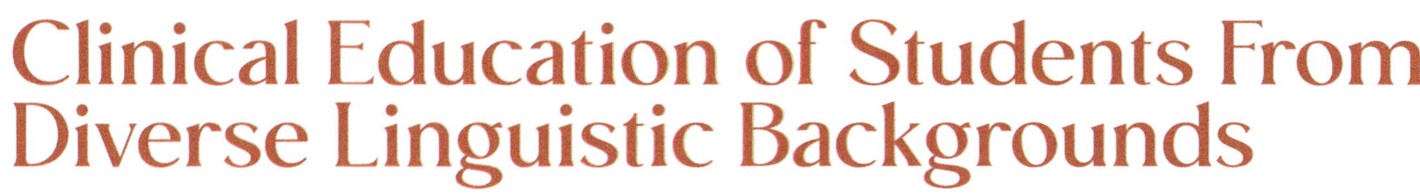

Clinical Education of Students From Diverse Linguistic Backgrounds

— Ensuring Appropriate Practices

Mariam M. Abdelaziz and Alicia Fleming Hamilton

PREBRIEF

Bilingual clinicians constitute a small population of the American Speech-Language-Hearing Association [ASHA] membership, as 6% self-identified as bilingual providers (ASHA, 2018) . However, there is documented need for bilingual service providers (ASHA, 2019b). To effectively support student clinicians, it is necessary for clinical educators to be sensitive to how linguistic differences can play out in clinician-client interactions as well as between a clinician and clinical educator. The following scenario outlines some negative experiences that students may experience in an academic and clinical setting.

OBJECTIVES

- Reflect on some of the potential challenges that students from diverse linguistic backgrounds may face during their clinical practicum.
- Understand the role of power differentials in a clinical educator-student clinician relationship.
- Consider the role of communication in the clinical educator-student clinician relationship.
- Reflect on how cultural biases (from a client or clinical educator) may negatively affect a student's clinical experience.

CASE SCENARIO

Fatima is a 30-year-old woman who is studying to earn her bachelor's degree in speech-language pathology. Fatima was born and raised in Cuba, where she was instructed in Spanish only from kindergarten to high school. She moved to the United States at 20 years old, with limited knowledge of English. Fatima enrolled in English as a second language classes at her local community college. After 1 year in these courses, she applied for and was accepted to an associate's degree program in mathematics. Fatima completed her program with highest honors, earning a 4.0 grade point average (GPA) and spent her extracurricular time working as a math tutor. Fatima was aware of her Spanish-influenced English and worked diligently to speak clearly and to check in with her tutees to ensure they understood her speech. No one ever mentioned difficulties un-

notes:

derstanding her. Fatima even looked into speech-language pathology services for accent modification. After an initial interview with the speech-language pathologist (SLP) and a brief phonemic assessment, she was told that her diction was very good, and there was no reason to pursue accent modification services.

Fatima was fascinated by the clinic and asked to shadow there. After shadowing a few sessions and speaking with the SLPs on staff, she applied to undergraduate programs in speech-language pathology. Fatima was admitted into a 4-year, private university, with a large scholarship to cover her tuition. Everything seemed to be going well for Fatima during her first year. She maintained a GPA of 3.9, was involved in research, and volunteered in a community aphasia support group. As Fatima approached her senior year, she prepared for her clinical practicum.

Fatima received an e-mail a few weeks before the beginning of her senior year, stating that to initiate her clinical practicum, she had to pass a 10-minute, informal verbal assessment for non-native English-speaking clinicians administered by a graduate student in her program. Fatima was not aware of this requirement but did not challenge the requirement because she wanted to do well. Fatima also feared a challenge to this requirement may decrease her chances of getting into her university's speech-language pathology master's program. Fatima completed the assessment and was told that she received a "borderline" score and was now on "probation" in her clinical program. If she did not pass the interview the following semester, she would be asked to leave. Fatima was crushed.

Fatima and another student in her cohort, a native English speaker, were assigned to an English monolingual pediatric client who was being treated for an articulation disorder. Fatima noticed that her clinical educator never provided direct feedback to her—only the student who cotreated with her. Fatima submitted her therapy plans at least 5 days in advance of her upcoming session (as requested) and frequently received corrective feedback just hours before therapy appointment. This gave Fatima insufficient time to implement all of the adjustments, but she always did her best to adapt the lessons on the basis of her clinical educator's requests. Fatima did not receive feedback on her SOAP notes or her performance during treatment, and she began to feel excluded by her clinical educator (Paul & Hasselkus, 2004). Her clinical educator constantly praised her partner's lesson plans and performance in front of Fatima.

Definition

SOAP—Subjective, Objective Assessment Plan. These are notes that clinicians often use to take data on sessions. They are common in graduate training programs.

Fatima shared her concerns and frustrations with friends outside of her department. Fatima's friend suggested that she share her concerns with her clinical educator or another teacher she trusted. Fatima considered this possibility, but she felt that she may be viewed negatively in her department. When pressed on this issue, Fatima told her friend that by speaking out against her clinical educator, a well-liked faculty member, her grade could be negatively affected, and she would be viewed negatively by her other teachers. Fatima stated that she did not want her teachers to think she could not cope with the demands of the program, and she did not want to be singled out among her peers.

During Fatima's midterm conference, her clinical educator asked her to list three of her personal strengths as a clinician. Fatima listed that she was bilingual, had come to the program through an alternative path, and that because she grew up in a different country she was able to apply culturally appropriate methodology to treatment and had an interest in fully understanding the cultural and language practices of the clients she served.

Her clinical educator told Fatima that she "struggled to understand how being bilingual was a strength when providing services to American clients, where English is spoken." Fatima was caught off-guard by the comments and did not pursue them further. She was also nervous that challenging this professor would affect her final grade. This lack of feedback and correction continued until the end of the semester.

Before Fatima's last session of the semester, she received a text from her treatment partner asking her why Fatima was not going to be at the therapy session that day. Fatima was confused, she had not told anyone she wasn't going to clinic. Her treatment partner explained that Fatima's clinical educator contacted her and said that Fatima was no longer providing intervention sessions in the clinic. Fatima's treatment partner shared that the client's mother did not want her child working with a clinician "like" Fatima. Embarrassed, Fatima did not ask any more questions.

At her final conference, Fatima's clinical educator told her that she had been penalized on her final grade for misarticulations and not adapting therapy plans based on the clinical educator's recommendations. When Fatima asked why she was not allowed to continue treatment with her client, her clinical educator explained that the client's mother did not want her child working with a clinician "like" Fatima because her child was getting confused by Fatima's accent. Fatima felt humiliated. Her clinical educator told her that what happened to her was "very common" and that it was probably best if Fatima applied to graduate programs with a high population of culturally and linguistically diverse students because she may feel more comfortable with students and clients "like her."

CRITICAL THINKING AND DEBRIEFING QUESTIONS

1. **What miscommunications occurred between Fatima and her clinical educator? What could the clinical educator have done differently to improve communication between him and Fatima?**
2. **What power differentials existed in this scenario?**
3. **The clinical educator recommended Fatima to pursue graduate programs with diverse student populations so that she may feel "more comfortable." Does a clinician need to be a native-English speaker to provide articulation services to an English-speaking client?**
4. **What biases were demonstrated here?**

COMMENTARY

A successful clinical educator-student clinician relationship includes many components. Most significantly, in the context of this case, are establishing a system of communication and navigating power differentials between the clinical educator and student clinician. The strength of a clinical educator's interpersonal skills can directly relate to the effectiveness of the student clinician (ASHA, 2008). Cultural background can also play a role in how communication is expected. Establishing when and how feedback will be provided should be established at the beginning of the clinical placement. In this particular situation, the student submitted her therapy plans 5 days in advance, as agreed on by her and her clinical educator. However, the clinical educator then provided corrective feedback only a few hours before the session, which reduced Fatima's ability to make any meaningful changes to her therapy session. Because she did not make the recommended changes, Fatima was penalized for this, setting her up for a system in which she would fail.

Recognizing the role of power differentials is a necessary part of culturally responsive service delivery (Purgason, Avent, Cashwell, Jordan, & Reese, 2016) and supervision (Gottlieb, Robinson, & Younggren, 2007). Power is relational in that it exists in and between people, as evidenced in interprofessional relationships that determine how collaboration or shared power is enacted (Engel, Prentice, & Taplay, 2017).

Recognizing the role of power differentials is a necessary part of culturally responsive service delivery (Purgason, Avent, Cashwell, Jordan, & Reese, 2016) and supervision (Gottlieb, Robinson, & Younggren, 2007).

In a clinical educator–student clinician relationship, power differentials present themselves in grading, approving clinical hours, and evaluating performance. In this scenario, there were moments in which Fatima felt uncomfortable, but she did not feel that she could say anything to her clinical educator. Many students, regardless of cultural and linguistic background, may have felt similarly to Fatima. However, it is important to note that perceptions and reactions to power differentials vary across cultural groups. In situations in which a clinical educator is unsure of how to effectively navigate power differentials to communicate with a student clinician in a culturally appropriate manner, the clinical educator may consider seeking an intermediary such as a cultural liaison who can provide information about how to communicate appropriately.

Finally, pay close attention to the clinical educator's response to Fatima's reported strengths. Fatima appeared proud of her bilingual abilities and connected her knowledge of two cultures to providing culturally responsive services in the future. In the case above, Fatima's linguistic abilities were not viewed as an asset but rather irrelevant to her abilities as a clinician. As the United States becomes more culturally and linguistically diverse, there is an urgent need for clinicians who can offer multilingual services. Only 5.3% of ASHA members identified as Latino (ASHA, 2019a), and 6% of ASHA members self-identified themselves as bilingual providers (ASHA, 2018). Therefore, Fatima's bilingual background will certainly serve as a strength in her future clinical practice. Furthermore, her clinical educator suggested that Fatima pursue further academic opportunities in more linguistically diverse environments. In an increasingly diverse world, the clinician's and client's cultural and linguistic backgrounds may not always align, but this does not mean that that clinician cannot provide culturally responsive services. Consider the impact of the statement and how it may have made Fatima feel.

As the United States becomes more culturally and linguistically diverse, there is an urgent need for clinicians who can offer multilingual services.

CRITICAL THINKING AND DEBRIEFING RESPONSES

1. **What miscommunications occurred between Fatima and her clinical educator? What could the clinical educator have done differently to improve communication between him and Fatima?**

Three general miscommunications occurred between Fatima and her advisor. First, there was a breakdown in how and when corrective feedback was communicated. Just as there was an expectation for students to submit therapy plans with 5 days of notice, student clinicians should also have concrete expectations for when their plans would be reviewed. Fatima received her feedback only hours before the session, which did not provide sufficient time for preparation. This was frustrating for Fatima, but it may have also been frustrating for the clinical educator, who wasn't seeing his suggestions implemented. Had the feedback been provided in a systematic and mutually agreed on manner, the frustration felt by both parties may have been alleviated.

Second, Fatima was not notified by her clinical educator about the parental request and that she was taken off the student's therapy team. In sensitive situations such as this one, the clinical educator should have scheduled a face-to-face meeting with Fatima about her performance. A plan should have been drawn up to address the mother's concerns before considering removal from the therapy team.

Third, to be compliant with the Family Educational Rights and Privacy Act of 1974 (FERPA), a student's performance and position within the clinic should not be shared with other students; this was the case for Fatima, who found out from her partner that she would not have any more interactive sessions on the clinic floor. By disclosing information about Fatima's situation with the therapy partner, the clinical educator was in direct violation of FERPA.

2. **What power differentials existed in this scenario?**

Two different power differentials presented themselves in this scenario: one between Fatima and her program at large, and another between Fatima and her clinical educator. First, the program required an evaluation exclusively to non-native speakers of English. Fatima did not want to "push back" against authority (i.e., her program) and complied. Fatima's speech was designated as "borderline" and was warned that she would be placed on probation if this did not improve. Fatima had previously sought accent reduction therapy and was informed by a licensed clinician that therapy was not warranted in her case. Something problematic in this scenario is that a graduate student in her program—or in other words, a peer—completed the evaluation. It is unknown what sort of training the graduate student had in this area.

Second, Fatima's clinical educator appeared to provide minimal and infrequent feedback. Fatima was aware that her clinical educator was more interactive with her classmate than her. However, she did not feel comfortable expressing her concerns because her clinical educator held greater amounts of power as the "teacher" in their relationship. Fatima feared negative repercussions, such as being estranged (feeling "pointed out"), being viewed as weak (feeling "like she couldn't handle the pressures of clinic"), and receiving poor grades.

3. **The clinical educator recommended Fatima pursue graduate programs with diverse student populations so that she may feel "more comfortable." Does a clinician need to be a native-English speaker to provide articulation services to an English-speaking client?**

Currently, there is very little research in the field of communication sciences and disorders that has investigated the outcomes of English-only articulation therapy provided by a non-native English-speaking clinician. However, there has been some research in recent years in the field of education about student outcomes when the instructor and student share a similar racial background (e.g., Egalite, Kisida, & Winters, 2015; Evans, Munson, & Edwards, 2018; Lindsay & Hart, 2017). Generally, these studies have found a very small, but positive, relationship in student outcomes (e.g., grades, disciplinary referrals) when both the student and teacher share the same race. No studies have advocated for students to strictly be taught by teachers of the same race; as diverse as the United States is, it is simply not possible to match the background of the clinician to the client. Consider that the majority of practicing SLPs identify as monolingual, English speakers, and they are not counseled to avoid working with students who speak languages other than English. Furthermore, the clinician's background does not diminish their ability to provide services.

4. **What biases were demonstrated here?**

The U.S. Department of Justice, Community Relations Service (n.d.) has defined implicit bias as "all of the subconscious feelings, perceptions, attitudes, and stereotypes that have developed as a result of prior influences and imprints. It is an automatic positive or negative preference for a group, based on one's subconscious thoughts" (p. 2). Although we cannot know for certain what was going on in the clinical educator's mind in this scenario, the U.S. Department of Justice, Community Relations Service has cautioned that implicit biases can inform explicit biases, which occur when "individuals are aware of their prejudices and attitudes toward certain groups .... Examples of explicit bias include overt racism and racist comments" (p. 2). Implicit bias is also defined as attitudes or stereotypes that unconsciously affect our understanding, actions, and decisions and that may go against the values we openly profess or believe (Arora, 2017).

In the therapy team, Fatima's clinical educator did not communicate frequently with Fatima but consistently provided feedback and praise to her partner. Her clinical educator also disparaged her strengths as a bilingual clinician and suggested that she may prefer a program with a more diverse student population where she would feel more comfortable. These behaviors and comments are examples of possible implicit bias toward Fatima. Consider how these actions and comments may further the power differential between student clinician and clinical educator. Are these interactions reflective of a constructive and supportive learning environment?

TAKE AWAYS

- Effective communication is necessary for a successful clinical educator-student clinician relationship.
- No individual should be discriminated against on the basis of race, ethnicity, sex, gender identity/gender expression, sexual orientation, age, religion, national origin, disability culture, language, or dialect.
- Power differentials can affect the dynamic of the clinical educator-student clinician relationship.

REFERENCES

American Speech-Language-Hearing Association. (2008). *Clinical supervision in speech-language pathology* [Technical report]. Retrieved from https://www.asha.org/content.aspx?id=10737450495

American Speech-Language-Hearing Association. (2018). *Demographic profile of ASHA members providing bilingual services, year-end 2018.* Retrieved from https://www.asha.org/uploadedFiles/Demographic-Profile-Bilingual-Spanish-Service-Members.pdf

American Speech-Language-Hearing Association. (2019a). *Highlights and trends: Member and affiliate counts, year-end 2018.* Retrieved from https://www.asha.org/uploadedFiles/2018-Member-Counts.pdf

American Speech-Language-Hearing Association. (2019b). *Self identify as a bilingual service provider (BSP).* Retrieved from https://www.asha.org/Members/Self-Identify-as-a-Bilingual-Service-Provider/

Arora, N. (2017). Look at your blind spots: Do unconscious preconceptions shape your clinical judgment? A school-based clinician offers ways to uncover—and address—implicit bias. *The ASHA Leader, 22*(11), 6–7.

Egalite, A. J., Kisida, B., & Winters, M. A. (2015). Representation in the classroom: The effect of own-race teachers on student achievement. *Economics of Education Review, 45,* 44–52.

Engel, J., Prentice, D., & Taplay, K. (2017). A power experience: A phenomenological study of interprofessional education. *Journal of Professional Nursing, 33*(3), 204–211.

Evans, K. E., Munson, B., & Edwards, J. (2018). Does speaker race affect the assessment of children's speech accuracy? A comparison of speech-language pathologists and clinically untrained listeners. *Language, Speech, and Hearing Services in Schools, 49,* 906–921.

Family Educational Rights and Privacy Act of 1974, Pub. L. 93-380, 20 U.S.C. § 1232g; 34 CFR Part 99.

Gottlieb, M. C., Robinson, K., & Younggren, J. N. (2007). Multiple relations in supervision: Guidance for administrators, supervisors, and students. *Professional Psychology: Research and Practice, 38*(3), 241–247.

Lindsay, C. A., & Hart, C. M. (2017). Exposure to same-race teachers and student disciplinary outcomes for Black students in North Carolina. *Educational Evaluation and Policy Analysis, 39*(3), 485–510.

Paul, D., & Hasselkus, A. (2004). *Clinical record keeping in speech-language pathology for health care and third-party payers.* Rockville, MD: American Speech-Language-Hearing Association. Retrieved from https://www.dhs.state.mn.us/main/groups/manuals/documents/pub/dhs16_158228.pdf

Purgason, L. L., Avent, J. R., Cashwell, C. S., Jordan, M. E., & Reese, R. F. (2016). Culturally relevant advising: Applying relational cultural theory in counselor education. *Journal of Counseling & Development, 94*, 429–436.

U.S. Department of Justice, Community Relations Service. (n.d.). *Understanding bias: A resource guide* [Community Relations Services Toolkit for Policing]. Retrieved from https://www.justice.gov/crs/file/836431/download

ADDITIONAL RESOURCES

Bolton-Koppenhaver, M. (2002, April 2). Serving diverse populations. *The ASHA Leader, 7*(6), 2. Retrieved from https://www.asha.org/content.aspx?id=13615

Multicultural Constituency Groups (MCCGs) https://www.asha.org/practice/multicultural/opportunities/constituency/

U.S. Department of Education, Office for Civil Rights. (n.d.). *How to file a discrimination complaint with the Office for Civil Rights.* Retrieved from https://www2.ed.gov/about/offices/list/ocr/docs/howto.html

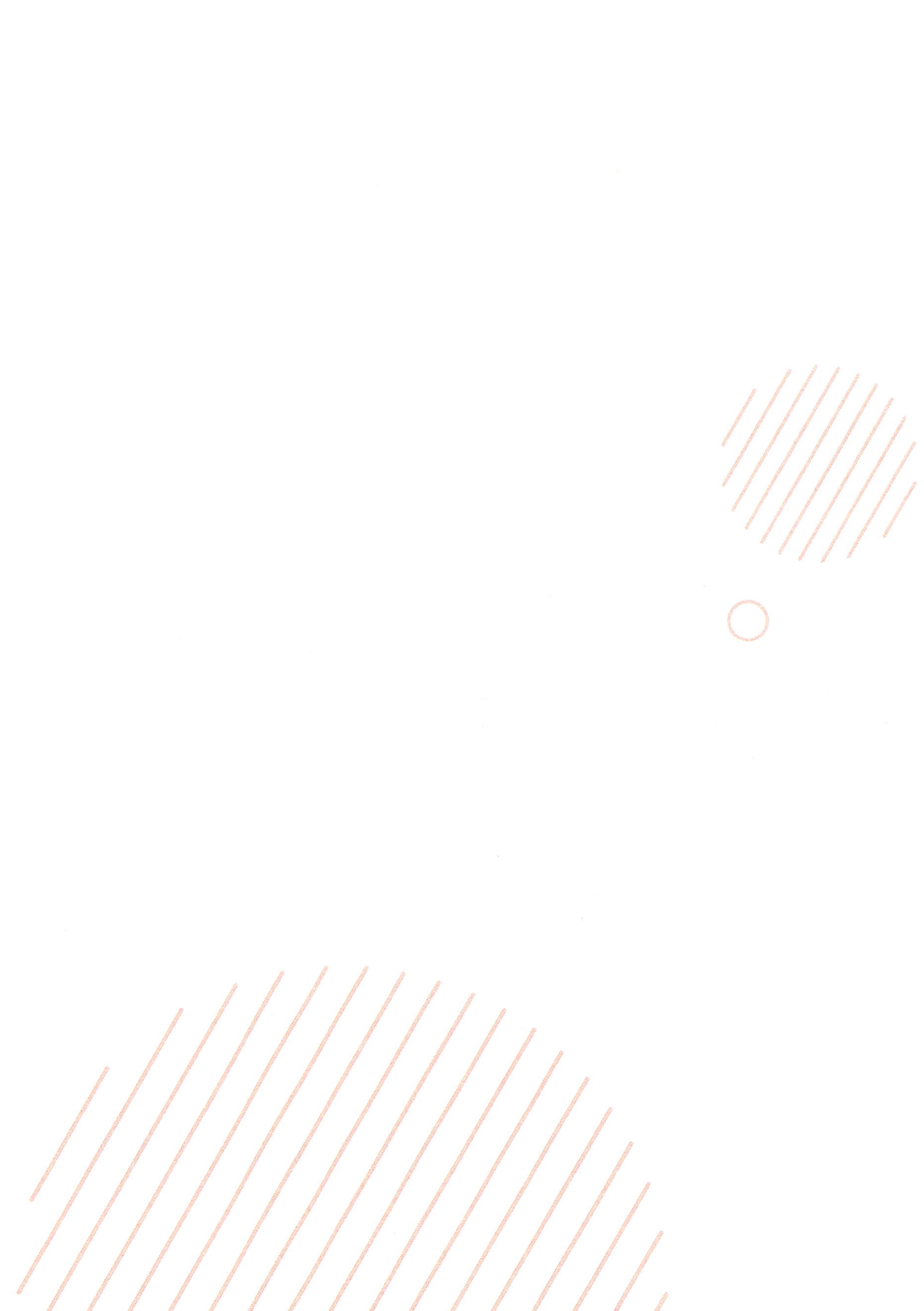

If These Walls Could Talk

— Professional Integrity and Cultural Responsiveness in the Workplace

Wendyliza González and Alicia Fleming-Hamilton

PREBRIEF

This scenario discusses ways to approach colleagues who are openly sharing discriminatory or offensive views. It reviews a situation that may be a common experience across multiple work environments. The scenario provides examples of possible solutions to address this type of behavior. As you read, pause and reflect on any situations you may have experienced that are similar to this one. Consider whether you were more like the speech-language pathologist (SLP) or the special education teacher, and what actions you could take in both situations

OBJECTIVES

- Identify effective approaches for addressing discriminatory or offensive behavior in the workplace.
- Understand the differences between harassment, "hate speech," and the first amendment protections for free speech.
- Become familiar with resources that are useful in instructing colleagues about diversity.
- Review Health Insurance Portability and Accountability Act of 1996 (HIPAA) requirements when talking about students or clients in an open environment.

CASE SCENARIO

Mrs. Rogers is a preschool special education teacher with 17 years of classroom experience. She coteaches with one general education teacher and two paraprofessionals. Both paraprofessionals are part of the special education team and are currently assigned to two students with individualized education plans (IEPs) for learning disabilities. Mrs. Rogers has five students with IEPs in her classroom, and all five students receive speech-language services. Her school also has another special education classroom for students with autism spectrum disorder (ASD) diagnoses.

During her duty-free lunch, Mrs. Rogers engaged in an informal conversation with other teachers in the staff lounge discussing concerns she had about one of her preschool

notes:

Definitions

Harassment–"Unwelcome conduct that is based on race, color, religion, sex (including pregnancy), national origin, age (40 or older), disability or genetic information" (U.S. Equal Employment Opportunity Commission, n.d., para. 2).

Hate speech–"Any form of expression through which speakers intend to vilify, humiliate, or incite hatred against a group or a class of persons" (American Library Association, n.d., para. 3).

Health Insurance Portability and Accountability Act of 1996 (HIPAA)–Privacy Rule standards used to "address the use and disclosure of individuals' health information–called 'protected health information' by organizations subject to the Privacy Rule –called 'covered entities,' as well as standards for individuals' privacy rights to understand and control how their health information is used" (U.S. Department of Health and Human Services, Office for Civil Rights, 2013, para. 2).

students. She mentioned the student, by name, indicating that she thought the student was presenting with characteristics of ASD. This student was from Ethiopia, and although not formally diagnosed with ASD, Mrs. Rogers explained that she showed some characteristics, including repeating phrases and self-directed play. Some observations Mrs. Rogers noted appeared to support her suspected diagnosis, including the child's difficulty moving from activity to activity, inability to answer a question on topic (if at all), and a low frustration tolerance for structured activities in the classroom. Mrs. Rogers went on to note that the student's social interactions were awkward and sometimes frightened other children. She finally shared how disgusted she was when the student ate using her hands and made a horrible mess.

Mrs. Rogers expressed how this child's behavior was "beyond frustrating" and that she just "didn't have any more patience for her inappropriate meltdowns or tantrums." When she asked her principal to evaluate the student for ASD and placement in the other classroom, she was chastised for "questionable cultural competence skills" and "lack of behavioral management techniques." Her supervisors also encouraged her to attend "diversity training" and to make adjustments to her classroom to support the child's culture by offering more student-directed activities and visual supports. She expressed loudly to all within ear shot that this child should just be taught to "follow the program, because this is where she lives now, and school isn't going to get any easier for her."

The SLP, Greg, was also present at the lunch table during this conversation, and he was personally offended by some of the comments Mrs. Rogers was making, but he said nothing to her. After their lunch break, Greg decided to compile a list of articles and other resources that he thought may help Mrs. Rogers work with this particular student. The resources included picture icons and visual supports to use around the classroom that would also support her other students. He added icons that would be especially helpful for the student Mrs. Rogers was describing. When he approached Mrs. Rogers with the tools, Mrs. Rogers looked at them, rolled her eyes, and said, "Thanks, but these things won't work; this little girl is just too retarded to learn all this, plus her parents can't even help her at home in English." Greg was stunned by her comment and reminded her that "retarded" is not a term used currently and furthermore not considered an appropriate way to describe children. Mrs. Rogers laughed off the comment and tossed the resources on her desk promising that she would "see whether she had time" to use them. As the SLP walked away, Mrs. Rogers said, "don't be so sensitive, everyone's entitled to free speech."

CRITICAL THINKING AND DEBRIEFING QUESTIONS

1. **What kinds of HIPAA regulations did Mrs. Rogers violate during her conversations in the lunch room? How could Mrs. Rogers have demonstrated better professionalism?**
2. **What are some other things the SLP could have done when he overheard Mrs. Rogers speaking in the lunchroom?**

3. What are some consequences that could occur as a result of this type of behavior in your work setting?
4. What kind of professional development resources could be useful for Mrs. Rogers to access to increase her cultural responsiveness?

COMMENTARY

In this case, we encounter a situation in which a teacher who is charged with the care and education of students is outwardly demonstrating a disregard toward this particular student and their disability. Additionally, the teacher is speaking in a way that could be offensive to a variety of other colleagues who are present in the lunchroom. Although seeking recommendations from colleagues is part of acceptable professional behavior, care should be taken when sharing information in public spaces. Sharing extensive identifying details—including the child's name, age, and country of origin—is in direct violation of HIPAA, which offers us guidance on the extent to which we can "consult" with other professionals.

One bystander was the SLP, who was offended by these statements and knew they were a violation of HIPAA. The SLP had many options to approach this staff member. The approach chosen, although an appropriate option, was a passive approach to correcting a colleague's overt discrimination. The SLP could have chosen to directly confront the teacher in the lunchroom and stop the continuation of her unprofessional dialogue. It is important to reflect on these situations and to have a plan in place for what to do if a situation like this occurs. Creating a plan of action can help professionals to be ready for volatile situations. Speaking out and stopping unprofessional behavior or pejorative speech helps all employees to behave in a more professional manner.

Creating a plan of action can help professionals to be ready for volatile situations.

As SLPs and audiologists, we frequently come into contact with a variety of professionals and populations, depending on our workplace. We maintain a professional responsibility to educate, advocate, and treat according to the American Speech-Language-Hearing Association's (2016) *Code of Ethics.* Workplace scenarios like the one involving Mrs. Rogers can be shocking, disheartening, and controversial. It is imperative to keep up to date on privacy regulations and procedures as well as best practices when working with all populations.

CRITICAL THINKING AND DEBRIEFING RESPONSES

1. **What kinds of HIPAA regulations did Mrs. Rogers violate during her conversations in the lunch room? How could Mrs. Rogers have demonstrated better professionalism?**

HIPAA privacy regulations were violated during this lunchroom interaction. The Privacy Rule under HIPAA protects all "identifiable health information" (U.S. Department of Health and Human Services, Office for Civil Rights, 2013, para. 2), including demographic information; any information regarding a person's physical, mental, or other health condition; and any plans for providing care to this individual. When Mrs. Rogers identified this student by name and proceeded to share information about the student's background and educational information, she was in violation of HIPAA privacy regulations. Aside from her questionable and derogatory comments, it would have been more appropriate for Mrs. Rogers to seek support for this student at another time in a more private, appropriate space—for example, in consultation with a pupil support team, special education committee, or trusted and qualified colleague. In addition, Mrs. Rogers may wish to seek out support services with managing the challenges of being a classroom teacher to special education students. This could include outreach to a union representative, a teacher mentor, special education teacher forum, or a content specialist within her school building or district. During these conversations, only nonidentifiable and pertinent information about the student would be shared.

2. **What are some other things the SLP could have done when he overheard Mrs. Rogers speaking in the lunchroom?**

The SLP had an appropriate response by providing resources that may have helped some of Mrs. Rogers's underlying complaints. In doing this, the SLP may have been attempting to establish himself as an educational ally and advocate while highlighting himself as a resource to Mrs. Rogers and the students in her class.

A more active approach to this situation would have been speaking out in the lunchroom. By not addressing Mrs. Rogers and stopping her offensive speech, Greg was participating in the "bystander effect" (Keltner & Marsh, 2006). He may have assumed that "someone else" would address Mrs. Rogers and he would not have to do it. Had Greg decided to address Mrs. Rogers in the lunchroom, he may have inspired others to do the same and to create an attitude among their staff that speech that denigrates others is not tolerated. Greg may have considered reporting her actions to a supervisor or administrator to ensure that they were aware of what occurred.

Although the SLP did try his best to be proactive with reframing Mrs. Rogers's thinking, she was not open to other suggestions. This SLP might use this experience to inspire a greater movement within his workplace, such as providing monthly newsletters or bulletin board presentations on culturally competent practices, providing workshops on culturally responsive intervention, or spearheading cultural competence initiatives. In addition, an experience like this reminds us as professionals that we must be vigilant with reflecting on our own biases and maintain our professional integrity by (a) ensuring that we are frequently educating ourselves about culture and practice and (b) holding ourselves and our colleagues to high standards of professionalism.

3. **What are some consequences that could occur as a result of this type of behavior in your work setting?**

Protocols and corrective practices differ on the basis of one's school district or work setting; however, there are several possible workplace "reactions" to the following scenario. Some employers may opt to see this as an opportunity to establish or "reinvigorate" cultural competence and implicit bias training for all staff members. Other employers may mandate cultural competence training as a corrective measure to avoid more stringent disciplinary action. Some work environments adopt a "zero-tolerance" policy regarding discriminatory language and outright violation of HIPAA laws, resulting in probationary action or removal.

In addition, someone like Mrs. Rogers may have a discriminatory complaint brought against her because of her lack of professionalism and violation of HIPAA laws. Although there is no formal international definition of hate speech, it is

> *understood as any kind of communication in speech, writing or behaviour, that attacks or uses pejorative or discriminatory language with reference to a person or a group on the basis*

of who they are, in other words, based on their religion, ethnicity, nationality, race, colour, descent, gender or other identity factor. (United Nations, 2019, "What Is Hate Speech?" section, para. 1)

Behavior like this does not create a positive work environment and is not supportive of students with disabilities or from different cultures. In fact, comments like those discussed in this scenario may contribute to a hostile work environment. This kind of behavior may send a direct message to colleagues that your professional practices and judgment are questionable, uninformed, and even harmful to the population you serve.

4. **What kind of professional development resources could be useful for Mrs. Rogers to access to increase her cultural responsiveness?**

Mrs. Rogers can take advantage of a variety of resources to enhance her cultural competence and responsiveness, including the following approaches:

- Learning about herself—for example, her historical and familial roots, beliefs, and values;
- Undergoing a deep self-reflection of cultural biases through the use of seminars, literature, and hands-on workshops;
- Taking professional development courses to learn and understand the most up-to-date diagnostic processes that are supported by evidence-based research;
- Educating herself on cultures and populations that are represented in her classroom;
- Reaching out to knowledgeable professionals in the building, including a union representative, professional development committee members, teacher mentors, and the SLP or audiologist; and
- Seeking out appropriate ways to manage personal and professional stress or "burnout," including support groups, counseling, exploring new hobbies, or volunteering in the community.

TAKE AWAYS

- Common areas in the workplace are never an appropriate space to discuss student or client information.
- Professionally competent clinicians understand and abide by HIPAA and workplace policies regarding sharing private information.
- Bystanders who witness problematic behavior from those charged with protecting and caring for vulnerable populations should feel comfortable seeking support to report or address these behaviors.
- Outdated, insensitive, and inflammatory comments are detrimental at the individual, company, and community level and are subject to disciplinary action.

REFERENCES

American Library Association. (n.d.). *Hate speech and hate crime.* Retrieved from http://www.ala.org/advocacy/intfreedom/hate

American Speech-Language-Hearing Association. (2016). *Code of Ethics.* Retrieved from https://www.asha.org/Code-of-Ethics/

Health Insurance Portability and Accountability Act of 1996 (HIPAA), Pub. L. 104-191, 42 U.S.C. § 300gg, 29 U.S.C §§ 1181–1183, and 42 U.S.C. §§ 1320d–1320d9.

Keltner, D., & Marsh, J. (2006, September 1). We are all bystanders. *Greater Good Magazine.* Retrieved from https://greatergood.berkeley.edu/article/item/we_are_all_bystanders

United Nations. (2019, May). *United Nations strategy and plan of action on hate speech.* Retrieved from https://www.un.org/en/genocideprevention/documents/UN%20Strategy%20and%20Plan%20of%20Action%20on%20Hate%20Speech%2018%20June%20SYNOPSIS.pdf

U.S. Department of Health and Human Services, Office for Civil Rights. (2013, July 26). *Summary of the HIPAA privacy rule.* Retrieved from https://www.hhs.gov/hipaa/for-professionals/privacy/laws-regulations/index.html

U.S. Equal Employment Opportunity Commission. (n.d.). *Harassment.* Retrieved from https://www.eeoc.gov/laws/types/harassment.cfm

ADDITIONAL RESOURCES

American Speech-Language-Hearing Association. (n.d.). *Health Insurance Portability and Accountability Act.* Retrieved from https://www.asha.org/practice/reimbursement/hipaa/default/

United Nations. (2019, May). *United Nations strategy and plan of action on hate speech.* Retrieved from https://www.un.org/en/genocideprevention/documents/UN%20Strategy%20and%20Plan%20of%20Action%20on%20Hate%20Speech%2018%20June%20SYNOPSIS.pdf

U.S. Department of Health and Human Services. (n.d.). *Health information privacy.* Retrieved from https://www.hhs.gov/hipaa/index.html

U.S. Department of Health and Human Services, Office for Civil Rights. (2020, January 10). *Disability discrimination resources.* Retrieved from https://www2.ed.gov/about/offices/list/ocr/disabilityresources.html

Open for Business

— Providing Culturally Responsive Support to Multilingual Patients

KAREN L. BEVERLY-DUCKER

PREBRIEF

notes:

There are many resources available to assist with setting up a private practice. With increasing access to information regarding a client's rights and options for health care services, consumers are becoming better informed and involved in their overall health care. When exercising their preferences, consumers take care when choosing their service providers. Careful consideration may be given to an environment where clients feel most culturally welcomed and comfortable. This may include environments that accommodate a client's unique needs, including interpretation and translation services. Providing these services is crucial in providing patient-centered care. It can be beneficial to business owners to understand the cultural needs of their clients to set them apart in a competitive field.

OBJECTIVES

- Understand the terms "patient-centered care" and "health literacy."
- Identify when cultural and linguistic differences indicate the need for modifications to service delivery.
- Identify appropriate alternatives in speech audiometry for non-English speakers.

CASE SCENARIO

Lynn and Marty are audiologists who have been in private practice for the past 7 years. They accept referrals from several sources, including self-referrals. Recently, their marketing efforts have included targeted outreach efforts via local community centers, churches, and other places of worship with the goal of reaching underserved and underrepresented populations. Demographic shifts in the area show a significant growth in the Spanish- and Portuguese-speaking populations. They distributed flyers, developed public service announcements, and placed newspaper advertisements that were translations of previously used marketing materials. The website for their practice included several downloadable consumer information brochures and handouts, such as "How to Recognize a Hearing Loss" and "How (and When) to Buy a Hearing Aid." These consumer information pieces were available in English only.

Lynn and Marty's practice provides comprehensive audiologic services, including administering diagnostic tests, hearing aid fittings, otoacoustic emission, tympanometry, central auditory testing, cochlear implant evaluations, aural (re)habilitation, and counseling services. Lynn and Marty are monolingual English speakers. Marty studied Spanish in high school and can participate in basic conversations and exchange pleasantries with Spanish speakers. Neither of them are familiar with Portuguese.

When preparing for the next day's schedule, Lynn and Marty noted that a new patient indicated during his initial phone call that he speaks Portuguese and has limited English skills. The office administrator shared that difficulties were encountered while communicating over the telephone during the scheduling process but was unsure whether it was because of a possible hearing loss and/or a language difference. In an attempt to be responsive to the patient's needs, Lynn and Marty decided to use a free, online language translation service to develop a case history form and test instructions in Portuguese. In addition, they used the service to translate several word lists for use during speech audiometry testing.

CRITICAL THINKING AND DEBRIEFING QUESTIONS

1. **What are some concerns related to translating materials?**
2. **What are some concerns associated with using an online translation software platform?**
3. **What are appropriate ways to meet the language needs of a diverse client population, including steps to help ensure that service providers are prepared to meet the language needs of their clients?**
4. **What are some factors to consider when evaluating the speech perception of bilingual speakers with hearing loss?**

COMMENTARY

The United States is becoming increasingly multilingual, and audiologists are called to serve populations who need hearing assistance. It is crucial when performing audiologic evaluations to separate an individual's difficulty communicating because of unfamiliarity with a language and a possible hearing loss.

At year-end 2019, The American Speech-Language-Hearing Association (ASHA) represented 201,961 audiologists; speech-language pathologists; speech, language, and hearing scientists; and audiology and speech-language pathology support personnel. Of that number, 31,211 (6.5%) indicated they met ASHA's definition of bilingual service provider, with 765 being ASHA-certified audiologists. Collectively, bilingual service providers reported 78 spoken languages other than English. In addition, 742 individuals indicated that they could communicate using American Sign Language, 141 use Manually Coded English (including Signed English, Signing Exact English, Cued Speech, etc.), and 26 use"other sign languages" (ASHA, 2020a).

Of the 13,211 individuals who self-identified on the basis of ASHA's definition of bilingual service provider, most (8,579 or 64.9%) were Spanish-language service providers. Of these, 290 were ASHA-certified audiologists (ASHA, 2020b). This information indicates that it is likely that many audiologists will need to use the services of interpreters at some point as they work with clients from a variety of cultural backgrounds. Audiologists should be prepared with resources for interpretation and translation so that they can accommodate a variety of languages and provide accurate testing practices with the help of interpreters. Providing accurate information in a variety of languages helps to increase a client's health literacy. For audiologists, this may encompass providing clear, comprehensible communication so that patients have access to appropriate information to help them better understand their conditions and make educated choices about their treatment. Patient information is best delivered in accessible formats using a wide range of modalities (Gilligan & Weinstein, 2014).

Definitions

Health literacy is defined by the U.S. Department of Health and Human Services as "the degree to which individuals have the capacity to obtain, process, and understand basic health information and services needed to make appropriate health decisions" (National Network of Libraries of Medicine, n.d., para. 1).

The Institute of Medicine defines **patient-centered care** as "care that is respectful of and responsive to individual patient preferences, needs, and values, and ensuring that patient values guide all clinical decisions" (Tzelepis, Sanson-Fisher, Zucca, & Fradgley, 2015, p. 831-835).

In addition to helping clients with their health literacy, clinics would benefit from designing their processes around patient-centered care. It involves educating patients/clients and their families/caregivers about a diagnosis, potential treatment, or healthy behavior. It means providing full, unbiased information and guidance from health care providers about options, benefits, and risks. It also means considering the individual's cultural traditions, personal preferences and values, family situations, social circumstances, and lifestyles. Effective communication is vital. Lynn and Marty may have benefited from seeking guidance about their community from community leaders and liaisons. They may also consider seeking guidance from other audiologist peers regarding how to access a variety of resources to enlist more patient-centered care delivery.

In this scenario, Lynn and Marty had good intentions, but their actions could have resulted in inaccurate and incomplete information for their client. It is inappropriate to provide services exclusively in English to non-English speakers or those with limited English proficiency. Speech tests should be used that have been specifically developed on the basis of target languages rather than those tests that have been simply and inappropriately translated (Nissen, Harris, & Dukes, 2008; Shi, 2014). Part of a complete audiological evaluation includes speech audiometry. Translating speech audiometry tests does not provide a tool that reflects the phonetic balance of the target language.

Another way to enhance Lynn and Marty's practice could include seeking out resources for increasing their cultural competence. Moxley, Mahendra, and Vega-Barachowitz (2004) have shared resources and suggestions for working with clients who speak a different language. Some suggestions include using available ASHA brochures in different languages; creating a binder or cue cards that include simple greetings and positive reinforcement phrases, accompanied by pictures, in commonly spoken languages at their facility; creating a laminated communication board with clear pictures of water, food, a toilet seat, wheelchair, a person sleeping, and a person in pain; and developing a directory of interpreters and interpreting resources, along with contact information that is readily available when interpretation needs arise. Moxley et al. also have cited general and specific strategies for enhancing cultural sensitivity. General strategies include becoming aware of differences in cultural attitudes regarding health, disability, and illness; asking explicit questions and seeking client input regarding appropriate treatment and expectations from the treatment process; validating a client's opinions as legitimate views of a situation; and respecting their autonomy in decision making. Specific strategies include conducting in-service trainings using case study approaches, emphasizing intercultural sensitivity, and becoming aware of other resources and experts available through ASHA and state associations (Moxley et al., 2004).

CRITICAL THINKING AND DEBRIEFING RESPONSES

1. **What are some concerns related to translating materials?**

Speech audiometry tests that have been specifically developed on the basis of target languages should be used instead of those tests that have been simply and inappropriately translated (Nissen et al., 2008; Shi, 2014). Different languages have different fundamental frequencies; therefore, a translation of words from one language to another would not account for these fundamental frequency differences. For some languages, certain frequency regions contribute to speech intelligibility more than others. Word lists are developed to reflect the phonemic balance of the target language. Additionally, some words and concepts are not readily translated.

2. **What are some concerns associated with using an online translation software platform?**

Online software translation platforms instantly translate words, phrases, and webpages between English and more than 100 other languages. Certain words, elements, and concepts are more difficult to translate, and their intent is lost in the literal translation of the word. For example, inviting someone to a "coffee" is typically understood to convey the message that a guest will be served a variety of beverages and possibly light appetizers/desserts, with the main emphasis being on the opportunity for conversation, sharing, and networking. A literal translation conveys the message that a guest will be served coffee. When using these platforms to translate medical information, one should take care and have their work reviewed by a native speaker of the target language to ensure clarity, account for possible regional dialect or vocabulary, and clarify that the original intent remains in the translation.

3. **What are appropriate ways to meet the language needs of a diverse client population, including steps to help ensure that service providers are prepared to meet the language needs of their clients?**

Advance planning and preparation are critical. Initial contact made during the scheduling process should include the opportunity and mechanism for the patient/client to share language-related information and needs. This would include the language(s) used by the patient/client/family and the need for an interpreter. The facility should have resources that include available translators and language lines.

Best practices utilize prerecorded materials to ensure consistency across trials (Mendel & Owen, 2011). Monitored live voice testing may be used, given a client's unique needs, such as age or ability. Careful consideration of accent, dialect, and linguistic background is given for the speaker used in live voice testing. Live voice administration of translated word lists by individuals who are unfamiliar with the language should not be used (Bokhove & Downey, 2018). Although audio-recorded tests are an option, consideration must be given to the impact of the tester's ability to discern the accuracy of the patient's response in their native language.

In addition to developing a pool of interpreter resources, test instructions that have been appropriately translated should be available. Creating resources such as informational packets and brochures that are multimodal can be beneficial to all clients, including those who are monolingual English speakers. Using photos and videos of testing procedures as well as instructional videos can also assist clients in understanding what will happen over the course of assessment and treatment.

4. **What are some factors to consider when evaluating the speech perception of bilingual speakers with hearing loss?**

Speech perception testing is an objective way to assess hearing technology benefit. It involves listening to sentences or words in quiet and with background noise while wearing hearing technology. Age of acquisition of the second language has been shown to influence speech perception results. Shi and Sánchez (2010) found that patients who acquired a second language at age 10 years or later performed more favorably on speech perception testing in their dominant language. The researchers recommended that patients who acquired a second language between ages 7 and 10 years should be evaluated in both languages. Mayo, Florentine, and Buus (1997) found that patients who acquired a second language before age 6 (i.e., early bilinguals) were better able to process speech in noise than patients who acquired a second language after age 14 (i.e., late bilinguals). This underscores the importance of language history questions during the patient interview/intake process.

Shi and Sánchez (2010) found that patients who acquired a second language at age 10 years or later performed more favorably on speech perception testing in their dominant language.

TAKE AWAYS

- Although convenient, online translation tools may fail to grasp the nuances of language and can contribute to miscommunications or inaccurate information.
- When serving any community, it is beneficial to engage with the community regarding their linguistic or cultural needs so that you can be prepared to provide any additional needed resources or personnel. Cultural values and preferences can influence how consumers respond to marketing strategies, products, practices, and communications related to their health care services. An approach that is successful in one culture may not be effective in a different culture. Effective communication is vital.
- Cultural audits examine current practices, programs, and processes to identify how culturally appropriate they may be for diverse populations. The information obtained supports the goal of culturally appropriate service delivery.

REFERENCES

American Speech-Language-Hearing Association. (2020a). *ASHA summary membership and affiliation counts, year-end 2019.* Retrieved from https://www.asha.org/uploadedFiles/2019-Member-Counts.pdf

American Speech-Language-Hearing Association. (2020b). *Demographic profile of ASHA members providing bilingual services, year-end 2019.* Retrieved from https://www.asha.org/uploadedFiles/Demographic-Profile-Bilingual-Spanish-Service-Members.pdf

Bokhove, C., & Downey, C. (2018). Automated generation of 'good enough' transcripts as a first step to transcription of audio-recorded data. *Methodological Innovations, 11*(2), 1–14. https://doi.org/10.1177/2059799118790743

Gilligan, J., & Weinstein, B. E. (2014). Health literacy and patient-centered care in audiology—Implications for adult aural rehabilitation. *Journal of Communication Disorders, Deaf Studies & Hearing Aids, 2,* 110.

Mayo, L. H., Florentine, M., & Buus, S. (1997). Age of second-language acquisition and perception of speech in noise. *Journal of Speech, Language, and Hearing Research, 40,* 686–693.

Mendel, L. L., & Owen, S. R. (2011). A study of recorded versus live voice word recognition. *International Journal of Audiology, 50,* 688–693.

Moxley, A., Mahendra, N., & Vega-Barachowitz, C. (2004). Cultural competence in health care. *The ASHA Leader, 9*(7), 6–22.

National Network of Libraries of Medicine. (n.d.). *Health literacy.* Retrieved from https://nnlm.gov/initiatives/topics/health-literacy

Nissen, S. L., Harris, R. W., & Dukes, A. (2008). Word recognition materials for native speakers of Taiwan Mandarin. *American Journal of Audiology, 17,* 68–79.

Shi, L. F. (2014). Speech audiometry and Spanish–English bilinguals: Challenges in clinical practice. *American Journal of Audiology, 23,* 243–259.

Shi, L. F., & Sánchez, D. (2010). Spanish/English bilingual listeners on clinical word recognition tests: What to expect and how to predict. *Journal of Speech, Language, and Hearing Research, 53*(5), 1096-1110. https://doi.org/10.1044/1092-4388(2010/09-0199)

Tzelepis, F., Sanson-Fisher, R. W., Zucca, A. C., & Fradgley, E. A. (2015). Measuring the quality of patient-centered care: Why patient-reported measures are critical to reliable assessment. *Patient Preference and Adherence, 9,* 831–835.

ADDITIONAL RESOURCES

American Speech-Language-Hearing Association. (2005, August). *Private audiology practice.* Retrieved from https://www.asha.org/Articles/Private-Audiology-Practice/

American Speech-Language-Hearing Association. (2014a). An "atypical" or a "new normal" day. *ASHA Audiology Connections,* 14.

American Speech-Language-Hearing Association. (2014b, May). *Get prepared: It's time for a culture audit!* Retrieved from https://www.asha.org/Articles/Get-Prepared-Its-Time-for-a-Culture-Audit/

American Speech-Language-Hearing Association. (2019a). *Frequently asked questions about business practices.* Retrieved from https://www.asha.org/practice/faq_business_practices_both/

American Speech-Language-Hearing Association. (2019b). *Private practice.* Retrieved from https://marketing.asha.org/work-settings/private-practice/

Ramkissoon, I., Estis, J. M., & Flagge, A. G. (2014). Digit speech recognition threshold (SRT) in children with normal hearing ages 5–8 years. *American Journal of Audiology, 23,* 182–189.

U.S. Department of Health and Human Services. (2015). *Health literacy online: A guide for simplifying the user experience.* Retrieved from https://health.gov/healthliteracyonline/

There are programs that provide tax benefits and funding for the provision of reasonable accommodations, including providing effective communication—for example, see the following:

Internal Revenue Service. (n.d.). *About Form 8826, disabled access credit.* Retrieved from https://www.irs.gov/forms-pubs/about-form-8826

U.S. Department of Justice, Civil Rights Division, Disability Rights Section. (n.d.). *ADA update: A primer for small business.* Retrieved from https://www.ada.gov/regs2010/smallbusiness/smallbusprimer2010.htm

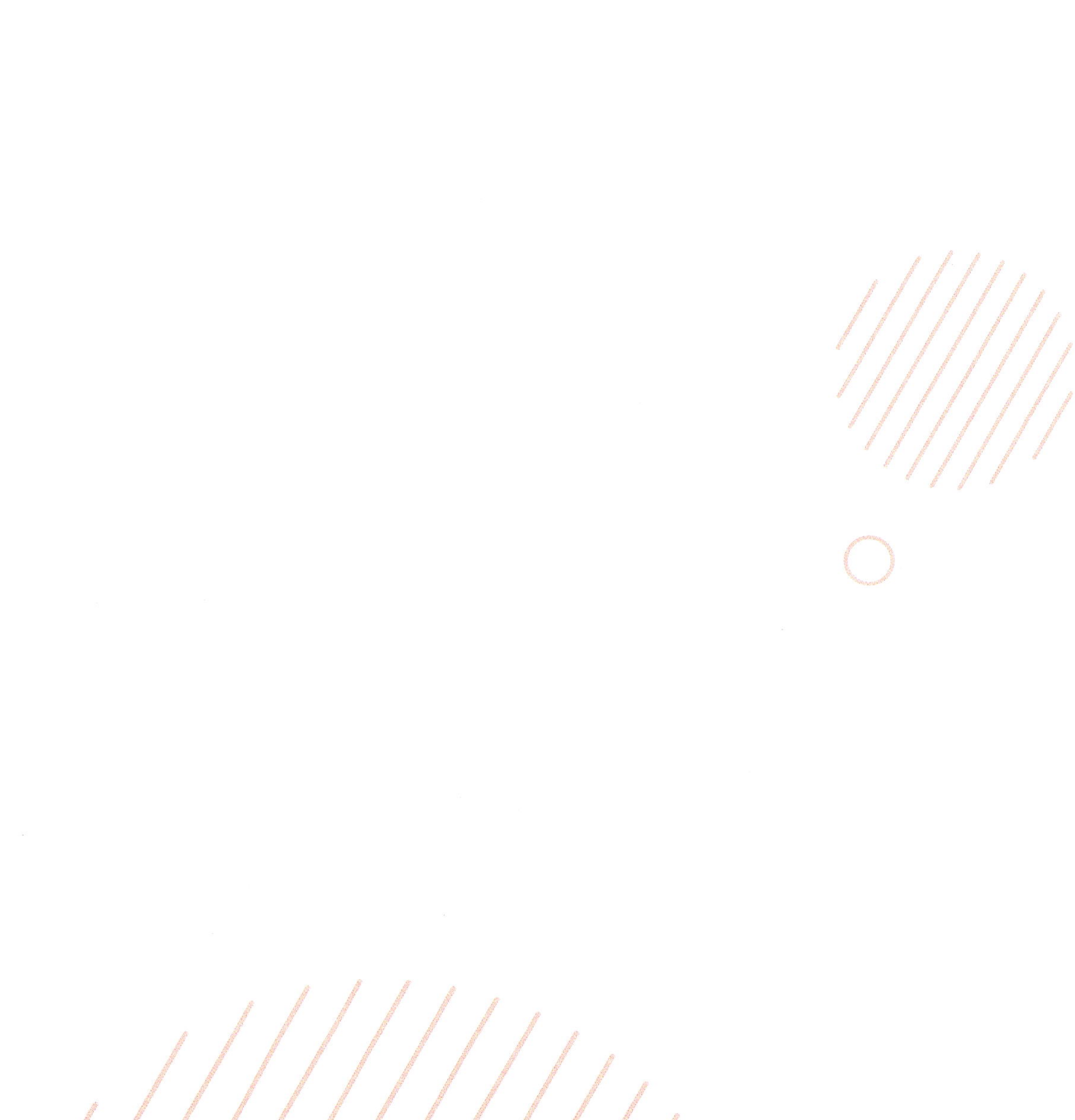

Cultural Responsiveness and Conscience Protection — Personal Beliefs, Discrimination, and Conscience Protection in the Clinical Setting

Alicia Fleming Hamilton

notes:

PREBRIEF

The American Speech-Language-Hearing Association's (ASHA, 2016) *Code of Ethics* reflects what we value as professionals and establishes expectations for scientific and clinical practice. It is based on principles of duty, accountability, fairness, and responsibility. It is intended to ensure the welfare of the consumer and to protect the reputation and integrity of the professions. Guidance is provided in several areas, including the avoidance of any form of bias or discrimination in service delivery. This case study highlights the difference between conscience protection, which protects an individual from performing or participating in specific medical services that interfere with a particular religious belief or practice, and discrimination that is based on another's perceived set of beliefs or expression.

OBJECTIVES

- Understand how ASHA's (2016) *Code of Ethics* guides professional practice in providing appropriate care for all clients who may present the need for therapy.
- Reference the final conscience rule and other antidiscrimination laws (e.g., Title VI) of the U.S. Department of Health and Human Services to better understand the rights of both clinicians and clients.
- Reflect on personal beliefs and professional responsibilities and how they may affect service delivery.

CASE SCENARIO

Sofia is a first-year graduate clinician completing her first clinical rotation in her university's voice clinic in her second semester of graduate school. The clinic serves members of the university and surrounding communities. The university's hospital also has a center for transgender health that conducts gender-affirmation surgery. One track of the graduate program's voice clinic has a focus to support patients at the center for transgender health. This track is prominently advertised in admission information for the program. Students are informed, after acceptance to the program, that they are expected to participate in a variety of practicum experiences that enhance their coursework. Students are given the option to choose specific tracks based on their area of interest. They are also notified that once a track is chosen, it is their responsibility to communicate any scheduling challenges or other applicable considerations that may affect their full participation in the track.

Sofia met with her faculty advisor and shared that she had an interest in voice therapy, specifically learning about intervention strategies for finding each client's target pitch and resonance. Sofia shared that she enjoyed singing in choirs and wanted to possibly use her knowledge of music and speech-language pathology to work with other singers, instructing them on appropriate vocal care habits. Sofia was assigned a client, Dani, who was seeking services to work on vocal feminization and learning ways to keep the voice healthy. During the intake interview, Dani shared that she is a transgender female, assigned male at birth, and uses "she/her/hers" pronouns. Dani stated that her goals in seeking voice treatment were to better align her voice and communication with her gender expression and identity. Sofia completed the initial interview and collaboratively established treatment goals and objectives with Dani. Dani made hour-long appointments for the following 6 weeks, at which point Sofia and Dani would reassess Dani's needs and review progress based on data obtained. According to her clinical educator, Professor Stevens, Sofia's initial meeting included all of the necessary components and focused on the client's needs and goals for therapy, successfully establishing a collaborative therapeutic partnership.

The following week, when Dani arrived for her first therapy appointment, she was notified that Sofia was absent due to illness. Fortunately, another clinician was available, and Dani agreed to have him carry out the treatment plan. Sofia arrived to clinic in the afternoon of the same day, informing Professor Stevens that she felt better. The following week, when Dani attended clinic, she was notified again that Sofia was absent due to illness. Dani was seen by the substitute clinician. Once again Sofia arrived at the clinic for her scheduled clients in the afternoon. This pattern continued for a total of 3 weeks, at which point Dani expressed her desire to continue therapy with the replacement clinician, given there were only three visits left. Professor Stevens, having noticed a pattern in Sofia's absences, scheduled a supervisory conference to discuss the absences.

During their meeting, Professor Stevens notified Sofia that Dani was reassigned to the substitute clinician who took over during her absences from clinic. She also addressed Sofia's absences and expressed curiosity as to why they only occurred for part of the day and in what appeared to be a pattern. Sofia, visibly upset, explained that she holds personal beliefs and faith practices that do not support Dani's gender identity. She concluded by stating that she cannot provide services to Dani, but she wants to continue working in the clinic and learning about voice therapy.

CRITICAL THINKING AND DEBRIEFING QUESTIONS

1. **If a student clinician has the clinical skills to provide a service, is it discriminatory for the student clinician to refuse provision of those services to a client?**
2. **Have you and a client ever had different values or beliefs? Did this affect your work? How did/could you respond to this?**
3. **In a clinical setting, are clinicians required to treat all clients who come to them, regardless of the clinician's beliefs?**
4. **Is it possible for Sofia to continue learning about voice therapy—specifically, pitch**

and resonance modifications and vocal care and treatment—if she refuses to see a specific population that seeks care within voice clinics?

COMMENTARY

Speech-language pathologists (SLPs) are professionals who are uniquely prepared to provide services to a wide range of clients who present with various communication needs. As individuals, SLPs have personal beliefs, cultures, backgrounds, and experiences that may differ from their colleagues and from the clients seeking their help. One instance of these differences was illustrated in the scenario. Sofia stated that she had religious beliefs that prevented her from being able to provide services to Dani. Sofia's stance raises a critical question: Should a student-clinician or clinician be required to provide services to a client if the provision of services is in contradiction to one's personal ethics, beliefs, or faith or be supportive of actions that are in contrast with one's personal ethics, beliefs, or faith?

ASHA's (2016) *Code of Ethics* provides guidance in Principles of Ethics I, Rule C, where it states that individuals may not discriminate on the basis of gender or gender identity. This rule also includes a protection against religious discrimination. In this case, the rule protects the client from discrimination based on gender or gender identity.

Expand Your Knowledge

"Conscience protections apply to health care providers who refuse to perform, accommodate, or assist with certain health care services on religious or moral grounds.

Federal statutes protect health care provider conscience rights and prohibit recipients of certain federal funds from discriminating against health care providers who refuse to participate in these services based on moral objections or religious beliefs."

https://www.hhs.gov/conscience/conscience-protections/index.html#conscience-rights

Current legislation for health care providers allows conscience protections that apply to health care providers who refuse to perform, accommodate, or assist with certain health care services on religious or moral grounds. This legislation may be interpreted in Sofia's case to allow her to refuse to provide gender-affirming voice and communication services. However, these protections may not necessarily be extended to all types of therapeutic interventions when Sofia is working with individuals who are transgender or gender diverse. Refusing all other therapies not directly related to gender-affirming voice and communication services may constitute as discrimination based on gender or gender identity.

Training programs have a responsibility to ensure that students complete their program with the appropriate knowledge and skills in the areas in which they are trained. To complete her program, on the basis of her desires, Sofia would still need to demonstrate mastery of voice competencies. It may be beneficial for Sofia and her supervisors to discuss her personal limits, or boundaries, for providing services and how those work with her clinical requirements for the completion of her program. The conscience protection law applies to health care providers who have conscience or religious objections related to performing, paying for, referring for, providing coverage of, or providing certain services—in this case, gender affirming voice and communication services (U.S. Department of Health and Human Services, 2019). The training program may consider offering Sofia an alternative option of completing clinical observation hours or simulated practice hours, dependent on her level of comfort, to receive appropriate exposure to the specified vocal techniques she will need to demonstrate the appropriate knowledge and skills in this area.

Students have the responsibility in their programs and as future professionals to communicate their needs in an appropriate and time-sensitive manner. Programs are encouraged to establish a process outlining how to exercise conscience protection and avoid situations like the one in this scenario. The university would benefit from a process that addresses possible clinical objections before clients are assigned and ensures the confidentiality of students when voicing any objections. Additionally, it may be beneficial to include cultural responsiveness training to the students, supervisors, and others who work at the clinic, focusing on specific groups who receive services, such as gender diverse individuals, to provide basic information to clinicians who will be working in this setting.

CRITICAL THINKING AND DEBRIEFING RESPONSES

1. **If a student clinician has the clinical skills to provide a service, is it discriminatory for the student clinician to refuse provision of those services to a client?**

Conscience protection states that if performing a medical treatment would go against a personal belief, it is not discriminatory to decline provision of that service. In this scenario, Sofia's beliefs were not in alignment with providing service to masculinize or femininize Dani's voice. Would this change if Sofia were providing vocal hygiene practices only? Although Sofia could have continued working with Dani on vocal hygiene techniques only, it may have been more appropriate to refer Dani to another qualified practitioner to provide both services to Dani in the clinical setting. Protections against discrimination apply to both clients and service providers. If a service provider's beliefs keep them from providing specific services, this must be disclosed to those who schedule and discussed with supervisors so as not to expose the client to undue stress as the result of improper scheduling. To the extent possible, clinicians and supervisors should have these conversations as situations present themselves before meeting with potential clients.

2. **Have you and a client ever had different values or beliefs? Did this affect your work? How did/could you respond to this?**

Personal response. If you have not faced a situation like this, reflect on what you may do in the future if this were to occur. Do you have full understanding of the protections of the law for both you and the clients you serve? In this example, Sofia's beliefs prevented her from providing gender-affirming voice and communication services. What if her belief system prevented her from working with individuals of the opposite gender alone in a room? Consider how this may affect staffing and exposure to a variety of diagnoses and treatment opportunities.

3. **In a clinical setting, are clinicians required to treat all clients who come to them, regardless of the clinician's beliefs?**

Although a provider may opt to exercise their conscience protection and refuse to participate in a client's care, this refusal of care should not compromise the client's health. Ultimately, a client should be able to access care without judgment or discrimination. It is imperative that all student clinicians are trained in cultural responsiveness, and it is highly recommended that training programs have a protocol in place if a student clinician wishes to exercise conscience protection.

4. **Is it possible for Sofia to continue learning about voice therapy—specifically, pitch and resonance modifications and vocal care and treatment—if she refuses to see a specific population that seeks care within voice clinics?**

Sofia is able to exercise her right to conscience protection under the law, but if the significant portion of the practicum involves gender-affirmation services, she may have less opportunity for voice hours or have a smaller voice caseload than her peers. This is something that should be discussed with her supervisors and the department chair in advance of starting her rotations. Additionally, it may be a useful reflective practice for Sofia to consider how her work with voice clients in the future may or may not be affected if her beliefs are not in alignment with some services provided at voice clinics. It is possible it could decrease her pool of clients, or she may choose to focus in another area of voice where this may not have a large impact on her caseload. All of these facts are things that Sofia should consider as she completes her training program. Clinical coordinators for the university program may develop alternative and parallel experiences to ensure that a student who is claiming conscience protection still meets ASHA's knowledge and skills standards.

TAKE AWAYS

- ASHA's (2016) Code of Ethics and guidelines for cultural competence guide the practice of audiologists and SLPs to provide appropriate services for all people regardless of race, ethnicity, sex, gender identity/gender expression, sexual orientation, age, religion, national origin, disability, culture, language, or dialect.
- SLPs are uniquely qualified to provide sensitive, skilled care to individuals who are seeking a more authentic voice that matches their gender identity.
- Although SLPs may exercise their right to conscience protection, they must also identify qualified referral sources to provide the needed service to the client seeking that service.
- When faced with an unfamiliar topic or clinical skill, clinicians can take that opportunity to reflect on their initial reactions and possibly seek further training to address possible bias or need for further cultural competence.

REFERENCES

American Speech-Language-Hearing Association. (2016). *Code of Ethics*. Retrieved from https://www.asha.org/Code-of-Ethics/

U.S. Department of Health and Human Services. (2019, May 2). *HHS announces final conscience rule protecting health care entities and individuals.* Retrieved from https://www.hhs.gov/about/news/2019/05/02/hhs-announces-final-conscience-rule-protecting-health-care-entities-and-individuals.html

ADDITIONAL RESOURCES

American Speech-Language-Hearing Association. (n.d.). *Voice and communication services for transgender and gender diverse populations*. Retrieved from https://www.asha.org/PRPSpecificTopic.aspx?folderid=8589944119§ion=Key_Issues

American Speech-Language-Hearing Association. (2017). *Issues in ethics: Cultural and linguistic competence.* Retrieved from https://www.asha.org/Practice/ethics/Cultural-and-Linguistic-Competence/

Deutsch, M. B. (Ed.). (2016, June 17). *Guidelines for the primary and gender-affirming care of transgender and gender nonbinary people* (2nd ed.). Retrieved from https://transcare.ucsf.edu/guidelines

L'GASP website: http://www.noglstp.net/LGASP/

Transgender Law Center website: https://transgenderlawcenter.org/

U.S. Department of Health and Human Services. (n.d.). *Conscience protections for health care providers.* Retrieved from https://www.hhs.gov/conscience/conscience-protections/index.html

U.S. Department of Health and Human Services. (2019, May 2). *HHS announces final conscience rule protecting health care entities and individuals.* Retrieved from https://www.hhs.gov/about/news/2019/05/02/hhs-announces-final-conscience-rule-protecting-health-care-entities-and-individuals.html

World Professional Association for Transgender Health. (2020). *Standards of care* (Version 7). Retrieved from https://www.wpath.org/publications/soc

Impact Versus Intent
— When "Trying to Help" Can Actually Be Harmful

Alicia Fleming Hamilton and Perry Flyn

PREBRIEF

notes:

Perceptions and beliefs regarding immigrant populations may influence referral practices for dual language learning (DLL) services. In this scenario, a professional's "attempts to help" may lead to inappropriate referrals of a specific population of individuals. It also highlights the impact of implicit bias on workplace interactions. Personal beliefs and perceptions about race, ethnicity, age, gender, gender identity, or any diversity factor can be addressed through self-reflection activities with the goal of identifying whether and how those beliefs and perceptions may be affecting professional services.

OBJECTIVES

- Identify patterns of prejudicial practices that can affect the trajectory of a student's academic career.
- Outline materials or resources available for colleagues and clinical professionals that can assist in constructing a more equitable referral process.
- Define the concept of implicit bias.

CASE SCENARIO

Joe is a speech-language pathologist (SLP) in a rural area and works for a middle school. The school secretary, Becky, has worked in this middle school for 25 years and is well liked in the community. Joe was at school the week before classes started setting up his room and volunteered to help Becky with new student registrations.

Joe was excited for the new school year and looked forward to meeting new families as they registered. During some down time, Becky explained to Joe that recently there was an increase in Vietnamese and Indian immigrants in their school district. She shared that she has heard from multiple sources that this might be due to the opening of a new health clinic and increased farming success in the community.

As the morning progressed, Joe started to notice that during the intake process, Becky was referring every Vietnamese student to special education and DLL services, but she did not make any DLL referrals for the Indian families who registered. After about five of these instances, Joe noticed a pattern, and he politely asked Becky why she referred the current student when the parents did not request DLL or special education help. Becky responded that, "The Indian families are able to speak English, and do it well. Plus their parents all work in the clinic. They've got good educations. The Vietnamese families can't communicate at all! They need all the help I can give them." Becky did not seem bothered by Joe's curiosity, as illustrated by her frank explanation.

As the day continued, Joe also noticed that Becky gave all of the Vietnamese families brochures with information on vocational schools, but she handed out "preparing for college" brochures to the Indian families. Additionally, when some of the Indian families noted they would like a screening for special education, Becky told them she was sure they didn't need it and that they would be just fine.

Joe felt uncomfortable with what he had observed. He believed that all families should have equal opportunities for learning–including special education referrals; DLL support; and options for vocational schools, trade schools, or higher education. He didn't think it made sense to group entire communities of people together and to make decisions on their behalf. Joe knew that their district practice was to screen all students using a survey for DLL services. By taking away that opportunity, Becky was limiting these families' options for appropriate and individualized educational opportunities. Joe was now unsure as to how he should proceed regarding his observations. He knew that Becky had a long history at the school and was well liked in the community, but he feared that these discriminatory practices would continue without intervention.

CRITICAL THINKING AND DEBRIEFING QUESTIONS

1. **What bilingual education services does your district offer to students who speak a language other than English? How are students typically referred for DLL services in your school district?**
2. **What are some alternatives this district or specific school could use when making student referrals?**
3. **What are some ways to approach a colleague who is speaking in a way that exhibits a significant bias toward certain racial, ethnic, or other groups?**
4. **Have you ever encountered situations in which you suspected that you had implicit bias against another race, age, or other demographic group? How did you manage to maintain fairness? Did you recognize your bias during the encounter, or afterward on reflection?**

COMMENTARY

Referral to DLL services may be initiated by concerned parents, guardians, family advocates, qualified school officials, or educational professionals. Potential candidates may include students who are explicitly identified as having a higher proficiency in a language other than English or a student who may benefit from DLL services. Generally, these determinations should be made using criteria that is applied consistently and equally across all students. Although Becky has years of experience at her job, the lack of a school-wide systematic strategy to generate the referrals is concerning. As the SLP, Joe is in a unique position to observe consistent behaviors and possibly provide some assistance in developing a referral checklist or questionnaire that can make the process more equitable and less susceptible to implicit bias. This may help to improve the accuracy of referrals and provide each family with the opportunity for services that are available to all students.

Biases toward a particular race or cultural group are at times not explicit and recognized by the individual (Staats, 2016). Studies have shown that the presence of implicit bias is not linked to age, gender, education, or political affiliation.

Researchers have noted that when a person becomes aware of their biases against specific races or genders, their own self-awareness may help to counteract the influence of those biases (Devine, Forscher, Austin, & Cox, 2012; Dovidio, Kawakami, Johnson, Johnson, & Howard, 1997). In other words, with effort, implicit bias can be "unlearned." Implicit bias is a commonality across all people, so the opportunity for implicit bias training for an entire staff will help everyone to recognize their biases and may positively impact the referral process in an effort to make it more balanced.

Definition

Implicit bias refers to attitudes or stereotypes that unconsciously affect our understanding, actions, and decisions. These biases may not align with the beliefs we declare ourselves to hold. We may believe we act objectively, but we are actually influenced by biases—toward people of particular races, genders, and linguistic or socioeconomic backgrounds—that pervade our society (Arora, 2017, p. 6).

A specific concern in this scenario is Becky's approach to special education referrals. Becky's outward validation of her biases and her prejudicial practices of distributing specific postsecondary education packets to specific ethnic groups demonstrated that not all families were being provided with the same opportunities. Her perception that she was "helping" the families may in fact be a demonstration of her desire to ensure the best for these children and families. This disconnect between her desires and her actions is precisely why educators should become aware of the concept of implicit bias: "the attitudes or stereotypes that affect our understanding, actions, and decisions in an unconscious manner" (Staats, 2016, p. 29).

Presenting specific groups with different information gave the impression that Vietnamese students were considered less likely to pursue higher education when compared with the Indian students. Although Joe's observations may indicate the presence of bias, Becky may not have even been aware that a bias was affecting the way she interacted with a specific group of people.

A way for Joe to address this issue may be to share it with a superior or offer to create training opportunities for the whole staff regarding implicit bias and its professional impact. Joe could talk to Becky about the process for qualifying for special education and explain that he works with students who are exhibiting true disorders—and not just differences because of a lack of exposure or the influence of other languages. He could illustrate the stages of second-language development (Krashen & Terrell, 1999) and note how many students are in different places on their journey to learning English. The teams could also work on educating colleagues about using dynamic assessment to measure the skills of English language learners. As an expert in language development, Joe has a lot of information that can be useful for colleagues across his job setting.

CRITICAL THINKING AND DEBRIEFING RESPONSES

1. **What bilingual education services does your district offer to students who speak a language other than English? How are students typically referred for DLL services in your school district?**

Personal/answers may vary. Possible DLL eligibility practices include the following:

- A registration process that includes a home language survey of all entering students to inform the possible need of DLL services;

- Parents or guardians explicitly requesting DLL services for their child(ren);
- Parent and teacher completion of "prescreening" language checklists assessing baseline language skills;
- Formal English language proficiency exams that include written, listening, reading, and writing assessments; and
- Eligibility measures that are administered by a bilingual or DLL-certified teacher.

2. **What are some alternatives this district or specific school could use when making student referrals?**

To make the process more equitable and to decrease personal bias, the district may consider creating a checklist that uses current research regarding students who qualify for DLL services. Districts could distribute information regarding home language practices, students' abilities in their native language and English, and an area for parent concerns. Policies to screen all students who identify as exposed to more than one language can be implemented, along with a formalized process for special education referrals that provides all students and families with the opportunity to share their concerns. Finally, trained professionals—including teachers who are bilingual or who have their English as a second language teaching certification—should be part of the student referral process. School community members who are charged with developing a screening process for DLL referrals may reference federal, state, and local requirements and would benefit from having experience working with students who learn, and who are exposed to, multiple languages.

3. **What are some ways to approach a colleague who is speaking in a way that exhibits a significant bias toward certain racial, ethnic, or other groups?**

In this case, Joe responded by asking Becky about what he was observing first. This step was appropriate because Joe did not assume that Becky was operating with ill intentions. When she shared her rationale, Joe was better able to understand her beliefs about the different groups they were interacting with. From this point, Joe has a variety of options. He could share his beliefs about different groups or engage Becky in a conversation about the possibility of bias affecting her decision making. He could share this information with a supervisor or someone who has more administrative responsibility to determine the next best steps. Joe may also take this opportunity to create or volunteer for a school-based committee that oversees the DLL referral process in his middle school or district. However, some sort of action is necessary in a situation like this. Implicit bias and cycles of discrimination cannot be stopped or changed if they aren't first interrupted.

4. **Have you ever encountered situations in which you suspected that you had implicit bias against another race, age, or other demographic group? How did you manage to maintain fairness? Did you recognize your bias during the encounter, or afterward on reflection?**

Personal/answers may vary. The authors encourage the reader to examine their own implicit biases. The reader may consider taking the Harvard Implicit Association Test online (https://implicit.harvard.edu/implicit/takeatest.html) and reflect on your results and feelings after the exercise.

Research from Devine et al. (2012) provides compelling evidence for the long-term effectiveness of an intervention focused on reducing implicit bias. The intervention was multifaceted and focused on prejudice habit-breaking interventions. The study lasted 12 weeks. The greatest reduction in implicit biases occurred in participants who also demonstrated concern about discrimination. The intervention increased both personal awareness of one's bias and a general concern about discrimination in society. Devine et al. suggested that the elevated concern about daily instances of discrimination may be due to an increased awareness of participants' own spontaneous biases. The authors' desires are that the intervention may help others to reduce persistent and unintentional forms of discrimination that arise from implicit bias.

TAKE AWAYS

- Referral to DLL and special education services should be consistent and systemized across settings to ensure the least amount of bias and the maximum opportunity for students to access services they need.
- Implicit bias is inherent across all cultures, races, ethnicities, and genders. Cultivating an awareness of implicit bias and working toward identifying and unlearning bias is a positive step toward cultural competence.
- It is recommended that SLPs and audiologists seek out resources to identify and diminish the impact of implicit biases that may directly affect their professional practices.

REFERENCES

Arora, N. (2017). Look at your blind spots: Do unconscious preconceptions shape your clinical judgment? A school-based clinician offers ways to uncover—and address—implicit bias. *The ASHA Leader, 22*(11), 6-7.

Devine, P. G., Forscher, P. S., Austin, A. J., & Cox, W. T. (2012). Long-term reduction in implicit race bias: A prejudice habit-breaking intervention. *Journal of Experimental Social Psychology, 48,* 1267-1278.

Dovidio, J. F., Kawakami, K., Johnson, C., Johnson, B., & Howard, A. (1997). On the nature of prejudice: Automatic and controlled processes. *Journal of Experimental Social Psychology, 33,* 510-540.

Krashen, S. D., & Terrell, T. D. (1999). *The natural approach: Language acquisition in the classroom.* Hertfordshire, England: Prentice Hall Europe.

Staats, C. (2016). Understanding implicit bias: What educators should know. *American Educator, 39*(4), 29.

ADDITIONAL RESOURCES

Eastern Stream Center on Resources and Training. (2003). *Help! They don't speak English* [Starter kit]. Oneonta, NY: State University College.

Kusimo, P., Ritter, M., Busick, K., Ferguson, C., Trumbull, E., & Solano-Flores, G. (2000). *Making assessment work for everyone: How to build on student strengths.* San Francisco, CA: WestEd.

Mandelbaum, E. (2016). Attitude, inference, association: On the propositional structure of implicit bias. *Noûs, 50*(3), 629–658.

Morin, R. (2015, August 19). *Exploring racial bias among biracial and single-race adults: The IAT.* Retrieved from the Pew Research Center website: https://www.pewsocialtrends.org/2015/08/19/exploring-racial-bias-among-biracial-and-single-race-adults-the-iat/

Multicultural Constituency Groups (MCCGs) https://www.asha.org/practice/multicultural/opportunities/constituency/

Bilingual Clients With Aphasia — Bicultural Perspectives When Interviewing, Assessing, and Treating

PEI-FANG HUNG, CARMEN ANA RAMOS-PIZARRO, AND ALICIA FLEMING HAMILTON

PREBRIEF

Speech-language pathologists (SLPs) focus on improving communication for individuals they serve. When working with clients, understanding their goals for communicating as well as their cultural communication practices and values helps tailor therapy for their unique needs. As a culturally responsive clinician, it is critical to provide culturally sensitive care by informing oneself about patterns of communication behavior that are accepted across cultures and within the specific culture of your client. It is important to understand practices that may be culturally offensive. This case discusses communication characteristics common in the Japanese culture and highlights register, age, and gender differences. Please note that each client may express their own cultural traditions in different ways. The characteristics listed in this scenario related to Japanese communication styles outline general practices and do not apply to all people of Japanese descent. Relying on generalizations and failing to recognize individual differences within cultural practices may be interpreted as cultural stereotyping and may lead to clinical interactions that do not feel welcoming or respectful to the client.

OBJECTIVES

- Describe how general verbal and nonverbal Japanese communication patterns may impact clinical assessment and intervention in the United States.
- Consider general strategies that clinicians can incorporate to ensure effective, culturally responsive communication with clients of Japanese descent.
- Access resources to improve understanding of diverse communication styles used within and across cultures.

CASE SCENARIO

Mr. Hiroji Kobayashi is a 62-year-old widowed, male patient who had a bilateral, ischemic middle cerebral artery stroke 2 years ago. Before his stroke, Mr. Kobayashi worked as a financial officer at a global company in Japan with plans to continue working until age 70 to maximize his pension. A few months after he was discharged from the hospital, Mr. Kobayashi's son encouraged him to move to the United States to be surrounded by

notes:

family and have access to rehabilitation services. Mr. Kobayashi agreed and has been in the United States for the last 6 months. His only prior experiences of the United States were several 2- to 4 week trips to visit his family.

Before his stroke, Mr. Kobayashi's dominant language was Japanese, and he could also understand and speak English fluently. Currently, he prefers to use Japanese for communication with family and caregivers who speak both Japanese and English. Mr. Kobayashi's stroke resulted in limited spoken and written expression, mild impairment of auditory comprehension, and left-sided hemiparesis that made him depend on others for his basic needs. Mr. Kobayashi was diagnosed with moderate apraxia of speech, dysarthria, and dysphagia. He has dietary restrictions pertaining to his dysphagia that have been difficult to accommodate because of his dietary preferences. Previous therapy reports noted that Mr. Kobayashi received occupational therapy, physical therapy, and speech-language pathology services in Japan, after his stroke, but the services were discontinued because of his move to the United States.

Recently, Mr. Kobayashi's family sought speech-language pathology services with the goal of securing a more effective way for him to communicate and possibly assist him in regaining skills to return to work. During the initial evaluation, Dr. Strome–the SLP–evaluated Mr. Kobayashi in English and concluded that he presented with both limb and oral apraxia and demonstrated limited spoken language expression, producing only stereotypic phrases (e.g., "hoy" and "hi") and vocalizations (e.g., "umm"). His comprehension showed significant deficits with compromised ability to respond to yes/no questions, only after moderate to maximum prompting. Reading and writing were also severely impacted, leaving him to rely exclusively on gestures, facial expressions, exaggerated changes in vocal intonation, and yes/no head nods.

Mr. Kobayashi and his son returned to the clinic to discuss the evaluation results. Dr. Strome sat at his desk as he warmly addressed Mr. Kobayashi's son by his first name, Minoru. The SLP insisted on being addressed as Bill and chatted about his extensive training and experience working with similar clients before beginning the discussion. Dr. Strome explained the testing results and patterns of impairment before he shared his guarded prognosis that it would be unlikely Mr. Kobayashi would be able to return to work, even with rehabilitation. When Dr. Strome inquired if there were any questions, Mr. Kobayashi and his son were silent. Dr. Strome interpreted this to indicate that Mr. Kobayashi and his son had no questions about the information he shared. He offered to shake their hands and escorted them out of his office.

CRITICAL THINKING AND DEBRIEFING QUESTIONS

1. What language(s) should have been evaluated in this case?
2. What assessment strategies could you implement if you are not fluent in your client's language?
3. How would you present and explain the diagnosis and the prognosis for recovery to the patient and his family?
4. What are strategies you can implement in your own practice to monitor your own communication styles and reactions from your clients? Where can you find information to inform and transform your practice?

COMMENTARY

Communication is vital across and within cultures; it is how we express our needs and wants and interact with others. Patterns of communication vary greatly depending on cultural values and practices. For example, European American culture often values openness, frankness, and directness. It relies on verbal expressions of meaning or nuance (low context) in lieu of nonverbal expression, or body language (high context; Park & Kim, 2008). SLPs focus on improving and maintaining communication in their clients, and care must be taken to understand the general communication styles and values that each patient brings to the interaction.

Misinterpretations of communicative intentions because of cultural practices or style differences can create confusion in patient and caregiver interactions and can make collaboration more challenging. In this case, we observed communication breakdowns between the Kobayashi family and Dr. Strome. The style used by Dr. Strome was informal and friendly, a common approach in the United States, whereas the Kobayashi family was accustomed to more formal, directive interactions when working with professional experts. This difference in expectations may have been perceived by the Kobayashi family as a lack of professionalism, disrespect, or lack of professional competence in Dr. Strome's subject area, leaving them questioning Dr. Strome's abilities and feeling as though he did not take their concerns and case seriously.

Definition

The Japanese culture has a rich history of communication practices that are high context (Park & Kim, 2008). **High context** indicates a communication style that relies on information that is expressed through physical contexts and inference; less emphasis is placed on direct communication. This contrasts with European American culture, which uses low context communication, relying on explicit messages and valuing clarity and effectiveness (Kim, 1994).

A general practice in Japanese culture is to hold formality in high esteem, emphasizing respect for and trust in trained professionals. This trust is paired with an expectation that highly trained professionals provide accurate assessments and offer treatment in a confident, decisive manner. The interactions between Dr. Strome and the Kobayashi family were casual and collaborative, which was in contrast to the communication styles and expectations of the Kobayashi family. Additionally, his informal use of first names may have been interpreted as insulting or disrespectful (Doutrich & Colclough, 2017). Clinicians may avoid this issue by discussing preferred ways of addressing clients and family members during the intake appointment. Unlike common European American practices in which adults remain autonomous, Japanese families value obedience, dependence on the family, formality in interpersonal relationships, and restraint in the expression of emotions (Battle, 2012).

Common communication practices in Japanese include silence as well as subtle gestures and facial expressions as a key way to convey attitudes and feelings when compared with European American culture. The preferred tone is often formal and deferential to experts. The reaction Dr. Strome received from the Kobayashi family as they concluded their session was consistent with this pattern. They may have had questions but did not ask because they did not want to offend Dr. Strome or question his authority as an expert. They also would not have wanted to express disagreement or disappointment with the findings, especially the information that Mr. Kobayashi was not able to return to work. Maintaining composure and control, or "saving face," can be another valued communication practice in this culture (Park & Kim, 2008) to avoid feeling shame or a threat to their social integrity.

Assessment results revealed that the area of nonverbal communication was relatively spared in Mr. Kobayashi. This finding could have been emphasized to the family, given that in their cultural tradition nonverbal communication is valued. Independent research done before the session about basic Japanese cultural values and communication practices could have been integrated into therapy to support Mr. Kobayashi's nonverbal skills that were preserved and to build on the limited verbal expression he currently exhibits. Finding a way to maintain effective communication with the family may have resulted in a more positive meeting and interaction.

A more comprehensive evaluation that included testing in both languages (Japanese and English) and involved a more robust family interview that included preferred cultural practices and values regarding communication would have provided a rich resource for Dr. Strome in working with the Kobayashi family and may have avoided some of the cultural disconnect.

Communication patterns and values vary across and within cultures. Caution should be exercised when interpreting the previous statements because there may be interpersonal variability in the values and patterns of communication exhibited by members of the Japanese community. Additionally, while observing cultural patterns that vary regionally across cultures, it's important to note the possibility that variation exists not only within groups and regions but across generations. Each generation within a culture may espouse its values in different ways.

CRITICAL THINKING AND DEBRIEFING RESPONSES

1. **What language(s) should have been evaluated in this case?**

In this case, a clinician should evaluate all modes of communication used by a client. The background information noted that the client primarily speaks Japanese with caregivers and that Japanese was the primary language for the client before his stroke. However, a more thorough background questionnaire or ethnographic interview could have provided useful information to personalize the language intervention and strategy approaches to optimally stimulate the various linguistic and cognitive processes to facilitate recovery (Centeno, 2010; Mahendra, 2006). As a result, obtaining information about the client's skill levels in Japanese should have been included as part of the initial evaluation. The client will likely want to target ways to communicate in Japanese, and omitting that language may separate the client from cultural connection and the ability to communicate effectively with caregivers. Because the assessment did not indicate whether Mr. Kobayashi's Japanese was compromised, a completed understanding of his communicative competence was not obtained. Treatment options may have included using both languages for communication, because some bilingual research suggests that cross-linguistic facilitation may occur between treated and untreated languages in bilingual aphasia therapy (Kohnert, 2009). The clinician could also complete an interview that highlights daily routines, outlining the ways in which Mr. Kobayashi communicates his needs throughout the day and working to repair breakdowns across his day, given the specific activity or routine.

2. **What assessment strategies could you implement if you are not fluent in your client's language?**

When assessing an adult client presenting with a brain injury and possible aphasia, it's important to complete basic cognitive functioning tasks that look at short- and long-term memory, attention, and executive functions in the client's dominant language (Lorenzen & Murray, 2008). It is also beneficial to conduct a thorough case history that provides detailed background information on the client's functioning before the incident. This could be completed with an ethnographic interview or bilingual questionnaire to provide information on daily routines of the client and how the client's communication across these functional contexts has been affected by the injury (Centeno et al., 2007).

Another key point in the evaluation is having access to an interpreter. The best scenario would be in-person, and the next best option may be via phone. If that was not possible, using a family member could be another option (American Speech-Language-Hearing Association, n.d.). This would be especially important when conducting any standardized testing. Using the BID (brief, interact, debrief) protocol includes taking the time to discuss expectations (brief) and a system for interpreting (interaction), along with time to debrief (Langdon, 2002). Because of different communication styles, expectations, and practices across cultures, it may be beneficial for the family to create a system to keep them informed and involved across the evaluation and treatment process, providing them with culturally appropriate opportunities to share concerns or ask questions. Directly addressing preferred cultural communication practices could be another opportunity for the family to discuss their expectations and goals.

When assessing an adult client presenting with a brain injury and possible aphasia, it's important to complete basic cognitive functioning tasks that look at short- and long-term memory, attention, and executive functions in the client's dominant language (Lorenzen & Murray, 2008).

3. **How would you present and explain the diagnosis and prognosis for recovery to the patient and his family?**

Explaining a prognosis can be difficult with any client. Taking the time to research and understand general cultural practices and expectations that your client may have is especially important. Although each person represents their culture in a unique way, identifying general practices and what is appropriate can help clinicians avoid offensive verbal or nonverbal interactions. Understanding the value that different cultures place on verbal communication, gestures, and nonverbal interactions—including facial expressions, tone, pitch, and proximity—may offer unexplored avenues for intervention because of relative saliency in their cultural communication patterns. Finally, understanding the view of disability within a culture may help influence how you approach sharing a diagnosis. It is common for Eastern cultures to view disability as a result of the wrongdoing of an individual's ancestors, resulting in guilt and shame. Disability may also be explained with spiritual or cultural beliefs, including imbalance of inner forces, also known as Qi (Battle, 2012, p. 46). Understanding a client's belief system regarding how a disability occurs may provide great insight in creating a personalized treatment plan.

4. **What are strategies you can implement in your own practice to monitor your own communication styles and reactions from your clients? Where can you find information to inform and transform your practice?**

Although answers may vary, some suggestions could include observations from peers, using online cultural competence tools, researching your own culture as well as a variety of cultures that are different from your own, and learning more about the nuances of communication across multiple cultures. Some of the resources included below are excellent places to start your learning. These topics would be considered excellent self-study or independent continuing education opportunities for any clinician. If a peer observation is not a possibility, a clinician could provide patients with anonymous feedback forms and surveys, or could videotape sessions, to analyze their nonverbal and verbal communication styles after a visit.

A study in the field of psychology training reviewed practical examples of cultural self-awareness assessments. The study concluded that it is "critical for all therapists to understand the impact of their cultural 'programming' on their development of self, their perceptions of others who are different, and their preferred theoretical orientation for interventions" (Roysircar, 2004, p. 665). It suggested that professionals engage in continued cultural self-assessment through a variety of options, including introspection, self-examination, reading, as well as quantitative and qualitative self-evaluations (Roysircar, 2004).

TAKE AWAYS

- Cultural practices and values should be considered when working with all clients, especially those who may be from a culture that is less familiar to the clinician or clients who speak multiple languages. When adapting tests to include a client's cultural practices and expectations, it is important to remember that modifications nullify the standardization and make standardized scores invalid. Instead, descriptions of performance can be used.
- Clients from cultures with more formal communicative registers may have different expectations regarding communication with health professionals, compared with standard practices in the United States. It is important for clinicians to ask about communicative styles and preferences and to research cultural values so that they can demonstrate cultural sensitivity when addressing and working with a variety of clients.

Cultural self-reflection is a critical tool to help inform and transform one's clinical practice (Roysircar, 2004).

- Clinicians should schedule time to self-assess and ask others for constructive feedback regarding cultural practices and different approaches to working with clients. Multiple perspectives can be invaluable in identifying areas of growth.
- The cultural practices and values of individuals can vary across and within cultures. Obtaining general information about cultural practices and beliefs can be useful in providing a basic understanding but cannot be applied to all people in a specific culture. Each individual is unique.

REFERENCES

American Speech-Language-Hearing Association. (n.d.). *Collaborating with interpreters.* Retrieved from https://www.asha.org/Practice-Portal/Professional-Issues/Collaborating-With-Interpreters/

Battle, D. E. (2012). *Communication disorders in multicultural and international populations* (4th ed.). St. Louis, MO: Elsevier.

Centeno, J. G. (2010). The relevance of bilingualism questionnaires in the personalized treatment of bilinguals with aphasia. *Perspectives on Communication Disorders and Sciences in Culturally and Linguistically Diverse (CLD) Populations, 17*(3), 65–73.

Centeno, J. G., Anderson, R. T., Restrepo, M. A., Jacobson, P. F., Guendouzi, J., Müller, N., . . . Marcotte, K. (2007). Ethnographic and sociolinguistic aspects of communication: Research-praxis relationships. *The ASHA Leader, 12*(9), 12–15.

Doutrich, D. L., & Colclough, Y. Y. (2017). Application of assessment and intervention techniques specific to cultural groups: Japanese Americans. In J. N. Giger (Ed.), *Transcultural nursing: Assessment and intervention* (7th ed., pp. 311-342). St. Louis, MO:

Elsevier.

Kim, M.-S. (1994). Cross-cultural comparisons of the perceived importance of conversational constraints. *Human Communication Research, 21,* 128–151.

Kohnert, K. (2009). Cross-language generalization following treatment in bilingual speakers with aphasia: A review. *Seminars in Speech and Language, 30*(3), 174–186. https://doi.org/10.1055/s-0029-1225954

Langdon, H. W. (2002). Language interpreters and translators: Bridging communication with clients and families. *The ASHA Leader, 7*(6), 14–15.

Lorenzen, B., & Murray, L. L. (2008). Bilingual aphasia: A theoretical and clinical review. *American Journal of Speech-Language Pathology, 17,* 299–317.

Mahendra, N. (2006). A multicultural perspective on assessing TW, a bilingual client with aphasia. *Perspectives on Neurophysiology and Neurogenic Speech and Language Disorders, 16*(3), 9–18.

Park, Y. S., & Kim, B. S. (2008). Asian and European American cultural values and communication styles among Asian American and European American college students. *Cultural Diversity and Ethnic Minority Psychology, 14*(1), 47–56.

Roysircar, G. (2004). Cultural self-awareness assessment: Practice examples from psychology training. *Professional Psychology: Research and Practice, 35,* 658–666.

ADDITIONAL RESOURCES

American Speech-Language-Hearing Association. (n.d.). *Working with bilingual clients with aphasia.* Retrieved from https://www.asha.org/practice/multicultural/bilaph/

Cheng, L. (2012). Asian and Pacific American languages and cultures. In D. Battle (Ed.), *Communication disorders in multicultural and international populations* (4th ed., pp. 37–60). St. Louis, MO: Elsevier.

Doutrich, D. L., & Colclough, Y. Y. (2017). Application of assessment and intervention techniques specific to cultural groups: Japanese Americans. In J. N. Giger (Ed.), *Transcultural nursing: Assessment and intervention* (7th ed., pp. 311–342). St. Louis, MO: Elsevier.

Gitterman, M. R., Goral, M., & Obler, L. K. (Eds.). (2012). *Aspects of multilingual aphasia* (Vol. 8). Tonawanda, NY: Multilingual Matters.

Associations outside of United States include the following:

- The Japan Society of Logopedics and Phoniatrics,
- The Japanese Association of Communication Disorders, and
- The Japanese Association of Speech-Language-Hearing Therapists.

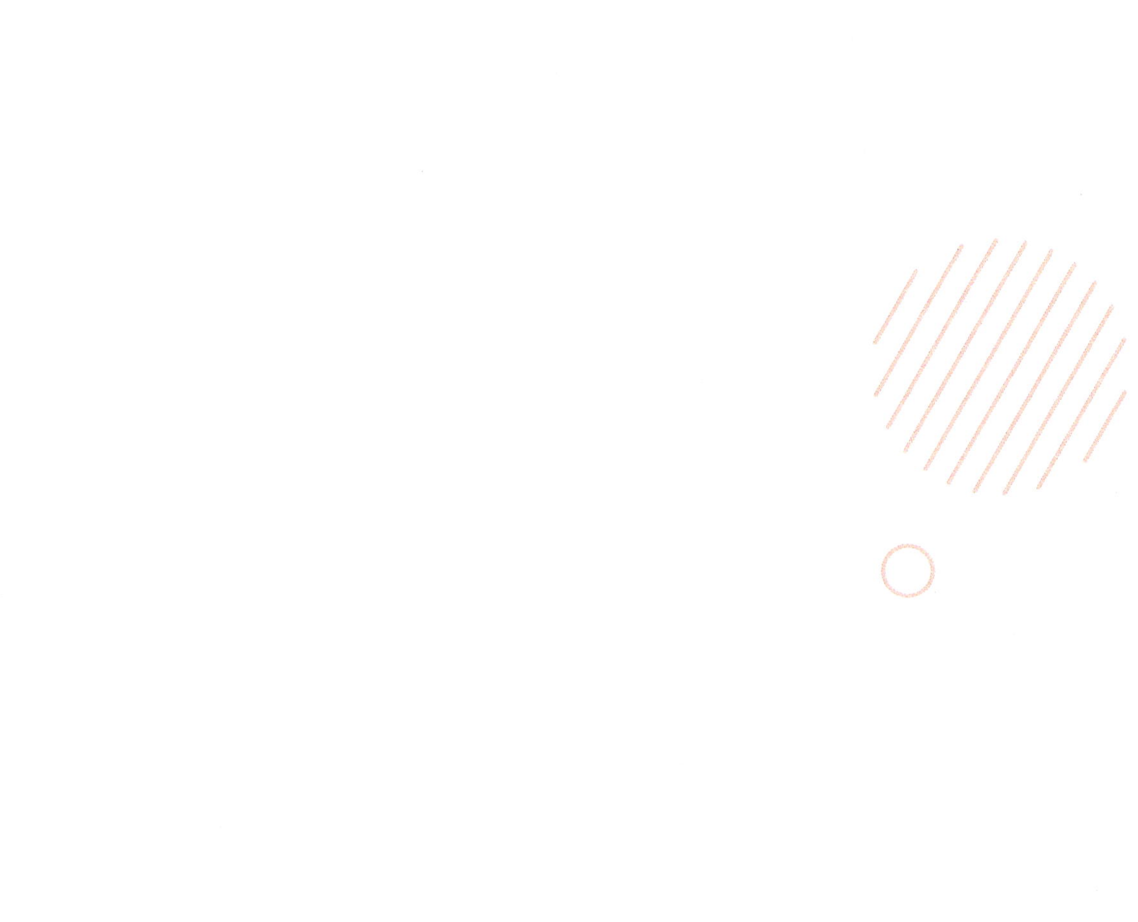

Can You Hear Me Now?

— Addressing Hearing Loss and Treatment in Aging Parents

Karen L. Beverly-Ducker

notes:

PREBRIEF

This scenario discusses some of the issues that arise when cultural and linguistic factors influence the treatment plan. Specifically, this scenario focuses on audiology services for a non-English speaker and addresses how family and gender roles vary across cultures and generations. While reading, consider how you might adapt your assessment and treatment practices when faced with a similar situation.

OBJECTIVES

- Understand the influence of gender and cultural expectations.
- Understand how cultural differences within a family (e.g., generational, nationality) can impact treatment expectations and acceptance.
- Identify approaches to align patient-centered care and language differences.

CASE SCENARIO

Mrs. Eshe Zegeye is a 72-year-old widow who recently left her home in Ethiopia and moved to the United States to live with her eldest son's family, which includes his wife and three teenage children. She has lived alone for the past 8 months since the death of her husband of 52 years. Mrs. Zegeye primarily speaks Sidamo and Amharic. She does not speak English. Although her son and daughter-in-law speak Sidamo and English, her grandchildren speak English only and have extremely limited understanding of either of the languages used by their grandmother. Mrs. Zegeye spends the majority of her weekdays at home alone. She typically refuses to use the telephone to talk with family members who are living in Ethiopia and becomes confused when presented with video chatting opportunities. She is often unaware that someone is knocking on the door or ringing the doorbell. During those times when she is aware, she is not comfortable with activities such as accepting packages delivered to the home, providing access to service workers who arrive for scheduled repairs in the home, or interacting with neighbors.

Mrs. Zegeye was seen in the ear, nose, and throat clinic on the basis of her son's "complaint" that she has hearing loss. Her son is her legal representative and has power of attorney. He served as the sole informant because there was no advance notice of the

Definitions

Multigenerational families–Families in which multiple generations of family members live with one another in the same household. Multigenerational families may share resources such as food, rent, and child/elder care(Muennig, Jiao, & Singer, 2018).

Sidamo–A language primarily spoken by individuals who identify with the Sidama ethnic group in Ethiopia. Approximately 4% of Ethiopians speak Sidamo (Central Intelligence Agency, 2020).

Amharic– The official language of Ethiopia spoken by 29.3% of Ethiopians (Central Intelligence Agency, 2020).

need for interpreter services, and this clinic does not have Sidamo or Amharic interpreters readily available. During the interview, her son answered all of the questions himself, without interpreting for his mother. He shared that his mother was a very private person and that he had no knowledge of any medical problems or use of any medications. He thought that both ears were "bad" and had been for some time. He denied that she experienced vertigo, otorrhea, otalgia, tinnitus, otologic surgeries, or a family history of hearing loss.

The evaluation from the ear, nose, and throat physician revealed normal external auditory canals with clear visualization of the tympanic membranes. A physical examination, laboratory tests, and imaging–which included a CT scan of the temporal bone and magnetic resonance imaging (MRI) with and without contrast– provided no remarkable findings or explanation for her reported hearing difficulties.

Instructions for the audiologic evaluation consisted of the use of gestures and an improvised sign system, the modeling of desired responses, and the son's translation of instructions. The audiologic evaluation showed a moderate to severe high frequency sensorineural hearing loss from 1500 - 8000 Hz. Word recognition scores were not obtained because of the language difference. Speech awareness thresholds were obtained at 55 dB and 65 dB for the right and left ear, respectively. Acoustic reflexes were present bilaterally. The results of immittance testing did not indicate concerns regarding the status of the middle-ear transmission system. The test results indicated a severe, bilateral, sensorineural hearing loss, and the audiologist concluded that Mrs. Zegeye was a hearing aid candidate.

The results of the evaluation were discussed with Mrs. Zegeye's son. He was very eager to obtain hearing aids for his mother. Several consumer information pieces that contained photos and diagrams of individuals using hearing aids were shown to Mrs. Zegeye and her son to prepare her for the hearing aids. While looking at the brochures, Mrs. Zegeye pointed to the pictures and shook her head as if to indicate "no" several times. The audiologist asked her son to clarify that she was truly interested in receiving hearing aids. Her son spoke to her in Sidamo, then turned to the audiologist and said, "Yes, she is very interested in getting hearing aids." Mrs. Zegeye's previously smiling countenance changed as she folded her arms and continued to shake her head.

CRITICAL THINKING AND DEBRIEFING QUESTIONS

1. Ideally, when working with non-English speaking patients, an interpreter would be present to interpret in the patient's native language. What are some options for working with a patient who comes to clinic without notifying you of interpreter needs? What are some ways to change an intake process to keep this situation from happening? If necessary, what are some ways to prepare or train a family member to serve as the interpreter?
2. As you are analyzing a situation and it appears, on the basis of body language and observation, that a patient's family member or spokesperson is making decisions

that go against the patient's wishes, how would you proceed?

3. What problems can arise when using family members as interpreters? What are ways to remedy these situations?
4. In general, how are age and gender roles defined in different cultures?

COMMENTARY

As professionals, we do our best to prepare for the unknowns in our work environments. Flexibility helps us tackle unplanned situations that may arise, without derailing our clinical objectives. This scenario presents a situation in which the clinic has prepared for the needs of multilingual clients but lacked appropriate information to plan for this specific language and client interaction. As a result, the clinician had to be flexible in approaching their communication with both the client and her son, who served as the interpreter.

As baby boomers age, multigenerational families are becoming more commonplace. Although this has been a cultural norm for some, more adult children are assuming responsibility for caring for their elderly parents and children simultaneously. Cultural factors such as gender roles have significant influence (Oláh, Kotowska, & Richter, 2018). For example, in Ethiopia, it is common for women to defer to their husbands or fathers when approaching care in medical settings. In the context of the present case study, Mrs. Zegeye is a widow. She has been accustomed to her husband making decisions and is now relying on her son. Additionally, we know that when adults present with hearing loss, outward symptoms may include depression, withdrawal, and a change in affect, which may be exacerbated by language differences (Jayakody et al., 2018).

During this appointment, it became clear that the son was in favor of his mother receiving hearing aids on the basis of his enthusiasm when agreeing to hearing aids after her evaluation. The clinician, while speaking to Mrs. Zegeye, observed that her son answered questions without consulting her or interpreting information to her, and he spoke about her hearing loss as it impacted his life (e.g., not being able to open the door for service workers or receiving packages). Mrs. Zegeye was also observed shaking her head side to side as she and her son looked at hearing aids.

When working with all clients, it is important to consider both verbal and nonverbal cues and to consider how they may vary across cultures (Cultural Atlas, n.d.). For instance, vocalizing "nee" in Afrikaans, "não" in Portuguese, "niet" in Russian, "nein" in German, "nahi" in Hindi, and "non" in French are the equivalent of "no" in English; therefore, care must be taken when attaching and interpreting gestures and body language. It is important to familiarize yourself with the meanings of different gestures that are common to different cultures. A gesture used in one culture may signal a greeting, whereas that same gesture may be offensive and obscene in another culture. Many Americans point their fingers to indicate something specific or for emphasis, but pointing can be viewed as rude across other cultures. For example, among the Navajo, it is considered rude to point; rather, they shift their lips toward the desired direction (Still & Hodgins, 2003).

At this point in the appointment, the clinician may have chosen to stop the appointment and present a process for interpreting that involved Mrs. Zegeye, noting that although her son indicated he was power of attorney and the medical decision maker, the clinician wanted to ensure that all of the information was being explained to her and that she was in agreement with the information. Because of the cultural practice of deferring to the eldest son, the clinician may not have been sure of Mrs. Zegeye's true feelings, but at least she would have been more aware of the process. The clinician also used gestures and models to explain the assessment process as well as diagrams and photos to illustrate the available hearing aids. These were good supports to offer Mrs. Zegeye and should be used with clients who do not speak English (Pratt & Searles, 2017). The clinician may have also considered online videos to demonstrate the evaluation process and placement of hearing aids. This may be a process the clinic can add to their "toolbox" to use for clarification when working with clients who speak different languages.

Although we can't control every situation that arises, clinics can implement processes and resources that can assist in ensuring professional practice in unpredictable situations. Multimodal presentations of assessment and treatment procedures, reviews of objectives, and asking consent are practices that can improve the treatment experience with all clients.

CRITICAL THINKING AND DEBRIEFING RESPONSES

1. **Ideally, when working with non-English speaking patients, an interpreter would be present to interpret in the patient's native language. What are some options for working with a patient who comes to clinic without notifying you of interpreter needs? What are some ways to change an intake process to keep this situation from happening? If necessary, what are some ways to prepare or train a family member to serve as the interpreter?**

The first step in this situation would be to review the intake procedures and ensure that the first contact with a client would include a question about the language services they may need and the offer for interpreter services. Systems should be in place to gather information about the patient's/family's linguistic needs during the appointment making process. For example, a specific question may be asked during the scheduling phone call or posted in multiple languages on the website if online scheduling is an option. If this occurs and the family does not divulge the need for language services, other options include (a) using interpretation services that are provided via phone, such as language lines for interpreting spoken languages (e.g., French to English); (b) using videoconferencing services/video interpreting platforms; or (c) using apps that are available via electronic devices, including tablets, computers, and smart phones. Information about how to access these different forms of interpretation services should be researched in advance and routinely updated. Although it is very common for family members, friends, cultural brokers, and so forth to accompany patients to appointments, they should not be expected to or relied on to translate for the patient.

However, if a situation arises and there is no trained interpreter, and a family member is present and willing, it may be useful to follow the brief, interaction, and debriefing (BID) procedure. Although this model is intended for professional interpreters, it can set up a simple framework to use in emergency situations.

2. **As you are analyzing a situation and it appears, on the basis of body language and observation, that a patient's family member or spokesperson is making decisions that go against the patient's wishes, how would you proceed?**

It is important to familiarize yourself with the meanings of different gestures that are common to different cultures. A gesture used in one culture may signal a greeting, whereas that same gesture may be considered offensive and obscene in another culture.

It is also helpful to be prepared to present appropriate options. In this instance, perhaps the patient would have been receptive to the use of some form of hearing assistive technology systems to support her needs. It may have been more appropriate and culturally responsive to show photos and videos of different options and ask the patient to point to these options demonstrating her preference. There are a variety of technological options that can be used to supplement an "experience" of hearing assistive technology, and using them could have helped Mrs. Zegeye be more involved in her health care decisions.

3. **What problems can arise when using family members as interpreters? What are ways to remedy these situations?**

Family or friends serving as interpreters may influence the reliability, accuracy, and effectiveness of the communication exchange and may present a potential for a conflict of interest. In this case, it was clear that Mrs. Zegeye's son was very interested in her being fitted with hearing aids. The son also shared that she would not answer the door for service workers or accept packages, which were likely services that benefited her son. He noted that she rarely participated in conversational speech with the family and did not like to participate in calls with extended family. In this case, Mrs. Zegeye's adult son may have made decisions in a self-serving manner that did not totally consider his mother's needs or input, as referenced by his lack of interpreting for his mother. Simultaneously, audiologists must balance respecting a client's family dynamics while adhering to the American Speech-Language-Hearing Association's (2016) *Code of Ethics,* which states that clinician must provide services that best fit the client's needs.

Definition

BID stands for "brief, interaction, and debriefing" (Langdon, 2002). This is a process in which the clinician can **"brief"** the family member on the purpose of the interaction, the steps of what will happen, and what the clinician expects in terms of information transferred back and forth. The **"interaction"** portion involves the family member/interpreter attempting to remain as neutral as possible and conveying information directly, instead of as a third party. For instance, the clinician would ask the client questions directly, which the family member would directly interpret, instead of saying, "please ask your mother . . . ." Finally, the clinician and the family member would **debrief**, reviewing the process and any other impressions.

When using family members or friends in this role, the clinician should consider the following factors:

- Intent of the message (e.g., sharing a diagnosis of a cognitive-communication deficit, which may be met with resistance or a strong emotional response, vs. modeling a therapeutic exercise);
- Age of the family member providing interpretation, the position and role of that individual within the family structure, and his or her overall linguistic ability; and
- The qualification of interpreters to provide services, be it in a school or health care setting.

Family or friends serving as interpreters may influence the reliability, accuracy, and effectiveness of the communication exchange and may present a potential for a conflict of interest.

A study comparing the roles of professional versus family interpreters indicated that the two types of interpreters viewed their roles differently (Rosenberg, Seller, & Leanza, 2008). Professional interpreters generally viewed their purpose as ensuring the accurate transfer of information. Family interpreters viewed themselves as participants in their family's care, explaining information as well as serving as a patient advocate. Best practice continues to recommend using professional interpreters whenever possible, but it does not exclude the addition of family members for patient support and advocacy (Rosenberg et al., 2008).

4. **In general, how are age and gender roles defined in different cultures?**

In many—but not all—cultures, greater respect for elders is shown because age is thought to indicate wisdom, knowledge, and experience. Although this is typical of the Ethiopian culture, gender roles are also clearly defined. Mrs. Zegeye comes from a patriarchal culture where her beliefs dictate that the men of the family typically provide financial support and make decisions, and where, in general, women are considered subordinate to their husbands and fathers. In the absence of a husband or father, the eldest son will usually adopt the role of the head of the household and hold more decision-making power than his mother. She may defer to him regarding her health practices, out of respect, even when she is not in agreement. In essence, a culturally responsive clinician should recognize the cultural influences on shared decision making and adapt clinical interactions accordingly to ensure a client's full agreement and participation (Hawley & Morris, 2017).

TAKE AWAYS

- It is important to be familiar with guidelines for appropriate interpretation and use of gestures as they vary across cultures.
- Patient-centered therapy includes providing multiple/alternate forms of communication. For example, translated self-report forms should be available so that every patient/client has the opportunity to contribute to his or her clinical picture.
- Be prepared to address instances when the patient/client and the family do not agree on the plan of care.

REFERENCES

American Speech-Language-Hearing Association. (2016). *Code of Ethics*. Retrieved from https://www.asha.org/Code-of-Ethics/

Central Intelligence Agency. (2020, March 2). Africa: Ethiopia. *The World Factbook*. Retrieved from https://www.cia.gov/library/publications/the-world-factbook/geos/et.html

Cultural Atlas. (n.d.). *Etiquette*. Retrieved from https://culturalatlas.sbs.com.au/greek-culture/greek-culture-etiquette#greek-culture-etiquette

Hawley, S. T., & Morris, A. M. (2017). Cultural challenges to engaging patients in shared decision making. *Patient Education and Counseling, 100*(1), 18–24. https://doi.org/10.1016/j.pec.2016.07.008

Jayakody, D. M., Almeida, O. P., Speelman, C. P., Bennett, R. J., Moyle, T. C., Yiannos, J. M., & Friedland, P. L. (2018). Association between speech and high-frequency hearing loss and depression, anxiety and stress in older adults. *Maturitas, 110*, 86–91.

Langdon, H. W. (2002). Language interpreters and translators: Bridging communication with clients and families. *The ASHA Leader, 7*(6), 14–15.

Muennig, P., Jiao, B., & Singer, E. (2018). Living with parents or grandparents increases social capital and survival: 2014 General Social Survey-National Death Index. *SSM–Population Health, 4*, 71–75.

Oláh, L. S., Kotowska, I. E., & Richter, R. (2018). The new roles of men and women and implications for families and societies. In G. Doblhammer & J. Gumà (Eds.), *A demographic perspective on gender, family and health in Europe* (pp. 41–64). New York, NY: Springer.

Pratt, M., & Searles, G. E. (2017). Using visual AIDS to enhance physician-patient discussions and increase health literacy. *Journal of Cutaneous Medicine and Surgery, 21,* 497–501.

Rosenberg, E., Seller, R., & Leanza, Y. (2008). Through interpreters' eyes: Comparing roles of professional and family interpreters. *Patient Education and Counseling, 70*(1), 87–*93.*

Still, O., & Hodgins, D. (2003). Navajo Indians. In L. D. Purnell & B. J. Paulanka (Eds.), *Transcultural health care: A culturally competent approach* (2nd ed., pp. 279–293). Philadelphia, PA: F.A. Davis.

ADDITIONAL RESOURCES

American Speech-Language-Hearing Association. (n.d.). *Collaborating with interpreters.* Retrieved from https://www.asha.org/Practice-Portal/Professional-Issues/Collaborating-With-Interpreters/

Chern, A., Rutherford, B., & Golub, J. (2019). Hearing loss and depression in the Hispanic/Latino population. *The Hearing Journal, 72*(4), 36, 38–39.

Golub, J. S., Brewster, K. K., Brickman, A. M., Ciarleglio, A. J., Kim, A. H., Luchsinger, J. A., & Rutherford, B. R. (2019). Association of audiometric age-related hearing loss with depressive symptoms among Hispanic individuals. *JAMA Otolaryngology–Head & Neck Surgery, 145*(2), 132–139.

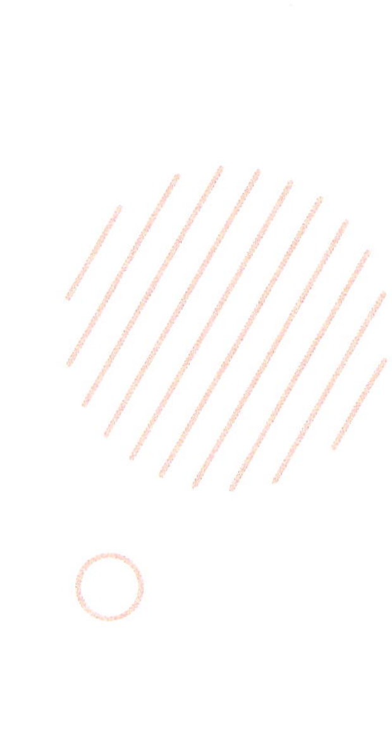

Cognition and Hearing Loss — Gender, Generational, and Multilingual Considerations in Differential Diagnosis

Ishara Ramkissoon

PREBRIEF

notes:

Culture is unique to each individual and shared across groups. Culture presents itself not only in the clients we serve but also in the way we practice as professionals. Our own cultural beliefs and attitudes are revealed through the way we practice as professionals. As you read this scenario, consider your own cultural values and attitudes and think about the ways in which they may impact your professional services.

OBJECTIVES

- Identify aspects of communication that may be due to generational and/or gender-related practices for the clients in this scenario (e.g., male spouse speaks for female client); explain how they are pertinent to the scenario and interactions.
- Develop procedures that can accurately determine whether a multilingual adult has sufficient English proficiency to complete traditional speech audiometry tests reliably.
- Increase awareness of client behaviors that suggest cognitive decline, and increase knowledge regarding interaction of cognition, hearing, and language background.

CASE SCENARIO

Mrs. Sabitha Kumar is an 82-year-old woman, who primarily speaks Hindi, who came to the ear, nose, and throat (ENT) clinic with a complaint of itchy ears. She was accompanied by her husband, 84-year-old Dr. Kumar. During the intake and evaluation, Dr. Kumar interacted with the ENT physician, Dr. Smith, and answered all of the questions regarding his wife's concerns. Dr. Smith examined Mrs. Kumar's ears and found irritation. She prescribed a mild cortisone cream to apply externally to the ear canal to relieve Mrs. Kumar's reported symptoms. Dr. Smith communicated with Mrs. Kumar in English, and she did not request the services of a spoken language interpreter for the patient's visit. During the assessment, Dr. Smith asked Mrs. Kumar if she had any concerns. Mrs. Kumar looked to her husband in response, and he answered for her. Dr. Kumar indicated that his wife often does not respond to him or to their friends when they speak to her in English. Dr. Smith referred Mrs. Kumar to the audiologist at the same clinic for a hearing evaluation.

The audiologist, Dr. Williams, completed a detailed case history. During the case history,

Mrs. Kumar appeared alert and made eye contact, but she rarely responded to questions in English. When Mrs. Kumar did not respond or appeared to pause, her husband spoke on her behalf. Dr. Kumar reported that they are both retired and spend most of their time at home or traveling to visit family. When asked about her communication interactions, Mrs. Kumar did not respond, but Dr. Kumar reported that she "hears okay most of the time." Dr. Kumar also noted that recently Mrs. Kumar has become more forgetful and less interactive, preferring to sit away from group gatherings. When Dr. Williams probed further, Dr. Kumar stated that his wife is sometimes confused when their American neighbor talks to her, shaking her head and appearing distressed. He also stated that she enjoys watching television, especially Zee-TV, a popular Indian channel that transmits programs in Hindi and Telegu. Dr. Kumar confirmed that his wife is fluent in three Indian languages and "does pretty okay" with English. Given these details, Dr. Williams suggested that Mrs. Kumar might not be able to complete speech audiometry with English words. After hearing concerns regarding her behavioral changes and considering the patient's age, Dr. Williams recommended that cognitive function be evaluated given research findings that suggest hearing impairment may be a marker for cognitive dysfunction in adults age 65 and older (Gurgel et al., 2014).

During the audiologic assessment, Dr. Williams observed that Mrs. Kumar seemed comfortable, and she demonstrated understanding of the test instructions. Her tympanograms were Type A, and distortion product otoacoustic emissions were within normal range, bilaterally. However, during speech audiometry, Mrs. Kumar faltered over several words and obtained speech reception thresholds (SRTs) of 45 dB bilaterally. Dr. Williams hypothesized that the words may have been unfamiliar, because they were in English, but wanted to complete a screening test for dementia.

The audiologist administered the Mini-Cog screening test (Borson, Scanlan, Chen, & Ganguli, 2003). Mrs. Kumar earned a score of 3/5, placing her at a borderline pass, because scores of <3 indicate higher risk for dementia. The audiologist noted that Mrs. Kumar performed poorly on the portion of the screening tool that uses English words such as "river, nation, finger, captain, season, sunrise" to assess registration and recall of single words. Dr. Williams repeated the SRT test using spondaic digits as stimuli (Digit-SRT; Ramkissoon, Proctor, Lansing, & Bilger, 2002) to counteract any unfamiliarity that Mrs. Kumar had with the English words. She obtained a Digit-SRT of 35 dB, bilaterally, which was consistent with her pure tone average (PTA). Word recognition testing at suprathreshold levels (WRS) in quiet and in noise using an English word list revealed scores ranging from 58% to 70%, indicating more severe hearing deficits than the SRTs or PTAs revealed.

Dr. Williams presented results of the audiologic assessment to Mrs. Kumar and her husband. Results indicated a mild, high-frequency, bilateral sensorineural hearing loss with disproportionately poor word recognition ability when evaluated with English stimuli. Dr. Williams informed that patient that her score of 3/5 on the cognitive screening test indicated the possibility that poor word recognition scores might be due to unfamiliarity with the English words used in the SRT and WRS tests. An annual hearing evaluation was recommended to monitor any change in the hearing loss to the point at which amplification, such as hearing aids, would be an option. It was also recommended that a diagnostic cognitive assessment be conducted by a gerontologist to rule out any early-stage cognitive changes.

CRITICAL THINKING AND DEBRIEFING QUESTIONS

1. What were your thoughts regarding Dr. Kumar's practice of responding to questions directed toward his wife? If this was a result of cultural practices, how do you incorporate those responses into your assessment? If these practices were different from your own cultural beliefs surrounding gender roles, what were your impressions?
2. What signs indicated the need for a cognitive screening?
3. How would an audiologist assess cognitive skills in an adult client whose first language is not English?
4. What other ways would you modify your speech audiometry protocols for a client with (a) limited English proficiency and (b) possible cognitive decline?

COMMENTARY

In American medical culture, clinicians often expect the adult client, not a family member or spouse, to respond to diagnostic questions. In this case, Dr. Kumar was likely responding for his wife, Sabitha, because of his cultural practices and her lack of English skills. Given their Indian heritage and their age, it may have been common practice for the male to serve as the speaker for all important matters, including his wife's health (Roopnarine, Krishnakumar, & Vadgama, 2013). Any confusion in this matter could have been alleviated by asking about preferred cultural practices or offering the services of an oral language interpreter.

The practice of the ENT to go along with Dr. Kumar's practice of answering for his wife could have been due to a shared communication style in which those who are educated at the doctoral level are more comfortable communicating with peers or accepting a man as the family spokesperson without further consideration. The audiologist made more concrete attempts to elicit information from the client by making eye contact with her, but when this did not produce the desired result, the audiologist relied on the husband as the spokesperson for his wife.

The last issue, not offering an alternate SRT test, may have been a contributing factor in Mrs. Kumar's difficulty with certain words during the SRT testing. When working with clients who speak languages other than English, it is important to have alternative assessments ready for their appointments that can measure true abilities that are not hindered by a lack of proficiency in English.

By failing to directly address cultural practices and offer alternate speech audiometry tests, both medical professionals disempowered Mrs. Kumar in her assessment and treatment journey. In the future, it would be appropriate to address Dr. Kumar's responses and to offer an interpreter at the beginning of any assessment to encourage Mrs. Kumar to respond during the case history interview. Overall, it is recommended that direct conversations occur with patients and families to optimize culturally sensitive practice as well as reliable assessment and treatment.

CRITICAL THINKING AND DEBRIEFING RESPONSES

1. **What were your thoughts regarding Dr. Kumar's practice of responding to questions directed toward his wife? If this was a result of cultural practices, how do you incorporate those responses into your assessment? If these practices were different from your own cultural beliefs surrounding gender roles, what were your impressions?**

This question necessitates personal reflection. When considering your answer, think about the communication styles from your culture: Do you have patriarchal communication styles? Direct? Indirect? Also, consider that your thoughts and impressions reflect your knowledge of culture (yours and a client's), any personal bias you may have, and your expectations for successful communication exchanges. Did you view the husband's responses a result of Mrs. Kumar's hearing loss and cognitive decline, or a patriarchal practice? Elaborate on your response.

2. **What signs indicated the need for a cognitive screening?**

In this scenario, the audiologist noticed possible memory loss, confusion, avoidance of communication during the intake, and faltering on responses during testing as possible signs of cognitive decline. This information, paired with Mrs. Kumar's case history, indicated that a cognitive screening was appropriate at this point. It was important that given these risk factors, the audiologist paused testing and screened for possible cognitive issues. Early recognition of cognitive decline is imperative in addressing issues and providing timely medical treatment and support (Zalewski, 2010).

3. **How would an audiologist assess cognitive skills in an adult client whose first language is not English?**

The first step in working with individuals who speak multiple languages is to offer interpreter services as part of the visit and intake. Because of the strong association between hearing loss and dementia, audiologists should be prepared to screen the cognitive skills of adults in their care (Loughrey, Kelly, Kelley, Brennan, & Lawlor, 2018). Practitioners should consider how a client's limited English proficiency might influence their performance on cognitive screening measures, especially in English. There are several screening tests available for cognitive evaluations. Best practice uses tests that are not linguistically loaded, normed on the target population, and preferably in the client's language, rather than tests translated from English.

4. **What other ways would you modify your speech audiometry protocols for a client with (a) limited English proficiency and (b) possible cognitive decline?**

Audiologists often modify test procedures but must take care to maintain validity while testing so that they can produce reliable information about a client's hearing ability.

(a) Deciding to eliminate the speech audiometric tests is not preferred practice. Instead, an audiologist may review some language-specific speech audiometry tests that are available. Audiologists should have access to tests in other languages that are readily available in the clinic. Some options include Spanish, Hindi, and Zulu. As an alternative to language-specific tests, the Digit-SRT test may be used irrespective of first language provided the client has a basic knowledge of English numbers.

(b) Clients with cognitive decline may be challenged to respond appropriately in speech and pure-tone audiometric procedures. Audiologists should include a screening test for cognitive function for older adults or any client who seems to not understand conversation or test instructions. Familiarize yourself with at least one cognitive screener.

TAKE AWAYS

- Clinicians should aim to identify preferred cultural practices and explore cultural family dynamics that may impact the intervention process to offer adequate support to the families, as needed, ensuring that their assessment is representative of their client's abilities.
- The benefits of involving oral language interpreters in clinical interventions with bilingual clients who might need them should be highlighted to them and their families ahead of their scheduled visit.
- Clinicians aiming to work with multicultural populations would greatly benefit from equipping their practice with materials and alternative assessments that can help more accurately measure their bilingual clients' true abilities.
- Given the link between hearing impairment and cognitive dysfunction, clinicians should be prepared to screen patients who demonstrate cognitive decline using appropriate language versions of the screening tests and an interpreter.

REFERENCES

Borson, S., Scanlan, J. M., Chen, P., & Ganguli, M. (2003). The Mini-Cog as a screen for dementia: Validation in a population-based sample. *Journal of the American Geriatrics Society, 51,* 1451–1454.

Gurgel, R. K., Ward, P. D., Schwartz, S., Norton, M. C., Foster, N. L., & Tschanz, J. T. (2014). Relationship of hearing loss and dementia: A prospective, population-based study. *Otology & Neurotology, 35,* 775–781.

Loughrey, D. G., Kelly, M. E., Kelley, G. A., Brennan, S., & Lawlor, B. A. (2018). Association of age-related hearing loss with cognitive function, cognitive impairment, and dementia. *JAMA Otolaryngology–Head & Neck Surgery, 144*(2), 115–126. https://doi.org/10.1001/jamaoto.2017.2513

Ramkissoon, I., Proctor, A., Lansing, C., & Bilger, R. C. (2002). Digit speech recognition thresholds for non-native speakers of English. *American Journal of Audiology, 11*(1), 22–27.

Roopnarine, J. L., Krishnakumar, A., & Vadgama, D. (2013). Indian fathers: Family dynamics and investment patterns. *Psychology and Developing Societies, 25*(2), 223–247.

Zalewski, T. R. (2010). Cognitive decline or hearing loss. *Perspectives on Gerontology, 15*(1), 12–18.

ADDITIONAL RESOURCES

Hanekom, T., Soer, M., & Pottas, L. (2015). Comparison of the South African Spondaic and CID W-1 wordlists for measuring speech recognition threshold. *South African Journal of Communication Disorders, 62*(1), a97. https://doi.org/10.4102/SAJCD.V62I1.97

Meulen, E. F. J., Schmand, B., van Campen, J. P., de Koning, S. J., Ponds, R. W., Scheltens, P., & Verhey, F. R. (2004). The seven minute screen: A neurocognitive screening test highly sensitive to various types of dementia. *Journal of Neurology, Neurosurgery, & Psychiatry, 75,* 700-705. https://doi.org/10.1136/jnnp.2003.021055

Ramkissoon, I., Proctor, A., Lansing, C., & Bilger, R. C. (2002). Digit speech recognition thresholds for non-native speakers of English. *American Journal of Audiology, 11*(1), 22-27.

Zalewski, T. R. (2010). Cognitive decline or hearing loss. *Perspectives on Gerontology, 15*(1), 12-18.